Leisure in a Changing America

SECOND EDITION

Leisure in a Changing America

Trends and Issues for the 21st Century

Richard Kraus

Temple University

Allyn and Bacon

Boston • London • Toronto • Sydney • Tokyo • Singapore

Publisher: *Joseph Burns*
Editorial Assistant: *Tanja Eise*
Senior Editorial-Production Administrator: *Joe Sweeney*
Editorial-Production Service: *Walsh & Associates, Inc.*
Composition Buyer: *Linda Cox*
Manufacturing Buyer: *Dave Repetto*
Cover Administrator: *Jennifer Hart*

Library of Congress Cataloging-in-Publication Data

Kraus, Richard G.
    Leisure in a changing America : trends and issues for the 21st century / Richard
Kraus.—2nd ed.
        p.   cm.
    Includes bibliographical references (p.) and indexes.
    ISBN 0-205-31456-2
    1. Leisure—United States. 2. Leisure—Social aspects—United States. 3. Leisure—United
States—Forecasting. 4. Minorities—Recreation—United States. I. Title.

GV53.K73 2000
790′01′35—dc21   99-053932

Printed in the United States of America

10 9 8 7 6 5 4 3 2 1   04 03 02 01 00

CONTENTS

11 Pastimes III: Popular Culture—Arts and Entertainment, Television, and Hobbies   270

12 The Commodification of Leisure   295

13 Environmental Trends and Issues   326

14 Charting the Future: Challenges for the Leisure-Service System   347

PREFACE

The first edition of this text, published in 1994, sought to provide a comprehensive picture of the role of recreation and leisure in American culture, with special emphasis on such factors as ethnic or racial identity, shifting gender roles, and the influence of socioeconomic class, disability, and environment on leisure pursuits.

This new edition is more broadly focused in several respects. First, it sets the stage for the beginning years of the twenty-first century by outlining a number of major trends, issues, and challenges for the leisure-service field as they have been ranked for importance by a large panel of recreation, park, and leisure-studies educators. Many colleges and universities offer courses and seminars with such titles as "Trends," "Issues," "Special Topics," or "Problems," and *Leisure in a Changing America* (2nd Edition) is designed to serve as a text in such offerings.

While retaining the strong emphasis on multiculturalism and issues of gender, disability, and social class, the book also places heavy emphasis on the growing role of technology, the commodification of leisure, and environmental needs and policies. Predictions for the future are examined in detail, including the trend in the American economy that threatens to create a society of leisure "have" and "have-nots" through business downsizing and technological job displacement. Given these varied emphases, it is expected that some departments may choose to use this second edition as a text in so-called "capstone" courses taken toward the end of undergraduate study, as students prepare for field work or internship. The book is also intended, like the first edition, to serve as a text in non-major courses to meet academic requirements in such areas as American Studies or Popular Culture.

Throughout, it is based on the principle that to understand leisure's role in society, it is essential to examine it from more than a conceptual or philosophical perspective or by learning practical principles of recreation management. Instead, emphasis is placed on correctly seeing leisure as an important part of total community and personal life, yielding immense benefits on many levels.

Organization of the Text

The book has essentially three sections:

1. An introductory section, Chapters 1 through 4, which presents basic concepts and values of leisure, an overview of its historical development to the beginning of the twenty-first century, and an analysis of the overall leisure-service system.
2. In Chapters 5 through 11, presentation of key trends and issues affecting leisure, including a detailed analysis of demographic influences such as population growth, racial/ethnic, gender-related, and age-group factors, and several major areas of

participation, such as sports, outdoor recreation, travel and tourism, television, and the arts.

3. In Chapters 12 through 14, examination of the impact of commercialism and commodification on leisure, issues related to both rural and urban environments, and a concluding discussion of challenges facing the recreation, park and leisure-service field in the twenty-first century.

Following the chapters are a comprehensive bibliography, two appendix sections providing fuller details of the 1998 Survey of Educators, and suggested class topics for discussion or assignments, and an index.

Sources and Credits

As in the first edition, extensive use was made of sources in the professional literature, including such general publications as *Parks and Recreation,* the *Journal of Physical Education, Recreation and Dance, Parks and Recreation Canada,* and more specialized research journals like the *Journal of Leisure Research, Leisure Studies, Leisure Sciences* or the *Journal of Applied Recreation Research.* In addition, journals in related fields, such as sports management, travel and tourism, or therapeutic recreation, were also systematically studied.

Many references in the text were drawn from major newspapers or news services, and from such newsmagazines as *Time* or *U.S. News and World Report* in order to gain an accurate, real-life picture of social and economic trends affecting leisure in the late 1990s. Numerous books by authors in the field, including John Crompton, Daniel Dustin, Christopher Edginton, Alan Ewert, Geoffrey Godbey, Thomas Goodale, Karla Henderson, Debra Jordan, John Kelly, Leo McAvoy, James Murphy, Ruth Russell, and H. Douglas Sessoms were also reviewed.

Gratitude must be expressed to a number of college and university professors who, in responding to the 1998 Survey of Educators, gave additional comments that were helpful to the author. They included: Karen Bibbins, State University of New York at Brockport; Judy Brookhiser, Murray State University, Kentucky; Willa Brooks, Catonsville, Maryland Community College; Gay Carpenter, University of Oregon; Mary Ann Chappell, University of Kansas; Robert Cipriano, Southern Connecticut State University; Robert Ditton, Texas A & M University; M. Jean Keller, University of North Texas; Douglas Kennedy, Virginia Wesleyan College; Annette Logan, York College of Pennsylvania; William McKinney, University of Illinois; D.R. Nichols, University of Victoria, British Columbia; Ernest Olson, California State University at Sacramento; Lisa Raymond, Chicago State University; Philip Rea, North Carolina State University at Raleigh; Stuart Schleien, North Carolina State University at Greensboro; Susan Weston, Montclair State University, New Jersey; and Brett Wright, George Mason University, Virginia. Other institutions responding to the survey are listed in the appendix.

The author also wishes to thank the following reviewers for their time and input: Lawrence Allen, Clemson University; Lynn Jamieson, Indiana University; Gail Vander-

rowth in Modern Society

he twentieth century that has just drawn to a close, recreation, parks, and leisure services ame increasingly powerful forces in the lives of North Americans. With the growth of time and a higher level of affluence, people of all ages and social classes became lved in varied forms of sport, outdoor recreation, artistic and hobby pursuits, social pas- es, and other forms of play. Volunteerism, community service, and membership in a t of civic organizations were widespread, and on every level of government in the ted States and Canada, parks, sports complexes, community centers, and other special- d recreational facilities were established.

The provision of organized forms of play became a major function of commercial inesses, nonprofit youth-serving organizations, the armed forces, private membership ups, therapeutic agencies, and other community organizations. Many universities estab- ed degree-granting programs in recreation, parks, and leisure studies, and leisure itself ame the focus of study by historians, philosophers, sociologists, and psychologists.

In the final years of the 1990s, economic and social conditions showed positive urns in a number of major respects. Economic growth had expanded and the poverty and less rates had both declined. Crime statistics and the number of welfare recipients were ch lower. Gym memberships and computer ownership had risen sharply, along with ritable giving, and the percentage of Americans who felt that things were going well dramatically during the mid- and late-1990s. Century's end was marked by national imism with the state of things.

to Recreation and
vice Agencies

he same time, a number of challenges and social problems confronted the managers of y governmental, nonprofit, cultural, and other leisure-service sponsors.

With sharp cutbacks in the budgets of many public recreation and park agencies in 1980s and early 1990s, along with a decline in the support of cultural and nonprofit anizations, reductions in programming, maintenance, and other services were widely erienced.

An escalating breakdown in family structure and stability, linked to the influence of y forms of popular entertainment, was believed to have an effect on the growth of gang vity and juvenile crime.

Racial antagonism and conflict, along with drug dealing and widespread vandalism, gued playgrounds, parks, and housing projects in many cities and invaded smaller com- nities as well.

In the area of sports, many members of the public became disillusioned by the relentless fit-seeking tactics of many team owners, agents, and sports stars that had resulted in strikes, ry holdouts, and the rapid flight of long-established teams from one city to another.

In environmental terms, while great progress was made in the recovery of wilderness s, waterways, and other ecological settings during the 1960s and 1970s, the decades

stoep, Michigan State University; Veda Ward, CSU Northridge; and Charles Yaple, SUNY Cortland.

It is hoped that this text will be of value both to non-majors and to students special- izing in the field of recreation, parks, and leisure studies, in terms of seeing their profession as an integral part of the larger society and of American culture itself. Throughout, the point is made that leisure not only reflects societal values and interests, but also helps to shape them significantly.

Finally, the author dedicates this book to the thousands of students that he has had the pleasure of teaching through the years, primarily at Teachers College, Columbia Univer- sity, Lehman College of the City University of New York, and Temple University in Philadelphia.

Leisure's

In
be
fr
in
ti
h
U
i

t
g

t

j

CHAPTER

1 Contemporai Trends, Conc and Values

An extremely high value in time, com been placed upon leisure experiences, force in the life of almost every indivi and leisure services movement is at ai tremendous opportunities, demands, a

After a century of unprecedented grow preparing psychologically to move int century hold for professionals in this fi addressed? What are the major opport establish an agenda for the 21st Centu services?[1]

Challeng Leisure-

From a narrow perspective, leisure may be thought of s or other pressing obligations and therefore available fo ation, and sociability.

From a broader perspective, leisure embraces a ho sonal and social possibilities. It may include varied forms lectual involvement that contribute to one's personal community's quality of life and economic growth. Outdoc sports all are linked to the nation's ecological concerns, a build family togetherness, neighborhood unity, and a bulv forms of deviant behavior. Artistic and cultural programs and reflect the contributions of many groups of different i

This chapter examines the role of leisure in contei the varied benefits that derive from its constructive use. inary picture of the challenges and opportunities that li park, and leisure-service organizations in the oncoming t that followed saw continued assaults on the natural environment in the United states and Canada.

Technology, which had been instrumental in expanding economic productivity and creating great amounts of free time, also evolved new forms of play—such as video games and other electronic entertainment or communications media—that threatened to diminish the face-to-face forms of play that had characterized much earlier leisure.

Time itself—the free time that is commonly regarded *as* leisure—appeared to be in shorter supply: Major studies in the 1980s reported that many people were working longer hours and under greater job stresses than in the past.

A continuing decline in traditional social values that had shaped public policy in regulating varied forms of popular recreation was evident in such examples as the widespread acceptance of legalized gambling as a means of economic advancement—without consideration for its negative impact on community life.

Given all of these concerns, what are the prospects for leisure and recreation in the twenty-first century?

Expectations of Leisure at Mid-Century

To fully understand the present and to plan constructively for the future, it is essential to examine the past. As Chapters 2 and 3 show in greater detail, the period following World War II in the United States and Canada was a time of dramatic economic expansion, population growth, and family mobility—all contributing to the growth of leisure in national life. It was widely expected that free time would continue to grow, that work would decline in relation to human satisfaction and personal values, and that leisure would become a source of the most significant kinds of positive social outcomes and cultural growth.

Growth of Discretionary Time

The 40-hour workweek was widely accepted in the United States after 1938, when the Fair Labor Standards Act, commonly called the Minimum Wage Law, came into effect. While many states had passed legislation having to do with work hours and wages before this law, it required employers to pay overtime wages to anyone who worked more than 40 hours a week.

Writing in the May 1965 *Occupational Outlook Quarterly,* Peter Henle, a U.S. Labor Department official, summed up some of the key developments leading to the growth of nonwork time. In 1940, for example, only about one-fourth of all union members and a smaller proportion of all employees had received annual vacations with pay; for most, the maximum period was one week. The average number of paid holidays was about two per year, although many workers received additional holidays without pay. By the mid-1960s, paid vacations had expanded greatly, with three-, four-, and five-week vacations becoming the standard for longer-service employees. The number of paid holidays had increased well beyond the six days that were recognized nationally; a number of holidays were rescheduled to permit three-day weekends. As a result, Henle reported that the average American now had more leisure hours than working hours in a year—2175 hours compared to 1960 hours of paid work.

In addition, early retirement, based on Social Security and company pension plans, had greatly increased leisure time for older workers. Another source of free time consisted of new labor-saving devices for the home, like power lawnmowers, automatic heating and air-conditioning systems, dish- and clotheswashers, and frozen foods that made daily chores less time-consuming.

Awareness of the "New Leisure"

As free time continued to expand, there was a growing awareness of leisure as a force in American life. Planning bodies like the Rand Corporation, the Hudson Institute, and the National Commission on Technology envisioned futuristic scenarios with such alternative possibilities as the lowering of the retirement age to 38, reduction of the workweek to 22 hours, or extension of typical paid vacations to as many as 25 weeks a year.

Some concluded that, thanks to the growing use of automation—highly sophisticated, self-governing, and electronically guided forms of production—it would soon be possible for only 2 percent of the population to meet all the material needs of society, thus providing an immense amount of new leisure. More conservatively, the U.S. Chamber of Commerce predicted that employers should expect a four-day, 32-hour workweek for most employees, along with new increases in vacations and holiday free time.

Emerging Leisure Ethic

Linked to the expansion of nonwork time was the confident expectation that leisure would give rise to a new set of values for society that would replace the old work ethic. Historian Daniel Rodgers pointed out that, while work had held moral predominance in society through the established Protestant work ethic, within the new industrial world it was easily possible to produce goods in great supply, and much manufacturing work had become increasingly repetitive and monotonous.

Increasingly, proponents of a new humanistic approach to leisure argued that it was rapidly becoming the focal point of our lives, playing a critical role with respect to work, family relations, education, and religion. Typically, the president of Yale University, A. Whitney Griswold, wrote:

> Now we stand on the threshold of an age that will bring leisure to all of us, more leisure than all the aristocracies of history, all the patrons of art, all the captains of industry and kings of enterprise ever had at their disposal . . . . What shall we do with this great opportunity? In the answers that we give to this question the fate of our American civilization will unfold.[2]

Similarly, in 1959, a year of great prosperity and boundless optimism, the editors of *Life Magazine* proclaimed that American civilization was on the brink of becoming more wise and powerful, responsible and happy, than all earlier societies—due largely to the emergence of the New Leisure. In part, this development stemmed from major shifts in twentieth century society. Peter Bramham and his coauthors wrote:

> . . . . urban life is increasingly concerned with non-work activities. The domination of the urban landscape by industrial forms of production, factories and office, is in many cities giving way to "consumption palaces" to accommodate the leisure consumer, with pavement cafes, museums, cultural events, and a wide range of entertainment facilities vying for the increasing disposable income and time of local citizens and tourists.[3]

"Fun Morality" versus Social Value

In the decades following World War II, the popular view of leisure and its uses had two sharply contrasting emphases—the idea of free time as an opportunity for personal pleasure and the notion that it should serve as a vehicle for achieving important social outcomes.

Sociologist C. Wright Mills pointed out that the public's "idols" had shifted from business, professional, military, or political figures to individuals who were successful in areas of leisure consumption—entertainment and sports. Similarly, Martha Wolfenstein confirmed this view, concluding that fun, from having been suspect if not taboo in American society, had tended to become obligatory. Instead of feeling guilty for having too much fun, one was now ashamed if one did not play enough.[4]

In contrast, during the 1960s and 1970s, many urban recreation and park agencies initiated socially purposeful programs, including specially funded services for disadvantaged populations and persons with physical or mental disabilities. Two influential writers, David Gray and Seymour Greben, summed up the views of many leisure-studies educators in urging the recreation and park profession to pursue the following goals:

> To adopt a humanistic ethic as the central value system of the recreation movement.
>
> To develop and act on a social conscience that focuses park and recreation services on the great social problems of our time and develop programs designed to contribute to the amelioration of those problems.
>
> To develop a set of guidelines for programs that emphasize human welfare, human development, and social action.
>
> To establish common cause with the environmentalists and other social movements that embrace a value system common to our own.
>
> To develop evaluation methods capable of measuring the contribution of park and recreation experience to human welfare, which can make us accountable for the human consequences of what we do.
>
> To develop an effective interpretation program capable of articulating to a national and worldwide audience the meaning of park and recreation experience in human terms.[5]

Economic Impact of Leisure

At the same time that scholars and practitioners expressed their own views of leisure's purpose and social contribution, it became increasingly evident that recreation as such as become a major source of economic growth and employment throughout the world.

In the 1980s, government economic reports showed that leisure spending involved hundreds of billions of dollars each year and was responsible for millions of jobs. This reality had profound implications, not only at home but throughout the world. American entertainment, for example, has "gone global" and is changing both those who consume it and those who create it:

> America is saturating the world with its myths, its fantasies, its tunes and dreams . . . . American entertainment products—movies, records, books, theme parks, sports, cartoons, television shows—are projecting an imperial self-confidence across the globe.
>
> Entertainment is America's second biggest export (behind aerospace), bringing in a trade surplus of more than $5 billion a year. American entertainment rang up some $300 billion in sales last year, of which an estimated 20 percent came from abroad. By the year 2000, half of the revenues from American movies and records will be earned in foreign countries.[6]

Today, government at all levels assists in the provision of varied forms of recreation by establishing national and state parks and other sites for outdoor recreation, local playgrounds, sports and arts complexes, senior centers, and other facilities and programs. Similarly, numerous nonprofit agencies have been developed to meet community needs for wholesome leisure activity. Major corporations, the armed forces, religious denominations, and real estate developers all sponsor recreation services to meet the needs of their constituencies. Within the fields of health care and rehabilitation, therapeutic recreation service has evolved as a recognized professional discipline.

It is now widely recognized that our free-time pursuits provide a major source of life satisfaction, healthful personal development, and rewarding social involvement. In the broadest sense, leisure helps to assure the quality of everyday life. It provides the opportunity for pleasure, relaxation, release from stress, and creative self-fulfillment.

When constructively used, leisure promotes a sense of community and civic pride and helps to build constructive relationships among people of different ethnic, racial, and religious backgrounds. Overall, it provides the space in which we come together as friends, family members, or neighbors to explore our talents and skills, compete and cooperate, celebrate our lives, and express our finest human qualities.

Leisure in North American society offers a diverse panorama of hobbies, rituals, fitness activities, competitive events, excursions, social groups, and other voluntarily chosen free-time pursuits. For those who think of it chiefly as casual relaxation and respite from work, it is instructive to recognize that millions of people engage regularly in strenuous sports or demanding outdoor recreation activities—not as work but as a form of play. Millions of others participate in community arts activities or volunteer in a host of community-service roles in their leisure hours.

All of our nation's traditions and values are clearly illustrated in such free-time involvements. In our hobbies, the games we play, the television shows or movies we watch, the tourist attractions we visit, and the toys and games we give our children, our character as a society is exposed. Our love of the land, sense of civic responsibility, aesthetic standards, attitudes toward winning and losing, and other traits all come into play in our leisure.

However, it would be wrong to assume that leisure represents a totally positive force in American life. Many forms of play—such as those involving compulsive gambling or drug abuse—degrade or injure those who engage in them. Beyond this, as a nation, Americans spend a great bulk of their free time in passive and unimaginative ways, often relying on stereotyped entertainment with an overwhelming emphasis on violence or other tawdry themes. Summing up, the case may be made that leisure in modern American life represents a blessing or a curse—with the potential for either enriching individual and societal well-being or for undermining and damaging it.

Key Concepts: Leisure, Play, Recreation

At this point, it will be helpful to briefly discuss—for the sake of those who may not have had earlier courses in this field—three terms that appear throughout this text: *leisure, recreation,* and *play.*

Meaning of Leisure

At its simplest level, leisure is usually thought of as time free of work commitments—generally available to one in the evenings, on weekends or holiday, or for more protracted periods during one's retirement.

A related meaning is that it is an attitude or state of being that is relaxed and free of care or obligation. The German philosopher, Josef Pieper, described leisure as:

> a mental and spiritual attitude . . . . not simply the result of external factors [such as] spare time, a holiday, a week-end or a vacation . . . . It is . . . an attitude of mind, a condition of the soul, and as such utterly contrary to the ideal of [work].[7]

It was usually assumed that leisure activities were relaxed and undemanding; Rom Harré suggests that they

> should be unhurried, idle, unstructured, perhaps even a mode of resting. They are thus defined in contrast to frantic, busy, structured, demanding activities in which time appears as some kind of discipline.[8]

Classical Perspective: Athenian Scholē. The earliest recorded references to leisure were in ancient Athens, where wealthy citizens did not work, but instead were free to engage in study, the arts, philosophical and literary discussion, and athletics. For them, leisure—or *scholē*, as it was called—was a way of life spent in the pursuit of virtue and civic contribution. It excluded the possibility of work, which was regarded as ignoble and unworthy of the Athenian citizen. Kelly comments that Greek towns were carefully designed to serve leisure needs:

> Not only did a central area for markets and government provide a "forum" for discussion and argumentation, but the town plan generally provided parks, baths, theaters, sports arenas, gymnasiums, and exercise grounds. Added to these were the academies for the learning and practicing of the arts and philosophy and music. Stress was placed on [enabling the free person to] develop both mind and body.[9]

Veblen's Leisure Class Theory.   Extending the idea of leisure as an aristocratic possession, social historian Thorstein Veblen concluded that throughout history, only the rich and powerful social classes had possessed leisure. In the modern era, members of royalty or wealthy industrialists engaged in what Veblen called "conspicuous consumption"; their elaborate homes and summer retreats and their ostentatious entertainment and pastimes all demonstrated their superior status.

Some critics have argued that the existence of a leisure class was essential to the development of culture through the ages. Clive Bell wrote:

> Civilization requires the existence of a leisured class and thus of slaves—of people, I mean, who give some part of their surplus time and energy to the support of others .... As a means ... to civility, a leisured class is essential.[10]

Veblen was less charitable in his view, considering leisure itself as a decadent example of economic exploitation. He deplored the extravagance of the rich in an era when vast numbers lived in hovels and toiled long hours in factories, in mines, or on farms.

At some points during the last decades of the nineteenth century and beginning years of the twentieth, the term "idle rich" was used as a form of angry ridicule by labor organizers or left-wing spokespersons who sought to arouse the resentment of poorly paid workers against the wealthy.

"Discretionary Time" Concept.   The most common understanding of leisure today is that it consists of time free from work or work-related responsibilities, such as study, travel, or union activity. Typically, when the workweek is shortened or when holidays or vacations are added, economists conclude that employees have gained increased leisure.

Other tasks required for self-maintenance, such as eating, sleeping, shopping, housekeeping, cleaning, or obtaining medical care, are also regarded as obligatory uses of time, and so are not considered to be forms of leisure. Thus, the French sociologist Joffre Dumazedier described leisure as time apart from the obligations of work, family, and society.

Free-Time Activity.   A related view is that leisure consists of the activities we engage in voluntarily during such periods of time. The *International Dictionary of Sociology* has defined leisure as the pursuits that people carry on in their free time, and many sociological studies of leisure have sought to identify and analyze the recreational involvements of different population groups.

Leisure activities range from games and hobbies to sports, creative pastimes, and varied forms of entertainment, outdoor play, and travel. They may also include volunteer activity and community service, education that is not career-directed, and religious involvement.

Leisure as Personal Experience.   A given activity may or may not constitute a form of leisure involvement, depending on the reasons for engaging in it and the circumstances under which it is enjoyed. An activity pursued primarily for gain—monetary or otherwise—is not usually considered leisure. Beyond this, leisure motivations may be listed by the dozen, including the need to achieve varied forms of emotional satisfaction—to gain a sense of accomplishment, pleasure, release or escape, self-discovery, excitement, mastery, or challenge.

In recent years, social psychologists have identified two basic characteristics of the leisure experience: (1) It must involve perceived freedom in selecting activities without compulsion or the hope for extrinsic rewards; and (2) it has the potential to involve all aspects of the individual's personality and, in its highest form, to reach a state of what has been called "self-actualization"—achieving one's fullest potential as a human being.

Any definition of leisure must be treated rather flexibly and must take into account the possibility of "semi-leisure"—that is, experiences that are chosen under certain constraints or pressure, or that may have practical or extrinsic purposes apart from pleasure or personal satisfaction. Religion might be an illustration of semi-leisure, in that it usually consists of a voluntarily chosen activity carried on in one's discretionary time. At the same time, many devout individuals might consider religious practice an important form of self-maintenance, essential to healthy living.

The claim that leisure provides the potential for creative self-actualization must be balanced against the reality that much free time is used in mechanical, superficial, or even self-destructive ways. This reality makes it all the more important that children and youth—as well as adults—be educated to recognize the value of positive forms of leisure, and that different societal institutions *provide* healthy and enriching free-time experiences.

The Leisure "Industry."   The most influential recent shift in our thinking about leisure has been to characterize it as an industry—a huge, diversified area of business opportunity, employment, and economic return. Butsch points out that two centuries ago, Americans purchased comparatively few leisure goods or services. They played their own games, created their own music, and made their own toys. Commercial amusements, while they existed, did not dominate daily life. Today, most of our leisure activities depend on some organized form of sponsorship or provision of service, must of it involving the purchase of commodities:

> a television set, a baseball, tickets to the theater. We spend much of our free time watching and listening to programmed entertainment distributed by large corporations; we use sports and recreational equipment distributed by oligopolistic industries. Toys, now a multibillion-dollar industry, are produced by major corporations and retailed through national chains. As we have become more and more dependent on purchased goods and services for our fun, so too has leisure become a source of profit for corporate enterprise, and an integral part of the economy.[11]

To illustrate, Table 1.1 sums up national expenditures on leisure goods and services in the United States extending over a recent twelve-year period. While impressive, these statistics do not report the full range of leisure spending, since they do not include a number of important areas of leisure activity, such as travel and tourism, casino gambling, alcohol consumption, adult education, or spending by government and nonprofit agencies on recreation and park facilities and programs. The actual amount, if it were possible to measure all leisure spending accurately, would be somewhere between $750 billion and a trillion dollars—rather than the *Statistical Abstract's* estimated sum of $420 billion spent annually.

Unlike other industries, leisure does not represent a single clearly identifiable service, manufacturing, or distributing process. Instead, it involves the provision of a remarkably diverse set of services and programs by several different kinds of sponsors: governmental, commercial, nonprofit, educational, and therapeutic.

TABLE 1.1   Annual Personal Spending on Recreation: 1985 to 1996

Type of Product or Service	1985	1990	1996
Total Recreation Expenditures (billions of dollars)	116.3	281.6	431.1
Percent of Total Personal Consumption	6.6	7.3	8.3
Books and maps	6.5	16.5	23.2
Magazines, newspapers, and sheet music	12.0	21.5	26.5
Nondurable toys and sport supplies	14.6	31.6	45.4
Wheel goods, sports, and photographic equipment	15.6	29.8	42.0
Video and audio products, computer equipment, and musical instruments	19.9	53.8	89.7
Radio and television repair	2.5	4.2	5.1
Flowers, seeds, and potted plants	4.7	11.1	14.9
Admissions to specified spectator amusements	6.7	15.1	22.1
Motion picture theaters	2.6	5.2	6.3
Legitimate theater and opera and entertainments of nonprofit institutions	1.8	5.6	9.3
Spectator sports	2.3	4.4	6.4
Clubs and fraternal organizations except insurance	3.1	8.9	13.0
Commercial participant amusements	9.1	23.0	46.2
Parimutuel net receipts	2.3	3.4	3.5
Other (includes lottery receipts, pets, cable TV, film processing, sports camps, video rentals, etc.)	19.4	62.7	99.6

Sources: *Statistical Abstract of the United States* (U.S. Department of Commerce), 1997 and 1998. See these sources for fuller explanation of product and service categories. See Chapter 12 for discussion of other major leisure expenditures not listed here.

For this reason, it should be clearly understood that, while the term "industry" may logically be applied to many forms of recreational services, others must be regarded as important social programs or environmental projects. As later chapters will show, to characterize them solely as entrepreneurial business ventures would mean that their constructive social purposes would not receive full recognition or priority.

Leisure: A Composite Definition

Since leisure may be conceptualized in several different ways, the following statement suggests its key elements, as it is presented in this text:

> Leisure is defined as that portion of a person's life that is marked by: (1) freedom from the necessity for carrying on paid work or other obligated tasks; and (2) the opportunity to engage in pursuits that bring a sense of pleasure and self-enrichment, or that meet other important personal or social needs.

Beyond this formal definition, Ruth Russell writes that there is a singular benefit that makes leisure unique among all other human experiences—the *intrinsic rewards* that it often provides:

> Leisure gives us a sense of living for its own sake. Cross-country skiers often exclaim about sensations of peacefulness and physical exertion while gliding along. Artisans may explain their interest in working with clay on the potter's wheel because of the elastic, smooth substance responding to their hands. Dancing could be described as moving to a rhythm. Hikers often stress the experience of being a part of the beauty of the natural environment. These are all intrinsic rewards.[12]

In addition to its important personal values, leisure also represents an important social institution. It is both a recognized function of government on all levels and a complex industry. It also encompasses the broad field of popular culture—the motion pictures, television, music, drama, video games and other free-time forms of entertainment or communication that dominate most individuals' nonwork lives.

Such experiences not only reflect the interests, customs and values of a people; they also transmit and shape them. For many centuries, it has been understood that leisure offers a means of acculturation. In ancient Athens, Plato argued that the laws of adulthood were taught through the games of childhood. In North America today, we have established numerous organizations, both sectarian and secular, that use recreation as a means of teaching responsible citizenship and moral values to children and youth. Similarly, we have established museums, libraries, theaters, art galleries, and opera and concert halls that carry on the cultural heritage of the past and contribute to new forms of creative expression.

Too often, however, we permit the private and commercial domination of leisure programming, particularly in urban ghettos where socially constructive forms of leisure opportunity are lacking. Three decades ago, economist John Kenneth Galbraith suggested that in well-organized communities with strong school systems, recreation programs, and other needed services, the diversionary forces operating on youth might do little harm. But, he wrote, in communities where public services failed to keep abreast of private consumption, things were quite different:

> Here, in an atmosphere of private opulence and public squalor, the private goods have full sway. Schools do not compete with television and the movies . . . . The hot rod and the wild ride take the place of more sedentary sports for which there are inadequate facilities . . . . alcohol, narcotics and switchblade knives [or today, semiautomatic weapons] are . . . part of the increased flow of goods, and there is nothing to dispute their enjoyment.[13]

To illustrate the power of popular entertainment to influence youth today, we find an incessant display of obscenity and often sexist violence displayed on the television screen or in the rock music that appeals to vast numbers of young people. It is widely believed that the growing incidence of violence against women and the mindless slaughter of the young by gunfire in inner-city slums are at least partly attributable to such causes. Certainly, when society fails to provide attractive and positive leisure outlets for disadvantaged youth today, it permits them to fall easy victims to the lures of drug culture, gang allegiances, and other forms of contemporary social pathology.

Related Terms: Recreation and Play

Recreation.   This term customarily is used to refer to activities carried on voluntarily in leisure, for pleasure, or to achieve other important personal outcomes. It is also described as a personal process or experience and in that sense is very similar to definitions of leisure. Gray and Greben define recreation as:

> An emotional condition within an individual human being that flows from a feeling of well-being and self-satisfaction. It is characterized by feelings of mastery, achievement, exhilaration, acceptance, success, personal worth and pleasure. It reinforces a positive self-image. Recreation is a response to aesthetic experience, achievement of personal goals or positive feedback from others. It is independent of activity, leisure or personal acceptance.[14]

A widely accepted principle in the professional literature holds that to be legitimately considered recreation, any free-time activity must adhere to generally approved social and moral values. This view is debatable, however, in that community standards change over time and vary from place to place, within such areas of involvement as gambling, drinking, or sexual behavior. One might argue that it is impossible to impose any universal set of rules with respect to approved forms of leisure activity—and that, therefore, all voluntarily chosen free-time pursuits should be regarded as recreation.

In general, however, the conviction that healthful forms of recreation contributed to social well-being led to the establishment of thousands of parks, playgrounds, community centers, nonprofit youth-serving organizations, and public recreation and park departments in the United States and Canada. Their facilities and programs were intended to help the children and families that immigrated by the millions to the new world to adapt to its customs and values and to counter the threat of growing juvenile delinquency. In time, recreation came to be viewed as an essential element in the well-designed community, contributing to mental and physical health, social cohesion, and the overall quality of life.

The term "recreation" tends today to be more widely understood and accepted than "leisure," which is often considered to be free time or a rather abstract state of being. Therefore, most public agencies serving leisure needs tend to have the term "recreation" in their titles—along with parks or other related services.

A final distinction between the two concepts is that leisure provides the opportunity for several other kinds of experiences, such as continuing education, community service, or religious worship, as well as passive forms of rest or relaxation—which are not commonly thought of as recreational. A brief definition of recreation, embodying these elements, would be:

> Recreation consists of free-time, voluntarily chosen activities or experiences, carried on for purposes of pleasure, sociability, creative expression or other significant motivations. It also refers to the network of community agencies or social organizations that provide such opportunities.

Play.   This term has frequently been used interchangeably with recreation, although it has an older history and has been studied more intensively by philosophers, psychologists, anthropologists, social historians, and other scholars.

The term itself has usually been applied to casual and informal free-time activities, such as simple games and contests, make-believe or dramatic pastimes, or just "fooling around." It was widely thought of as an essentially purposeless form of activity, engaged in chiefly by children and—within the strict Puritanical moral code and Protestant work ethic that dominated much of North America for many years—morally dubious.

Over the past century and a half, however, we have come to recognize that play represents quite a different kind of purposeful experience. A number of European and American scholars developed theories of play which saw it as a means of: (1) expressing surplus energy, (2) restoring oneself after work, (3) preparing the young for the tasks or challenges of adulthood, or (4) maintaining emotional balance. Still other community leaders argued that play offered an invaluable means of promoting positive social relationships and values, or strengthening community life.[15]

Recent studies by ethologists and biologists have confirmed the value of play in the lives of various animal species, showing how it contributes to developing survival skills, cementing social bonds, and courtship rituals. Summarizing evidence showing that play is nearly as important to many kinds of animals and birds as food and sleep, Shannon Brownlee writes:

> These new findings have important implications for the most playful species of all—our own. Without play, particularly imaginative games, children fail to gain a sense of mastery and are less adept at social interactions than their more playful counterparts. [One psychiatrist concludes] "I think we get in trouble socially, physically, and culturally, if we neglect [play]."[16]

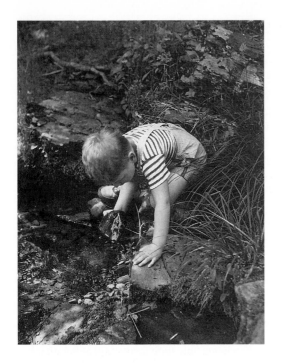

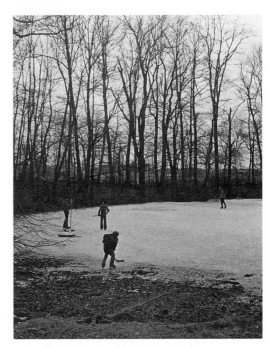

In the past, many forms of play were relatively simple and unstructured, making use of the natural environment, as in these scenes of children and youth playing hockey on a frozen pond or exploring playground equipment and a little stream.

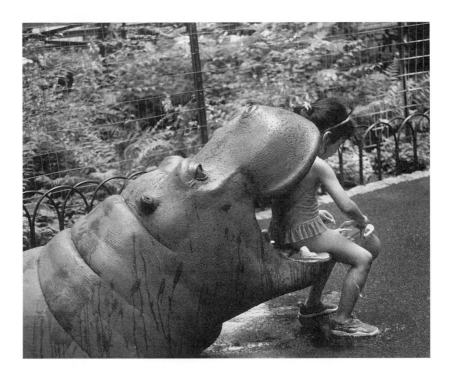

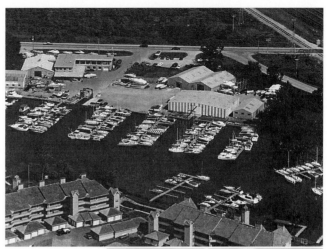

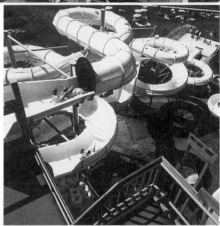

Today, many activities make use of more complex and expensive resources. In aquatic play, for example, millions of participants enjoy home-based swimming pools, impressive water-play parks, or huge marinas for boating recreation.

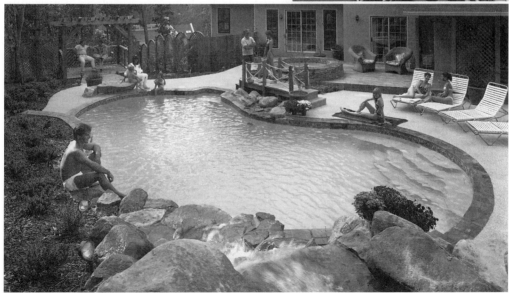

Other psychological analyses of play stress two primary kinds of play impulses: *stimulus-arousal*, meaning the need to experience risk, excitement, surprise, and pleasure; and *competence-effectance*, which involves the player's need to solve problems, explore new environments, and gain a sense of mastery and accomplishment.

Play may be defined simply in the following terms:

> It is a form of animal and human behavior, engaged in at all ages to meet developmental or other important life needs. It ranges from casual and spontaneous to highly structured and organized activity, and often incorporates such elements as competition, play-acting, creative problem solving, or environmental exploration. It may also be viewed as a behavioral style marked by improvisation and often humor.

Contrast Among Terms

Of the three concepts just discussed, the linkage between play and recreation is obvious: (1) The play impulse underlies many recreational activities, in that we play at games, cards, sports, or with musical instruments; (2) the early recreation movement was known as the "play movement," with children's playgrounds an early feature; and (3) in daily conversation, the two terms are often used interchangeably.

Play and recreation differ in that play customarily involves some form of activity—physical or mental—while recreation incorporates many more passive pursuits, such as reading a book, watching a film, or listening to music, which would not normally be thought of as play. Similarly, as later chapters will show, recreation agencies or other leisure-service organizations often provide various forms of social-welfare or human-service activities that have nothing to do with play.

From a professional perspective, the term recreation is more widely used and accepted than play, and leisure is used more frequently by economists, sociologists, philosophers, or other social or behavioral scientists.

Values and Outcomes of Leisure Experience

At several points in this chapter, reference has been made to the important personal and social benefits of participation in organized recreation programs.

What are these benefits? Do they represent more than the untested views of leisure enthusiasts or practitioners?

Initially, there were relatively few documented efforts to prove recreation's worth. Most of the early statements of leisure's value were essentially philosophical, or based on anecdotal observations. During the 1920s, as community recreation programs expanded rapidly, a number of municipal judges and law enforcement figures testified that playgrounds and other organized leisure services had resulted in sharp reductions in juvenile delinquency. Other sociologists and child guidance experts supported the value of constructive play and youth-serving organizations in building character and preventing deviant behavior.

However, it was not until the decades after World War II that fuller evidence was gathered to document recreation's values. Accelerating over the past several years, there now is a wealth of research that confirms the value of play and recreational experiences and organized recreation services.

Many of these values have been documented in two recently published sources: a text by Driver, Brown, and Peterson on the benefits of leisure[17] and a compilation of research findings by the Parks and Recreation Federation of Ontario, Canada.[18]

Personal Values

Numerous studies have shown the importance of children's play in terms of physical, social, and intellectual development. For example, in a review of varied research findings, Lynn Barnett found convincing evidence of play's contribution to creative problem-solving and other areas of cognitive growth.[19] Other reports show recreation's value for other age groups. To illustrate, J. R. Kelly and M. W. Steinkamp confirmed its benefits in contributing to the life satisfaction, social integration, and feelings of competence and self-worth of older adults.[20]

Still other studies document the outcomes of specific kinds of leisure experiences for children and youth. Alan Ewert, for example, compiled a summary of findings of the benefits of outdoor adventure recreation in terms of improved self-concept, confidence, feelings of well-being, group cooperation skills and respect for the law, and improved academic performance.[21] Numerous research studies show the value of recreation in helping individuals resist stress or improve work performance.

Health Benefits.   Even moderate forms of exercise, such as walking, gardening, or other outdoor or sports activities, reduce the risk of heart disease, high blood pressure and diabetes, according to a U.S. Surgeon General's report on physical activities issued in July 1996. Based on a concept of health as personal wellness, involving more than the absence of disease, Leonard Wankel points out that to experience leisure with the characteristics of perceived freedom, competence, self-determination, and improved quality of life contributes significantly to personal well-being.[22]

Concrete evidence of such benefits is found in the reports of many major corporations that have initiated employee recreation and fitness programs, with sharp reductions in employee absenteeism, turnover, and health-care costs for workers who participated regularly.

Social Values

Elsewhere, the author has cited a number of the important functions of organized recreation, park, and leisure-service agencies in cities throughout the United States and Canada. Beyond the purposes of contributing to the quality of life and the personal development of participants, these include the following:

> Making the community a more attractive place to live by improving the physical environment, providing a network of parks and open spaces, and incorporating leisure attractions in the redesign and rehabilitation of rundown urban areas.

Helping to prevent or reduce antisocial or destructive uses of leisure, such as drug abuse, delinquency or gang activity.

Improving intergroup and intergenerational relations among residents of different racial, ethnic or religious backgrounds through shared recreational and cultural experiences.

Strengthening neighborhood and community life by involving residents in volunteer projects and service programs and events.

Meeting the needs of special populations, both in segregated and integrated settings that help individuals with physical or mental disabilities become part of the mainstream of community life.

Enriching cultural life, both through the direct provision of music, drama, dance and literary programs and through assistance to agencies offering such activities.[23]

A vivid example of such social benefits directed specifically at youth may be found in a listing of program services offered by its member agencies, published by the California Park and Recreation Society. These include such elements as: programming for "latch-key" children; juvenile curfew support; gang prevention and intervention; academic support, career development, and training; youth mentoring and youth leadership; substance abuse prevention; individual and family counseling; teen pregnancy; and physical and mental rehabilitation programs—all linked to other youth recreation activities.[24]

Documented evidence of the value of sports and other youth-centered programs in combatting juvenile delinquency is cited in the Ontario, Canada, Parks and Recreation Federation report on recreation benefits. Similarly, a 1994 study of nineteen small towns and large cities throughout the United States, sponsored by the National Recreation and Park Association and the National Recreation Foundation, confirmed that public recreation services offered more than "fun and games." Instead, there was compelling proof of the cost-effective value of recreation and park services in reducing crime, improving health and the quality of life, and creating safer communities.[25]

Environmental Values

Clearly, both public recreation and park agencies and other nonprofit outdoor recreation or conservation-oriented organizations play an important role in preserving the natural environment. As later chapters show in detail, national, state, and local park agencies maintain and protect millions of acres of wilderness, including extensive forest areas, spectacular scenic attractions, and historic monuments.

The functions of government agencies in managing these natural resources range from regulating multiuse operations that include grazing, lumber, mining, and intensive outdoor recreation visitations to keeping wilderness areas as untouched as possible.

Over the past forty years in both the United States and Canada, government agencies and environmental organizations have cooperated in acquiring huge amounts of new open spaces through land and water fiscal assistance programs, as well as promoting the recovery of damaged land and water resources. Improving wildlife habitats, protecting threatened species, and enforcing stronger air and water quality standards have contributed significantly to environmental health, and many local recreation and park agencies today promote conservation education and mobilize their citizens in volunteer efforts to improve natural environments.

Beyond such efforts, as Chapter 13 points out, the term "environment" means more than wilderness protection. Instead, hundreds of millions of citizens today live in congested urban and metropolitan areas, and concern must be paid to *their* environments. The provision of well-maintained, attractive parks, nature reserves, zoos, picnic grounds, sports facilities, and other resources for outdoor recreation represents a key environmental concern. Similarly, the conversion of rundown or abandoned waterfront or factory sites into appealing settings for popular recreation, residential redevelopment, shopping, or cultural programs has become an increasingly high priority in many communities over the past two decades.

Economic Values

A fourth major area in which recreation and leisure provide important benefits to communities throughout the United States and Canada involves their contribution to economic prosperity.

Obviously, the massive sums spent on leisure goods and services each year, as shown in Table 1.1, translate into hundreds of thousands of successful businesses large and small and into employment for millions of men and women.

As a single dramatic example of the economic benefits of recreation and leisure within the area of tourism, the New York City Convention and Visitors Bureau found that the city had played host to 32 million visitors who spent close to $14 billion and provided employment for many thousands of city residents, in a recent year.

Sports have offered a major attraction that draws tourists to many cities. Denver, Colorado, for example, has traditionally been a popular center for many winter sports, including skiing and snowboarding, as well as mountain biking and rock climbing. When the city's professional football team, the Broncos, won the 1998 Superbowl, it gave Denver an immense boost in morale and visitor appeal. Some cities have deliberately set out to maximize their sports involvement by building expensive new stadiums. Indianapolis, Indiana, for example, set out to carve a niche for itself as the nation's amateur sports capital, building new stadiums for soccer, tennis, track and field, a world class pool, a velodrome, and the 60,500-seat Hoosier Drome. In the 1980s and 1990s hundreds of national and international sports events were hosted in Indianapolis, with substantial income to the city.

Cultural attractions have been widely promoted in other cities. Toronto, Ontario, Canada, for example, noted for its colorful, diverse population makeup, has developed numerous national and ethnic festivals, as well as museums, restaurants, and musical and stage attractions—such as a highly successful Shakespeare festival—that appeal to visitors. In the same province, Ottawa offers skating, skiing, and other winter competitions featuring the Rideau Canada, the world's longest ice-skating rink. In the United States, cities like Des Moines, Iowa or Sarasota, Florida, have relied on symphony orchestras, opera companies, community theaters, and world-class art museums to build their own quality of life, image, and tourist appeal.

Strikingly, when *U.S. News and World Report* sought to identify a number of cities that were flourishing in the modern era, it found that the most successful cities—such as

Vancouver, British Columbia, Minneapolis, Minnesota, or Chattanooga, Tennessee—had made major effects to provide appealing waterfront settings, park systems, aquariums, children's museums, day-care facilities, walking trails and bicycle paths, and other leisure-related attractions.[26]

Summing up, the economic contribution made by recreation, park, and leisure-service programs is greater and more diversified than simply the money spent on recreation. There are a number of important, separate areas of economic benefit, including the following:

1. Employment opportunities in varied public, private, and commercial recreational facilities and programs that improve the economic standing of communities. Linked to this, tax revenues derived from admissions or the sale of goods and services linked to sports, entertainment, and other leisure attractions.
2. The value of recreation and parks in the revival of older cities, both in providing attractive new settings that join environmental, business, and residential functions and in attracting new residents. These may include elderly persons who retire in cities, returning middle- or upper-income suburbanites, and young professionals or business employees who value the city's culture and social opportunities.
3. The appeal of similar leisure-related elements to companies that are planning to relocate and are seeking communities that will be attractive to their employees. Similarly, communities in more rural or scenic regions may find outdoor recreation and sports attractions appealing to "footloose" companies or "telecommuting" workers.
4. The increased value of residential properties close to cultural arts centers, beautiful parks, and waterfront areas, or similar leisure facilities. This represents a key factor in maintaining economic stability and encouraging new real estate development or the redevelopment of older neighborhoods.
5. Finally, the direct income gained from tourist spending, either simply for sightseeing purposes, or for attending sports events, festivals, theater, music, or cultural programs and facilities.

Taken all together, the values and outcomes of leisure and organized recreation services that have just been described affirm the importance of this field in community life. They lead one to ask two questions: What is the present state of leisure at the end of the twentieth century? and What will the changing role of recreation and leisure be in the new century that lies ahead?

Retrospective at Century's End

Given the glowing forecasts and optimistic expectations regarding leisure's societal role that were voiced at mid-century, one must take a hard look at the state of leisure in the United States today.

Has nonwork time actually expanded, as predicted at that time? Have the uses of discretionary time contributed richly to the quality of national life?

Has leisure become an effective tool in combatting many of the social problems that affect the poor, racial and ethnic minorities, persons with disabilities, and other populations in North American society?

Are recreation and park professionals committed to furthering environmental causes, promoting neighborhood and community development, and expanding the arts and other cultural pursuits?

What trends, issues, and challenges face leisure-service practitioners today and are likely to become more pressing in the early decades of the twenty-first century? What conditions will encourage or limit participants of all ages and socioeconomic classes as they seek to find fulfillment, pleasure, and growth in their uses of leisure? Recognizing that we live in a time of immense social and technological change, how will the shifts in job settings and business practices affect leisure motivations, participation, and outcomes?

All of these questions are explored in the chapters that follow, which deal with the early and recent history of leisure in the United States, with an overview of recreational participation and the organized leisure-service system.

Following that, the text will examine a number of major economic, social, and environmental trends that influence leisure patterns today and will present both opportunities and challenges for the leisure-service field in the years ahead. These will be placed within a forecasting perspective that seeks to describe the framework in which recreation and leisure will function.

Futurist Predictions: An Overview

While it is not possible to state definitively what *will* occur in the early decades of the twenty-first century, social scientists, futurologists, and other authorities tend to agree on a number of major predictions, including the following.

Among the present-day trends that are likely to accelerate in the years ahead are:

1. The emergence of an "interactive society," with the sophisticated development of electronic information processing affecting every aspect of life.
2. The growth of other new forms of technology in manufacturing, communications, health care, agriculture, and other societal processes.
3. The globalization of the business and entertainment world.
4. Increased emphasis on a high level of education needed to succeed in varied career fields.
5. The shifting of value structures, in terms of gender, race or ethnicity, and other demographic factors, which will result in a vastly different social environment.
6. Environmental issues becoming increasingly important, both nationally and internationally.
7. Radical shifts in the world of work, both in terms of job availability and demands, and potentially in work locations and leisure allocations.

Linked to such predictions, but with more direct applicability to the concerns of leisure-service agencies are the following trends:

- The steadily increasing aging population, the impact of electronic forms of play, the commodification of sports, and the growing fascination with "extreme" physical pursuits.
- Increasing concern about family stability and the need to provide alternatives to negative leisure attractions, such as substance abuse, gambling dependency, or commercialized and exploitive sex.
- Fuller need to link the recreation and park profession with environmental organizations, with emphasis on such programming thrusts as "ecotourism."
- Efforts to promote recreation and leisure as important vehicles for improving personal wellness, along with increased emphasis on serving over 45 million persons with disabilities in the United States, and proportionately comparable groups in Canada.
- The goal of achieving fuller public awareness of the value of recreation, parks, and leisure services as a key contributor to community well-being, along with emphasis on developing cooperative relationships and partnerships among different segments of the human-service field.

Carter, Keller, and Beck support the last of these needs, as recreation and park providers strive to provide significant forms of involvement that serve important community needs. They write:

> If we refocus our mission and leadership to address common social issues, we can ally professionally with other community change agents. These alliances result in safety nets that ensure service continuity to increasingly limited resources. We must take a stand along with those health and human services agencies in our communities to contribute to the betterment of our citizens and enhancement of [overall] community welfare.[27]

Accepting Social Responsibility: Providing More Than "Fun" and "Games"

Some readers may question whether the trends, issues, and challenges just described represent legitimate concerns of recreation, park, and leisure-service agencies and practitioners. In their view, recreation should be seen primarily as a source of personal pleasure or other private values—rather than as a social welfare instrument.

However, as this chapter has shown, leisure has far broader impacts than simple individual needs. To offer a single example within the huge realm of international tourism, Donald Holecek writes:

> International tourism in the 21st century will be a major vehicle for fulfilling the aspirations of mankind in its question for a higher quality of life [and] hopefully laying the groundwork for a [more] peaceful society through global touristic contact. Tourism also has the potential to be one of the most important stimulants for global improvement in the social, cultural, economic, political, and economic dimensions of future lifestyles.[28]

Many comparable statements might be made regarding other important goals and elements of leisure services today. The benefits-based movement that has become immensely popular among recreation, park, and leisure-service managers in recent years is based on the firm conviction that recreation will become an even more important source of societal well-being in the years ahead.

Finally, some readers may feel that North American society does not really need improved social services and that its economy, standards of living, and social relationships are among the best in the world today. Given this view, why should recreation and park educators seek to contribute to social progress?

Tom Goodale, at the time President of the Society of Park and Recreation Educators, offered a sobering response to such views. Summarizing the message of a recently published book by Derek Bok, formerly president of Harvard University, that compared the United States to six other advanced, industrialized, and democratic nations, he found that this country scored favorably on such measures as per capita income, housing quality, technical quality of health care, and average retirement income.

However, Goodale continues, the United States was *last* or *next to last* on such measures as affordability of housing for the entire population, degree of segregation by race, percent of waste recycled, and

> . . . infant mortality, percent of children living in poverty, life expectancy, health care cost, health insurance coverage. We were last or next to last on three of four measures of job security, three of three measures of crime, three of three measures of providing for the poor and disadvantaged. Though it may seem impossible to us . . . the fact is that we, as a nation, are underachievers on a grand scale, and that should not be tolerated . . . . [Therefore,] should we not address ourselves to the gap between our aspirations and quite extraordinary resources on the one hand and our lack of achievement on the other?[29]

The inescapable message that Goodale's question presents is the need for recreation, park, and leisure-service practitioners, planners, and educators to commit themselves to the task of delivering programs and services that will have a significant positive impact on public life, today and tomorrow. This need will be more sharply defined in the chapters that follow, which deal with the recent and current history of recreation and leisure, the nature of public involvement in leisure pursuits, and the structure and role of the diversified leisure-service system.

Summary

This chapter presents an overview of the growth of leisure availability, interest, and participation in the United States over the past century.

It discusses the meaning of three related terms—leisure, recreation, and play—and summarizes research documenting their value with respect to personal, social, environmental, and economic benefits. It concludes with a brief discussion of major trends that are predicted to occur within the years ahead and the issues and challenges they will present for the organized recreation, park, and leisure-service field.

Key Concepts

1. While the growth of leisure in modern society has led to an expansion of participation in organized activities on every level, it has been accompanied by a variety of social changes that pose serious challenges for this field.
2. In the post-World War II period, two conflicting views of leisure emerged: the "fun morality" emphasis on personal pleasure and the "social value," or humanistic, view that stressed its social contribution.
3. Varied definitions of leisure have ranged from its social-class identification, to considering it free or discretionary time; the latest concept regards it as a huge, complex industry.
4. Leisure may be seen both as reflecting social values and traditions and, in a more proactive sense, helping to shape them.
5. Recreation has traditionally been defined as a form of voluntarily chosen free-time activity, but is now often regarded as an emotional or social experience.
6. Play, once regarded as a purposeless and often negatively viewed form of children's behavior, is today respected as a significant activity carried on by all age groups, marked by characteristic themes and behavioral styles. Particularly for children, it has important developmental purposes.
7. The values of organized leisure programs fall into several categories, including personal, social, environmental, and economic benefits, which are briefly detailed in the chapter.
8. While some may feel that American society provides the best possible quality of life for its citizens, in several respects the United States falls short of the standards met by other nations. Recreation, parks, and leisure services should play a meaningful role in helping to overcome these deficiencies.

Endnotes

1. Mobley, T.A., and T.F. Toalson, eds. 1992. *Parks and Recreation in the 21st Century (Conference Report)*. Arlington, VA: National Recreation and Park Association, p. 8.
2. Griswold, W.A. 1959. *Life Magazine* (December): 59.
3. Bramham, P., I. Henry, H. Mommaas, and H. van der Poel, eds. 1989. *Leisure and Urban Processes*. London and New York: Routledge, p. 1.
4. See articles by Mills, C.W. and M. Wolfenstein in Larrabee, E., and R. Meyersohn, eds., 1948. *Mass Leisure*. Glencoe, IL: Free Press, pp. 28, 56.
5. Gray, D., and S. Greben. 1974. Future Perspectives. *Parks and Recreation* (July): 53.
6. Bernstein, C. 1990. The Leisure Empire. *Time* (December 24).
7. Pieper, J. 1952. *Leisure: The Basis of Culture*. New York: Pantheon, 52.
8. Harré, R. 1990. Leisure and Its Varieties. *Leisure Studies* 9: p. 187.
9. Kelly, J.R. 1982. *Leisure*. Englewood Cliffs, NJ: Prentice-Hall, pp. 43–44.
10. Bell, C. 1958. How to Make a Civilization. In *Mass Leisure, op. cit.*, p. 32.

11. Butsch, R., ed. 1990. *For Fun and Profit: The Transformation of Leisure Into Consumption.* Philadelphia: Temple University Press, p. 3.

12. Russell, R.V. *Pastimes: The Context of Contemporary Leisure.* 1996. Dubuque, IA: Brown and Benchmark, p. 48.

13. Galbraith, J.K. 1958. *The Affluent Society.* Boston: Houghton Mifflin, pp. 256–257.

14. Gray and Greben, *op. cit.,* p. 49.

15. Kraus, R., 1997. *Recreation and Leisure in Modern Society.* Menlo Park, CA: Addison Wesley Longman, pp. 24–27, 201–203.

16. Brownlee, S. The Case for Frivolity. 1997. *U.S. News and World Report* (Feb. 3): 45.

17. Driver, B.L., P. Brown, and G. Peterson, eds., 1991. *Benefits of Leisure.* State College, PA: Venture Publishing.

18. *The Benefits of Parks and Recreation: A Catalogue.* 1992. Gloucester, Ontario, Canada: Parks and Recreation Federation of Ontario.

19. Barnett, L. 1990. Developmental Benefits of Play for Children. *Journal of Leisure Research* (22/2): 138–153.

20. Kelly, J.R., and M.W. Steinkamp, 1986. Later Life Leisure: How They Play in Peoria. *The Gerontologist* (26): 531–537.

21. Ewert, A. 1986. Values, Benefits, and Consequences of Participation in Outdoor Adventure Recreation. *A Literature Review: The President's Commission on Americans Outdoors.* U.S. Govt. Printing Office: Values, p. 71.

22. Wankel, L. (1994). Health and Leisure: Inextricably Linked. *Journal of Physical Education, Recreation and Dance* (April): 29. *See also* Siegenthaler, K.L. 1997. Health Benefits of Leisure. *Parks and Recreation* (January): 24.

23. Kraus, *op. cit.,* pp. 136–155.

24. Parks and Recreation Goes Beyond "Fun and Games." 1995. *Phoenix Report.* California Park and Recreation Society: IV-37.

25. New Study Reveals Recreation, Parks' Impact on Serious Social Issues. *Dateline: NRPA* (December 1994): 1–2.

26. Koerner, B. 1998. Cities That Work. *U.S. News and World Report* (June 8): 26–36.

27. Carter, M., M.J. Keller, and R. Beck. 1996. A Vision for Today's Recreation and Leisure Services. *Parks and Recreation* (November): 49.

28. Holecek, D., in van Lier, H.N., and Taylor, P.D., 1993. *New Challenges in Recreation and Tourism Planning.* Amsterdam: Elsevier, p. 17.

29. Goodale, T. (1997). Editorial. *Society of Park and Recreation Educators Newsletter* (January): 1–2.

2 Leisure in America: The Post-War Years

It enriches us in many ways . . . . The great outdoors is a great health machine, toning up our minds and bodies. The engineer kayaking through a cataract and the assembly-line worker hunting in quiet woods are both recharging themselves for more productive work. Our economic health benefits more directly. Recreation products and services are a [multi] billion-dollar industry, and the economic web does not stop there. The clothes we wear, the automobile that takes us to recreation areas, and the photographic equipment that records the highlights all derive in part from the outdoor use of leisure time.

Open space is a silent social worker as well, in its ability to reduce crime and delinquency. A drop in vandalism accompanied the building of a small park in Trenton, New Jersey, prompting Mayor Arthur Holland to tell the commission, "You don't throw stones when you've got basketballs to throw around."[1]

In the early years of the twentieth century, leisure became increasingly available for many Americans as a consequence of the shortened work week and the development of labor-saving devices. Government on all levels established recreation and park agencies, and popular entertainment, sports, and travel and tourism reached a new peak of involvement during the 1920s. While the Great Depression of the 1930s shattered national confidence, the federal government under President Franklin Roosevelt's New Deal employed great numbers of recreation leaders, artists, writers, and cultural performers in order to restore public morale and provide emergency employment. Thousands of community sports and cultural facilities were built at this time.

Then, after World War II, a wave of economic prosperity led to rapid expansion of recreation and leisure in the United States. Commercial recreation businesses and new public recreation departments were both established, and varied technologically based pursuits captured public interests. At the same time, the nation became more aware of growing problems of crime, poverty, and social breakdown in many impacted central cities, and the need to reverse the tide of environmental decay that had threatened its open spaces, wilderness areas, and waterways.

In the 1960s, youth-led counterculture groups mobilized resistance to the Vietnam War and challenged traditional standards of sexual morality, the work ethic, and other established social values. Rapid progress was made in overcoming discriminatory practices against racial or gender minorities and in providing improved leisure opportunities for elderly persons or those with disabilities.

Growing Affluence in the Post–World War II Years

A critical factor in promoting the growth of recreation and leisure in the United States in the late 1940s and 1950s was the nation's economic prosperity. The Gross National Product rose from $211 billion at the war's end to over a trillion dollars annually by 1971. In the late 1950s, it was reported that Americans were spending $30 billion a year for leisure—a sum that seemed astounding but was just one-tenth of what it was to become in the 1980s.

Millions of young families moved from city neighborhoods to new suburban single-family developments. Suburban townships or villages established recreation and park departments and shopping malls offered a host of new consumer possibilities. Most families in the post-war environment followed the traditional model of Mom staying at home with the children, while Dad went off to work. Family recreation became a primary focus, with Little League, PTA programs, summer camping, and other shared pastimes contributing to the new ideal of "togetherness." Television entered most American homes, and with it a barrage of advertising that promoted a vast array of consumer-directed products and services.

Involvement in varied forms of recreation exploded during this period. Visits to national forests increased by 474 percent between 1947 and 1963, and to national parks by 302 percent during the same period. Overseas pleasure travel increased by 440 percent and attendance at sports and cultural events also grew rapidly. Sales of golf equipment increased by 188 percent, of tennis equipment by 148 percent, and use of bowling lanes by 258 percent. Hunting and fishing, horse-racing attendance, and copies of paperback books sold all gained dramatically and—most strikingly—the number of families with television sets grew 3500 percent over this sixteen-year period.

Recreation and leisure experiences of every sort were marketed by expanding conglomerates that offered theme parks, cruise ships and land tours, toys, sports events, video games, and a host of other free-time products and services. With this immense expansion as a form of economic enterprise, organized recreation also evolved into an impressive field of public service and career involvement.

Major Trends and Events Affecting Leisure Services

During this period, seven major trends or events influenced public participation and the delivery of recreation, park, and leisure programs in the United States:

1. The *growing professionalization* of large numbers of men and women working in different segments of the field, including public, nonprofit, military, therapeutic, commercial, and other specializations.

2. A wave of concern over the environmental degradation that had imperiled the *nation's natural environment,* accompanied by legislation and federal, state, and local action to protect and recover open spaces, wilderness, waterways, and other ecological resources.

3. Realization that affluence had not reached millions of Americans, both in central cities and rural areas, leading to a *"war on poverty"* that incorporated major elements of recreation and leisure services.

4. An explosion of *poverty- and race-related rioting* in a number of major cities that stimulated federal action, accelerated efforts to overcome past discrimination and segregation, and bring racial or ethnic minorities into the mainstream of national life.

5. Linked to the preceding trends, a *counterculture movement* that had its roots in protests against the Vietnam War in the 1960s, but also incorporated rebellion against traditional social codes, promoted permissive new attitudes regarding drugs and sex, and led to what has been called the "Me Decade."

6. New drives to promote social and economic quality for *other minorities*: girls and women, persons with nontraditional sexual lifestyles, individuals with physical or mental disabilities, and the elderly.

7. At the end of a period of steady economic expansion, a period of fiscal cutbacks that led to *new marketing approaches* in public and nonprofit leisure-service organizations, as well as a new emphasis on work and productivity that was reported to have sharply reduced free time for many.

Professionalism in Recreation, Parks, and Leisure Services

During the early decades of the twentieth century, as growing numbers of public recreation and park agencies were established, most recreation leaders were drawn from the fields of education and physical education. Park personnel were trained in fields like forestry, agriculture, and, in some cases, civil engineering. Schools of education offered courses in playground leadership, and the National Recreation Association sponsored one-year graduate training for recreation and park administrators. With the expansion of federally funded recreation programs during the Great Depression of the 1930s, there was increased awareness of the special role of leisure in society.

The American Association for the Study of Group Work published an important report in 1939 stating that the "leisure of the American people constitutes a central and crucial issue of social policy." Its author, Eduard Lindeman, a key federal official during the Depression, pointed out that American workers were gaining a huge "national reservoir" of leisure amounting to hundreds of billions of hours a year. If this free time was not to become "idleness, waste, or opportunity for sheer mischief," Lindeman urged that a national plan for leisure be developed, including the widespread preparation of professionally trained recreation leaders.

Beginning in the late 1930s and accelerating shortly after World War II, a number of major universities around the United States began special courses and degree programs in recreation leadership and park management. By the mid-1960s, there were several dozen such curricula—most housed in departments or schools of physical education, but others administratively attached to agriculture, social work, or other higher education subjects.

At the same time, a number of professional organizations that had had their beginning in the early decades of the century—including the National Recreation Association, American Recreation Society, American Institute of Park Executives, National Conference on State Parks, and American Association of Zoological Parks and Aquariums—merged into the new National Recreation and Park Association. This large body, with separate branches and divisions concerned with specialized leisure-service functions or administrative responsibilities, served to promote public awareness of the field, support needed legislation, hold conferences, sponsor research and publications, and provide field services.

Environmental Programs

Through the post-war years, a strong linkage developed between the recreation and park movement and environmental organizations and causes. In the 1950s, many Americans came to realize that the nation's wildlands had been despoiled by uncontrolled lumbering, grazing, strip-mining, and oil drilling; that breeding grounds and wetlands for wildlife had been destroyed or ravaged by pesticides or herbicides; and that there had been a steady loss of ocean frontage to private development and commercial exploitation.

Although we had set aside huge tracts of federally owned parkland for outdoor recreation, the bulk of these were in the western states and Alaska, far from the urban populations who needed them. In 1958, the Outdoor Recreation Resources Review Commission was appointed by Congress to review the situation and develop recommendations. Its extensive report, presented to President John F. Kennedy in 1962, documented the seriousness of the situation and offered major recommendations for legislation and new agencies to reclaim and protect the environment—with outdoor recreation a key priority.

With stimulation and fiscal support from the federal government through the new Land and Water Conservation Fund, states and communities throughout the nation acquired, developed, and rehabilitated major new tracts of land for outdoor recreation. Lakes, streams, and formerly wild rivers and trails were all revived; new national parks, seashores, and recreation areas were established, many close to crowded cities; and environmental beauty became a major concern in American life and public policy.

This positive trend continued until the 1980s, when conservative political policies that were closely linked with powerful business interests sought to roll back much of the progress that had been made. Through the 1990s, environmental organizations and citizen groups fought such efforts with growing success (see Chapter 13). At the same time, it became evident that many of the outdoor recreation pursuits that millions of Americans had been engaging in, including off-road travel, and overuse of wilderness areas, were clearly harmful to the natural environment and needed to be more carefully regulated.

Recreation and the War on Poverty

Another major thrust for the recreation and park movement came during the 1960s, when the Lyndon Johnson administration initiated a War on Poverty that embraced a range of programs designed to provide job opportunity, improve living conditions, and bring the poor—particularly those in the inner cities—more fully into the mainstream of national life. The Office of Economic Opportunity was created in 1964 to coordinate all antipoverty programs on the federal government level.

Among the innovative programs begun at this time were Job Corps, VISTA (Volunteerism in Service to America), CETA (Comprehensive Employment and Training Act), Model Cities, and a host of other housing and human-service programs designed to provide employment to poor people, improve the quality of life, particularly in urban slums, and give disadvantaged residents the opportunity to make decisions and work to improve their own neighborhoods. Recreation played an important role in each of these federal initiatives, which were generally coordinated through state agencies and carried out on the local level.

Why did poverty become an important national concern at this point? The reality was that the prosperity that had reached most Americans in the post–World War II years had not improved the condition of many citizens. As millions of families, primarily young, white, and middle-class, moved from central cities to new suburban communities at this time, the neighborhoods they left began to be populated by increasing numbers of economically disadvantaged people—many of them black or Hispanic workers and their families from the rural South, Central America, and the Caribbean. Within a complex economy where manual and other low-level jobs were disappearing, unemployment rates were high, resulting in growing welfare dependency, crime and delinquency, deteriorated housing, and other severe forms of social pathology.

The suburbs and small towns of the nation generally moved ahead to develop rich park and recreation resources and programs, with swimming pools, golf courses and tennis courts, recreation centers, and other facilities. However, the urban sector of the nation was far less fortunate. Living chiefly in cities, the poor suffered from inferior municipal services, including recreation and parks. With increased costs of welfare, law enforcement, and health services, budgets to support other human services were cut. Parks and recreation centers were often poorly maintained, and leadership staffs were slashed.

Beyond this, it became apparent that in many American cities, park and recreation acreage and facilities were more unevenly distributed than personal income. Based on an analysis of a sample of cities across the nation, Clawson and Knetsch found that in comparison to low-income areas, which often had impacted housing neighborhoods and few parks and playfields,

> the higher income sections had relatively generous parks and recreation areas. This situation is made still worse by the racial pattern of urban living . . . . The low-income central city areas so deficient in recreation space are likely to be Negro; the suburban and outer city ring areas, generously supplied with recreation, are likely to be white. One of the great myths of the outdoor recreation field is that free public parks are a boon to "poor" people; actually it is the poor who frequently lack them.[2]

This disparity between the recreation and park opportunities accessible to Americans of different racial backgrounds had come about initially as part of the process of urban growth. As cities expanded, they tended to add parks on their periphery, where land was inexpensive and available and where new housing was being built. In the central areas of cities where old industrial plants and run-down tenements existed side-by-side, there were few parks.

Given these conditions, the rationale for supporting recreation as part of the nation's antipoverty programs had several components. It was believed that recreation was particularly important to poor people, who were unable to pay for private or commercial forms of play. It was also recognized that past patterns of discrimination in providing adequate inner-city public facilities had deprived disadvantaged persons—particularly members of racial minorities—of adequate leisure opportunity. Beyond this, recreation offered a useful alternative to socially destructive forms of play, and both cultural enrichment and job training for many young people.

Civil Rights and Leisure

Despite other forms of social progress, racial segregation actually increased in the United States during the early twentieth century. It took a concentrated drive by many groups and individuals from the 1940s through the 1960s to begin about both federal legislation and Supreme Court decisions to end segregation in education, housing, public accommodations, and other areas of public life.

The first breakdown in recreational segregation came about during World War II, when army hospitals and armed forces centers moved toward desegregation. Based on presidential executive orders in the late 1940s, living quarters and schools for dependents, bars, clubs, athletic fields, and swimming pools were all gradually desegregated. The cracking of the color line in professional baseball shortly after World War II had a major effect on both professional and amateur sports. Not only did large numbers of black athletes join major league teams in baseball, football, and basketball, but increasing numbers also became active in college athletics.

Throughout the southern and border states, places of public accommodation, including libraries, museums, parks, and beaches, began to be opened to integrated participation. In some cities, black artists, entertainers, and speakers appeared before unsegregated audiences. Private lawsuits, sit-ins, demonstrations, and boycotts were all used to open up public and private facilities to integrated use. In some situations, African American college students who entered segregated facilities in the face of angry opposition were beaten, attacked by police dogs, and arrested. However, they persisted and, ultimately, in three 1963 decisions the Supreme Court affirmed that no municipally owned and operated facilities might be segregated, and that this practice must be promptly reversed.

Throughout the late 1950s and early 1960s, southern and border states responded to such pressures in varied ways. In some cases, all municipal areas were thrown open to use by African Americans. In other cases, cities closed down swimming pools or golf courses rather than integrate them. In still others, publicly owned facilities were changed to pseudo-private ownership and operated in this way. However, gradually the majority of publicly owned bathing beaches and tennis and golf facilities that were formerly legally segregated were quietly opened to general use, and the principle of desegregation became generally accepted.

The 1964 Civil Rights Act stipulated that places of public accommodation (such as theaters, sports arenas, or other places of public exhibition or amusement) or publicly supported facilities like parks or libraries might no longer be racially segregated. Some ambiguity remained with respect to privately operated amusement parks, dance studios, bowling alleys, billiard parlors, or skating rinks.

Urban Riots as Racial Protest

However, despite such areas of progress, racial discrimination remained widespread throughout the United States in economic, social, and educational terms. In the 1960s, the country was torn by a series of major urban riots. Protesting against discriminatory forms of education, justice and law-enforcement practices, health and welfare services, and limited job opportunity, rioters burned building, looted stores, and had violent confrontations with police and National Guard units in dozens of inner-city areas—in Los Angeles, Newark, Chicago, Cleveland, Detroit, and many other communities. In a number of such cases, the flash point came when African Americans were denied access to adequate recreation opportunities during the long, hot summer months. For example, an account of one of the first riots, in Jersey City, New Jersey, in 1964, reported:

> Three recreation centers are being reopened today in the riot-scarred Negro areas of Jersey City as the start of a civic effort to ease racial tensions there . . . . The play-grounds opening today are at housing projects [that] were at the center of several riot incidents. They were among several the city had decided not to open this summer for economy reasons. Lack of recreational facilities was one of the grievances cited by Negro leaders as contributing to the bitterness behind the rioting.[3]

Within a Chicago slum area where over 300,000 African Americans were crowded into 800 square blocks, the lack of adequate recreation facilities was one of the key factors that led to bloody rioting in July 1966. The rioting began when police turned off a fire hydrant being used by black children during a particularly oppressive and sustained heat spell.

> The park district has twenty pools on the West Side, four of them within walking distance of the hydrant over which the first disorder began. Officially, none of the pools has a racial restriction. But practically, authorities concede, only one of the four has been readily available to Negroes because of hostility in white neighborhoods near the others.[4]

In numerous other cities, the demand for improved recreation was an important element in ghetto dissatisfaction. As a consequence, Congress voted hundreds of millions of dollars each year at this time for community action programs to keep the summers "cool." The bulk of these emergency funds were granted to special antipoverty neighborhood programs to provide new jobs, light playgrounds, provide portable swimming pools, and support recreational programs for blacks and Hispanics in impacted inner-city areas.

Recreation was widely recognized as a useful means of encouraging residents to take responsibility for upgrading their own communities and for reducing delinquency, tension, and gang violence. However, as the riots declined during the late 1960s and 1970s, national concern diminished and federal support for most such programs was sharply cut.

Youth Rebellion and the Counterculture

During the same period in which the urban riots occurred, but extending beyond them well into the 1970s, there was also a widespread protest movement among the nation's young. Fueled by resistance to the Vietnam War, this rebellion took the form of a broad attack on establishment values and the powerful institutions of society.

The young people who spearheaded it challenged what they saw as the artificial constraints and values that governed their lives—the rigid curricula and lack of opportunity for self-governance in schools and colleges, the materialistic values that made money and economic success the keystone of success in life, and the traditional but often hypocritical sexual values that adults professed. Many young people became involved with drugs; rock music became increasingly popular, and the Beatles and the Rolling Stones helped to create an atmosphere symbolized by such popular slogans as "Do your own thing," "Let it all hang out," and "Don't trust anyone over thirty." Even younger teenagers were caught up in the rebellion, and many naive "flower children," wearing beads and long hair, flocked to neighborhoods like the East Village in New York City or Haight-Ashbury in San Francisco, where they often were preyed on by pimps, drug pushers, and other hardened slum residents.

Older students led antiwar and curriculum-change demonstrations in schools and colleges through the country, in some cases occupying administrative offices and sometimes shutting down entire universities. As a result, curriculum requirements were abandoned in many institutions and more flexible and "relevant" courses and requirements substituted; social-life restrictions, including those on sexual behavior, were also widely relaxed, and students were given a fuller role in campus governance.

Much of the impulse underlying the counterculture movement stemmed from Charles Reich's immensely popular book, *The Greening of America,* which bemoaned the destruction of the environment, the artificiality of work, the reliance on unlimited technology and the rigidity of the ruling bureaucracy. As Reich saw it, an era that he called "Consciousness III" would be spearheaded by the young leaders of the counterculture, and human society would evolve into more loving, less competitive, and ecologically sensitive state.[5]

While *The Greening of America* turned out be somewhat mystical and unrealistic as a prediction of things to come, it had a powerful impact on many individuals who sought a new, freer, less competitive, and more natural way of life. One of the counterculture's immediate effects was that it sharply undermined the faith of many young Americans in the nation's economic system and caused many of them to question the dominant work ethic. While many individuals simply turned off or joined rural communes, others took jobs but regarded them simply as "selling their time," rather than meaningful life experiences.

Decline in Acceptance of Work Values

The belief that work was a critical element in the moral and religious life of the nation came under increasing attack at this time. The instinct of "workmanship" no longer motivated employees in boring and uncreative jobs. A nationwide study of work attitudes in the United States showed that college students voiced growing resistance to authority and to being "bossed around" on the job. In 1968, 60 percent of respondents accepted the view that "hard work will always pay off," but in 1971 only 9 percent supported it. In offices and factories, absenteeism increased dramatically and growing numbers of employees refused overtime work. In *Work and Its Discontents,* Daniel Bell had concluded that if "conspicuous consumption" had been the badge of a rising middle class, "conspicuous loafing" was now the hostile gesture of a tired working class.[6]

By 1971, a Harris Poll revealed that:

- 78 percent of all working Americans felt that "people take less pride in their work than they did 10 years ago."
- 73 percent believed that the "motivation to work hard is not as strong today as it was a decade ago."
- 69 percent felt that workmanship had declined significantly, and 63 percent felt that people did not work as hard as they had in the past.[7]

The ultimate expression of the Protestant ethic, what psychiatrists had begun to call *workaholism,* was now widely scorned as neurotic behavior. Instead of commitment to work, Bell wrote, many employees had embarked on a desperate "drive for leisure":

The themes of play, of recreation, of amusement are the dominant ones in our culture today. They are the subject of the "hard sell." Sports clothes, travel, the outdoor barbecue, the portable TV set, all become the hallmarks of the time.[8]

Leisure's Relationship with Work

A number of investigators examined the changing relationship between work and leisure. In one study, Spreitzer and Snyder explored what they called a "compensatory" hypothesis—that when work failed to provide self-actualization and the opportunity for rewarding self-expression, leisure would tend to take on enriched meaning. They found that, while leisure activities may be useful in compensating for job dissatisfaction, they were not as psychologically encompassing as work experiences that were fully self-actualizing. Other studies examining the relationship between leisure and work were carried out by John Kelly at the University of Illinois. Kelly suggested two contrasting concepts: (1) the *dualist* view, which sees leisure as a sphere of human activity that is distinctly separate from work; and (2) the *holistic* view, which sees a close relationship between leisure and work. He developed an analysis of leisure that took into account both societal constraints and pressures that affect it and also its degree of work-relatedness. Based on these variables, there were four ways of defining leisure:

1. Unconditional leisure: carried on for its own sake, and for intrinsic satisfaction, with a minimum of expectations related to family or community values.
2. Coordinated leisure: freely chosen, but similar to the participant's involvement in work, in its form or content.
3. Complementary leisure: strongly influenced by work; may be either role-related (similar to work) or compensatory (contrasting with work).
4. Required activities carried on in nonwork time: not really regarded as leisure, but done to prepare for work, maintain household, etc.[9]

Throughout this period, accompanying the decline of interest in work, Americans showed a steadily growing fascination with play—both in the search for pleasure and other personal values and as a means of asserting their own individuality.

Leisure and the Search for Happiness

In a special seventeen-page feature in May 1977, *Newsweek* described the economic impact of the "dazzling world of play" that Americans had embarked on:

> Almost unnoticed, leisure-time activities have become the nation's No. 1 industry, as measured by people's spending. Latest figures . . . show that Americans will spend more than 160 billion dollars on leisure and recreation in 1977. By 1985, the total is expected to climb to 300 billions. The expenditure is a clear indication, sociologists say, of how avidly Americans pursue "the good life" beyond the bounds of work and home.[10]

As examples of the growth in leisure involvement, *Newsweek* reported that sports activities—including boating, tennis, football, archery, jogging, hunting, bowling, and others—drew more than 700 million participants a year. Attendance at sporting events had risen during the past decade to 314 million, and participation in cultural activities also had climbed by leaps and bounds; 78 million Americans visited museums each year, and 62 million attended at least one performance of live theater. Active hobbies were also growing, with 36 million households involved in gardening, 16 million participants in stamp collecting, and 10 million in bridge and chess. An estimated 40 million Americans were spending leisure time in volunteer and religious activities.

Individuality versus Conformity in Play

Some critics were skeptical about the impact of the nation's growing involvement in leisure pursuits. Daniel Bell, for example, felt that much of the new American lifestyle represented the influence of relentless advertising and pressure to consume lavishly. He wrote:

> The American citizen, as *Fortune* once noted, lives in a state of siege from dawn until bedtime. "Nearly everything he sees, hears, touches, tastes, and smells is an attempt to sell him something . . . . Advertising is the handwriting on the wall, the sign in the sky . . . ."[11]

Similarly, psychiatrist Erich Fromm argued that many individuals were passive, alienated, and controlled by others in their free time, just as they were in their work:

> [The individual] "consumes" ball games, moving pictures, newspapers and magazines, books, lectures, natural scenery, social gatherings, in the same alienated and abstractified way in which he consumes the commodities he has bought . . . . Actually, he is not free to enjoy "his" leisure; his leisure-time consumption is determined by industry, as are the commodities he buys; his taste is manipulated . . . . entertainment is an industry like any other, the customer is made to buy fun as he is made to buy dresses and shoes. The value of the fun is determined by its success on the market, not by anything which could be measured in human terms.[12]

Certainly many forms of play were marked by mass conformity and passivity at this time, just as they were in earlier periods. However, given the impact of the consciousness-raising period of the 1960s and 1970s, growing numbers of Americans were determined to assert their own individuality through leisure. So, instead of relying on mass-produced toys or free-time gadgets or the world of electronic entertainment that had become increasingly popular, a sizable segment of the population sought out unique hobbies in their leisure:

> Retired individuals who live in travel trailers and go south in the winter and north in the summer, backpacking enthusiasts, scuba divers, antique collectors, swamp buggy racers, body builders, craftsmen and craftswomen, snowmobile racers, skydivers, folk music performers and fans, tailgating fans at professional football games, collectors, artifact searchers who use metal detectors, mummy dusters who volunteer in archaeological museums, hang gliders, performers in little theaters, people who practice "creative anachronism" (enacting lives of past or mythical cultures)—all illustrate such absorbing hobbies.[13]

Harvard sociologist David Riesman concluded that the herd instinct had largely disappeared when it came to lifestyle behaviors, and the director of the values-and-lifestyle program at SRI International, a California think-tank agency, summed it up: "The trend is that there is no trend. We're in the midst of a celebration of diversity."

Search for Self: The "Me Generation"

Sociologist Robert Bellah concluded that individualism had been encouraged to "run rampant" in the society by the mid-1980s. He attributed much of this to the role of psychologists in emphasizing almost exclusively the needs, interests, and feelings of the individual, rather than those of the broader society. John Hewitt agreed, writing that the "self" is omnipresent in contemporary life. Everyday conversations are filled with references to identity, self-concept, self-esteem, self-image, self-fulfillment, self-actualization. He continued:

> Therapists and best-selling books promise to teach assertiveness, raise consciousness, enhance self-esteem, or improve relationships. Celebrities parade their psychic

wounds before television audiences, and the language of self-reference has become a widely acceptable part of popular vocabularies of motive. Men and women . . . speak of "finding themselves" and of their "real" selves, as if the self could lose itself or be mistaken for another self.[14]

Inevitably, the 1980s became known as the "Me Decade." While work was no longer viewed as a moral imperative, to be successful and make money became increasingly important. So-called Yuppies (Young Urban Professionals) became the model for many young people. These success- and career-oriented individuals were out to make a killing by whatever means, including junk-bond speculation, leveraging companies, making high-flying deals, and enjoying a flashy, hedonistic lifestyle.

Other Effects of Counterculture:
Emergence of Minority Groups

Beyond these changes in public values and behavior, the counterculture also served to draw attention to the needs of different kinds of minorities—including gender-based, disabled, and elderly groups—that had formerly been poorly served in terms of leisure opportunities.

Within the larger society, the youth rebellion stimulated other groups in the population to initiate drives for fuller recognition and societal status. Feminists became increasingly active in the fight for equality in all spheres of American life. Women formed support groups and established national organizations and lobbying mechanisms to attempt to overcome male dominance in government and politics, the job world, and family life. For the first time in America, homosexuals began to demand fuller civil and political rights and to lobby successfully for the decriminalization of alternative forms of sexual behavior.

Similarly, in the 1960s and 1970s, there was growing social concern about persons with mental and physical disabilities. The first important step in the United States came when President John F. Kennedy supported new legislation to serve developmentally disabled persons, and when organizations like Special Olympics and the Kennedy Foundation began to provide needed community programs for this population. There was a massive drive toward deinstitutionalization—getting hundreds of thousands of mentally retarded and mentally ill persons out of long-term custodial institutions into community-based residential facilities where they might become more fully functioning members of community life. Public Law 94-142, the Education for All Handicapped American Children Act, resulted in sharply improved services for disabled persons, including support for physical and occupational therapy, along with recreation as a "related service." Section 504 of the Rehabilitation Act of 1973, often called the "Nondiscrimination Clause," made it clear that schools and colleges were required to provide interscholastic athletics and extracurricular programs for disabled students, in "least restrictive" settings, and mandated that athletic, cultural, and entertainment events be made more fully accessible to all persons.

The elderly, who had long been demeaned and economically vulnerable in American society, also began to mobilize to improve their status in community life. Led by such individuals as Maggie Kuhn of the Gray Panthers, older Americans joined organizations like the American Association of Retired Persons, lobbied vigorously for fuller community services, and gained, through the Older Americans Act, new federal and local programs to assist the aged in terms of health care, retirement and housing assistance, and other social services.

For each of these special populations, one of the battlegrounds in which greater opportunity was a target was the broad area of leisure. Women, for example, sought support for fuller involvement in sports, outdoor recreation, and career employment in recreation. Advocates for physically and mentally disabled persons pressed for the integration of special populations in recreation on all levels in community life. Homosexuals began to present themselves openly in gay social clubs on university campuses and in community settings and exerted pressure to gain a more positive image in the mass media of communication and entertainment.

Implications for Leisure and Recreation

What did these radical changes in values and behavior have to do with leisure and recreation? Obviously, they sharply challenged many of the traditional beliefs and shibboleths that had governed past recreational practices. For example, most youth sports programs had typically been conducted within a highly competitive, gender-segregated structure that strongly emphasized winning as a goal and ignored the needs of less-skilled youngsters. Under the impetus of the humanistic thinking that gained popularity at this time, greater efforts were made to promote play for all, within a noncompetitive, corecreational framework.

For adolescents and young adults, as sex became more acceptable, pornography gained semilegal status (with adult videos and VCRs entering millions of respectable middle-class households) and drug use became endemic. The hedonistic leisure possibilities that beckoned made the traditional social activities of earlier generations seem pallid and boring.

For example, at the height of the counterculture movement, college courses were added that dealt with new lifestyle values and interests. Students at the University of Connecticut at Storrs established an Experimental College that sought to be responsive to the "real" needs of youth. Instead of courses, it offered "learning collectives," and instead of teachers it had "resource persons." Its curriculum included sessions in how to grow marijuana, build an atomic bomb, and play the banjo, as well as other collectives in massage, welding, yoga, automobile electrical systems, belly dancing, Chinese cooking, guitar playing, bread baking, vegetarian cooking, sewing, and stargazing.

Many women who faced lives as single parents because of divorce took courses or joined support groups that helped them deal with their need for economic independence, roles as working women and mothers, and other challenges in the rapidly changing society. Both men and women by the millions joined support groups dealing with assertiveness training, stress management, weight loss, and dozens of other themes linked to consciousness-raising. One critic commented that whatever the motive—"pleasure, profit, or paradise now"—America in the mid-1970s had embarked on the biggest "introspective binge" any society in history had experienced.

Summary

The three decades after the end of World War II were a period of affluence and national optimism, as well as a time of profound social change. Spending on various forms of play exploded, and those working in the recreation, park, and leisure-service field became increasing professionalized. Environmental programs gained support, and recreation was a key element in the nation's "war" on poverty, as well as in the accelerating Civil Rights movement.

However, in the 1960s, the nation was torn apart by opposition to the Vietnam War. This in turn was linked to a larger, countercultural rebellion that challenged many established values with respect to work, social and sexual relationships, and the role of authority in educational and civic institutions. It gave rise to demand by groups that had formerly been poorly served in American life—including racial and gender minorities, the elderly, and those with disabilities—for fuller opportunities and access to community services. At the same time, many formerly disapproved forms of play gained widespread acceptance.

Key Concepts

1. Among the key changes of the 1950s, 1960s, and 1970s was a dramatic expansion of interest in leisure activities, less emphasis on the Protestant work ethic, and the acceptance of "fun morality" in American society.

2. During the 1960s and 1970s, the nation became aware of the growing threat to the natural environment, and major pieces of legislation and funding programs were established to curb pollution, acquire additional open space, and provide fuller access to outdoor recreation environments for millions of Americans.

3. At this time, major federal programs were put in motion to include recreation as part of the effort to overcome both urban and rural poverty and respond to urban riots protesting racial discrimination in the United States.

4. With the growth of many new suburban communities and the merger of the park and recreation movements, professionalization in the leisure-service field accelerated, linked to the emergence of new or expanded professional organizations serving leisure needs.

5. The counterculture led by youth activists during the 1960s and 1970s represented challenges to established social values, traditional moral codes, and restrictions against racial, gender-related, and other minorities in terms of leisure roles and opportunities.

6. Many social critics argued that individualism had been allowed to run rampant at this time, with both youth and adults becoming over-absorbed with their own, rather than community-based needs, leading to what became known as the "Me Generation."

Endnotes

1. *Report of President's Commission on Americans Outdoors,* 1987, Washington, DC, p. 1.
2. Clawson, M., and J.L. Knetsch, 1960. *Economics of Outdoor Recreation.* Baltimore: Johns Hopkins Press and Resources for the Future, Inc., pp. 256–257.
3. *New York Post* (August 6, 1964), p. 50.

4. *New York Times* (July 18, 1966), p. 17.

5. Reich, C. 1970. *The Greening of America.* New York: Random House.

6. Bell, D. 1958, 1988. Work and Its Discontents. In *The End of Ideology.* Cambridge: Harvard University Press, p. 239.

7. Yankelovich, D. 1982. The Public Mind: The Work Ethic Is Unemployed. *Psychology Today* (May): 6.

8. Bell, D., *op. cit.,* pp. 257–258.

9. Kelly, J. 1975. Leisure Decisions: Exploring Extrinsic and Role-Related Orientations. *Society and Leisure* 4: 45–61.

10. The Boom in Leisure: Where Americans Spend 160 Billions. *Newsweek* (May 23, 1977): 62.

11. Bell, *op. cit.*

12. Fromm, E. 1955. *The Sane Society.* New York: Fawcett, p. 124.

13. Summarized from Jury, M. 1977. *Playtime: Americans at Leisure.* New York: Harcourt, Brace, Jovanovich.

14. Hewitt, J. 1989. *Dilemma of the American Self.* Philadelphia: Temple University Press, p. 3.

3 Challenge and Change at Century's End

By most objective standards, the last half century in our national life has been enormously successful. Americans have achieved unprecedented levels of material prosperity and personal freedom. We are healthier, work at less exhausting jobs, and live longer than at any time in our history . . . and government provides a safety net for the poor, disabled, and elderly that never before existed. Many old discriminations—based on race, sex, or religion—have diminished dramatically, even if they haven't entirely disappeared.

In short, America today is a far wealthier and more compassionate society than fifty years ago, and on a personal level, most Americans appreciate these achievements. When surveyed, about four-fifths of us say we are satisfied with our own lives.[1]

Following the turbulent post-war years described in Chapter 2, the decades of the 1980s and 1990s represented a retreat from the counterculture period, as well as a time of retrenchment and growing conservatism.

First, work began to gain a new degree of respect in society, and reports indicated that Americans were working longer hours and possessed less leisure than in the years after World War II. Job pressures were intensifying, linked to heightened business competition, employee downsizing, and the use of technology that speeded communication and decision making. Widespread budget cuts in many fields of government led to the need for growing numbers of recreation and park agencies to rely on self-generated revenues and adopt an entrepreneurial, marketing identity. So-called recreation "apartheid" appeared, symbolizing the contrast between wealthy communities with rich resources and poorer neighborhoods with skeletonized recreation and park facilities and programs.

Beyond these changes, there was an era of increasingly conservative policy making in such areas as the justice system, public support of the arts, or race-related issues such as affirmative action or immigration policy. As many members of the public withdrew from the use of community programs and resources, privatization began to represent a threat to the popular support of public recreation and parks. At the same time, at the very end of the twentieth century, the national economy was booming, unemployment hit a new low, recreation spending continued to rise, and most Americans expressed satisfaction with their lives and confidence in the future.

Work and Free-Time Shifts in the 1980s

In the early 1980s, it was apparent that a retreat from the era of the counterculture was in order. As part of an overall trend in public thinking, work began to regain its earlier positive image—and research reports indicated that Americans *were* working longer hours than they had a decade or two earlier. For some time, economists and political scientists had pointed out that America's shorter-hours movement was selective in its impact. Sebastian de Grazia had reported that, while average weekly hours of work had declined in the post–World War II years, this was due to the increase in holidays and paid vacations—and that professionals and business executives were now working disproportionately long hours.[2]

In 1987, pollster Louis Harris reported that the number of hours the average American was working had risen from 40.6 hours weekly in 1973 to 48.4 in 1985, and that the leisure hours available to most Americans had declined from 26.2 hours to 17.7. The number of weekly work hours was particularly high for professional people, those with incomes of $50,000 a year and over, and for women, who often have both jobs and home-based responsibilities. Harris concluded:

> Clearly, a phenomenon has emerged among the country's most affluent sectors: They work the longest hours and have the least time for leisure. This trend toward longer work hours and shorter leisure time runs counter to all the predictions that were made 10 to 20 years ago, when it was widely assumed that automation and technology would shorten the workweek and would give most people more and more leisure time. Precisely the opposite has happened.[3]

A number of other reports supported the Harris Poll findings. A *Wall Street Journal*/NBC News survey in 1986 showed that, however Americans defined leisure, twice as many claimed to have less of it than those who claimed to have more, than in the past. The survey found that professionals and managers had less vacation time—two weeks a year on the average—than in any other industrial nation but Japan.

In the early 1990s, Juliet Schor, a Harvard economics professor, wrote a book that summed up the trend—*The Overworked American: The Unexpected Decline of Leisure.*[4] In an article in *Newsweek*, Schor concluded that from the end of the 1960s to 1992, Americans had increased the amount of time they spend at work by about 160 hours, or nearly one month per year. This was equally true, she wrote, for workers in service jobs and those in "glamour" positions, and for both women and men. In part, Schor felt, the change had occurred because of employment practices within the competitive capitalist system:

Businesses would rather employ fewer workers and pay overtime than hire more and pay fringe benefits. And as productivity increases, business would rather give employees more money than more time off.[5]

Leisure's Decline: Reality or Myth?

This reported trend represented a sharp reversal of the economic and employment statistics and expectations of the past one and a half centuries and the predictions at mid-century that work hours would be lessened and leisure increased as part of the "good life" for all. But *was* the reported expansion of work and decline of leisure a reality? A number of reputable authorities challenged the Harris Poll findings on several grounds. For example, economist Robert Samuelson concluded that the Harris statistics were unreliable, citing the data drawn from elderly respondents as evidence:

> Although few of them hold jobs, they recorded the largest drop in leisure in the latest survey. And they say they have only about an hour more of daily leisure than working-age Americans. How can this be? It can't. People don't offhandedly know how much free time they have and Americans are reluctant to admit they spend too much time relaxing.[6]

Samuelson went on to point out that the Harris data on work and free time were drawn from two questions taking about a minute to administer, in a 72-question telephone interview on another subject entirely. Asked to give information of this type, respondents can easily provide subjective, inaccurate responses. Similarly, in a critique of Schor's book on the overworked American, Robert Sobel concludes that she had oversimplified the problem, in drawing inferences about the decline of leisure: "Schor ignores this matter [complexity of the country's population], preferring instead generalization, stereotype, and recourse to aggregate statistics followed by [carefully selected] anecdotes."[7]

The most effective approach to gathering valid statistics in this field is to collect precise information from employees using daily diaries of time use. The most systematic and comprehensive studies of this type have been carried out by sociologist John Robinson of the University of Maryland. Based on surveys conducted in the 1960s, 1970s, and 1980s in cooperation with the University of Michigan and funded by the National Science Foundation, Robinson found that free time—defined as everything that excluded work, self-maintenance, or family care—had actually risen about 10 percent over this period.[8]

Increased Job Stresses for Many

Robinson also suggested several reasons why many Americans feel that they have less leisure—including the growing number of working women, single parents, latchkey children, and parents working separate shifts—all of which create time pressures.

The likelihood is that the so-called time famine is in part a reality, stemming from the increase in workload for individuals in companies that were downsizing during difficult economic times and from the pressure on many wealthy and successful professionals and business executives to compete in a heightened work climate.

Certainly time pressures have increased for many Americans, particularly in the child-rearing, career-building, debt-assuming years. Fax machines, E-mail, computers and the Internet, car phones, and other technological innovations may have made life easier, but they also tend to wipe out time that is spent waiting for things to happen, or simply for reflection and thoughtful decision making.

Particularly in the transition from an industrial to a post-industrial, global, information-based economy—to be discussed later in this text—many professionals such as lawyers, bankers, and accountants must work harder than ever to meet their clients' needs.

Leisure as a Source of Pressure

A paradox of the current work-leisure relationship is that leisure, which was traditionally supposed to contribute to a sense of relaxation and escape from work pressures, today provides pressures of its own. Despite the findings that leisure time declined during the 1970s and 1980s, numerous sources have documented the continuous *rise* in spending on sporting goods, travel, recreational reading, music cassettes, electronic entertainment, and other leisure pursuits.

The very nature of much modern play has made it worklike, writes Witold Rybczynski in *Waiting for the Weekend*. Once free time was intended to be just that: freedom from the need to be busy, from commitments and pressure. With a new emphasis on fitness and health, many adults commit themselves to regular workouts in jogging, aerobics, or racquetball. There has been an evolution from casualness to intensity, from the simple to the intricate, in almost every form of contemporary play, whether it's bicycling, roller skating, cross-country skiing, or boating. Technical gadgetry and advanced play equipment, often becoming obsolete within a year or two, emphasize not only the marketing of leisure as an industry, but also the serious meaning we assign to play. Rybczynski suggests that the reason we place so much energy and effort into play is because we do not believe that our work is really significant. But what it means in the long run is that leisure itself contributes to the sense of pressure in daily life and to the contemporary belief in the time famine.[9]

Summing up, while reports of declining leisure may have been seriously exaggerated, they reflect the fact that for many individuals there is a clear sense of pressure and a real overload in work. The predictions of the post–World War II years about the future growth of leisure have not been realized for the society as a whole. They were dependent on the assumption that all groups would share the new leisure equally; instead, one segment of the population continues to work long hours, while others—with marginal job skills—struggle to *find* work.

Fiscal Cutbacks and the Leisure "Industry"

Following a sustained period of steady expansion for the organized recreation, park, and leisure-service field, the 1980s and 1990s saw a mounting wave of tax protests throughout the United States—leading to severe slashes in many governmental agency budgets. In part,

Crompton and McGregor point out that cutbacks reflected the public's growing distrust of government effectiveness. Opinion polls showed that:

> There was a growing perception that governments wasted money, taxes were too high, government employees were highly paid and lazy, welfare services were fraudulently consumed, and that many services were nonessential or inefficiently provided. A sizable proportion of the electorate believed that taxes could be cut without endangering "basic" or "essential" services.[10]

The response to reduced budgets varied greatly, according to the economic capability of the communities involved. In the late 1970s, a study of municipal recreation and park agencies by Kraus found that in U.S. cities with a population over 150,000, 59 percent had imposed manpower freezes on new hiring, 35 percent had discharged personnel because of budget cuts, 35 percent were forced to eliminate significant programs, and 25 percent had bond issues rejected or facilities maintenance was either reduced or entirely eliminated in some areas.[11]

In cities, small towns, or suburban communities composed chiefly of middle-class or wealthy residents with a strong tax base, public recreation and park authorities began to depend more fully on self-generated revenues such as fees and charges for the use of facilities, enrollment in classes or leagues, the rental of equipment, or similar services.

Crompton and McGregor found that between the mid-1960s and early 1990s, there was in real dollar (inflation-adjusted) terms, a 259 percent increase in the self-generated income of local public recreation and park agencies. In Illinois, a study of such departments found that they had an average self-generated revenue of 32.7 percent of total operating budgets through fees and charges in the late 1980s, compared to a total figure of about 10 percent in past decades.

Effect on Poorer Communities

However, in many economically disadvantaged communities and neighborhoods, it was not possible to impose new or increased charges for recreational participation. Typically, in such communities—marked by high welfare rates, school dropouts, drug and alcohol abuse, juvenile crime, and gang violence—there is a high level of need for positive, organized recreation programs and facilities.

Playgrounds and community centers in such settings tend to be poorly staffed and maintained, often subject to vandalism and delinquency. Often, such neighborhoods lack other, nonprofit youth-serving organizations that might compensate for the lack of public recreation programs and youth services. Foley and Ward describe South Los Angeles as an area, for example, in which organizations like Little League, AAU swimming, or track-and-field or gymnastic clubs that often use public facilities simply do not exist. They write:

> Boys and Girls Club, YMCAs and YWCAs, Scouts, and so forth, which rely on business and community support, are underrepresented and [under]financed in poor communities. A market equity policy (one gets all the recreation one can buy) has created a separate, unequal, and regressive City of Los Angeles recreation system.

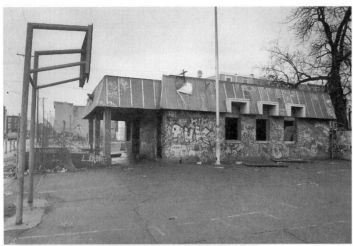

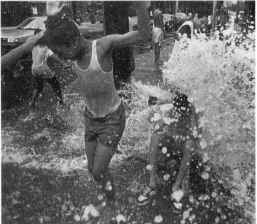

In many inner-city neighborhoods, the 1970s and 1980s saw a decline in the support of public recreation and park programs and facilitates serving the poor. Recreation centers were often vandalized or offered limited activities and leadership, with children and youth forced to rely on their own resources for play—such as using street hydrants to keep cool during the hot summer months.

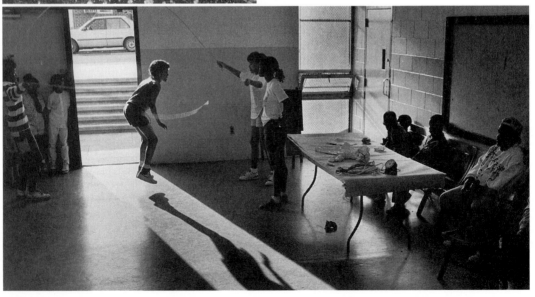

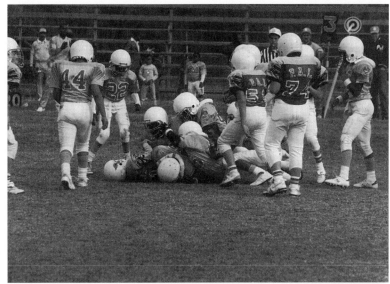

On the other hand, many youth-serving nonprofit organizations, such as the Police Athletic League, expanded programs designed to serve primarily disadvantaged or at-risk youth. Archery programs in Odessa, Texas, youth football in Denver, fishing outings in Milwaukee, and ski trips sponsored by the Fresno, California, PAL, illustrate such services.

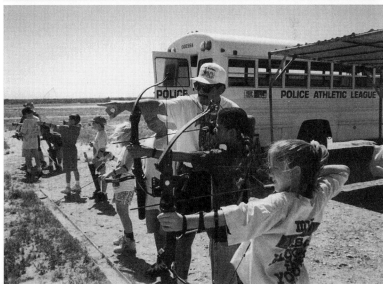

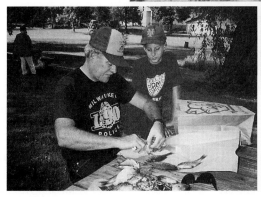

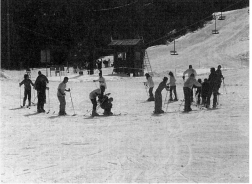

Many city parks [in wealthier neighborhoods raise huge sums] annually from user fees and donations for state-of-the-art services, while recreation centers in South Los Angeles exist on small city subsidies and what money they can squeeze out of the parents of poor children.[12]

The contrast between recreation, parks, and leisure services in poorer and wealthier communities—which some have termed *recreation apartheid*—is dramatized by the trend in the late 1980s and 1990s for many municipal and county recreation and park departments to build huge, lavishly equipped recreation and fitness centers. Andrew Cohen describes the pattern in which fast-growing suburban communities are developing such expensive centers, along with:

> . . . pool complexes, in-line and ice skating rinks, batting cages, miniature golf courses, basketball, volleyball and tennis courts, skateboard facilities, ballfields, soccer pitches, and [other indoor and outdoor recreation facilities].[13]

Often, membership in such publicly built fitness centers as those described by Cohen may cost families several hundred or more dollars a year.

Entrepreneurship and Leisure's "Marketing Identity"

In simple terms, the recreation and park movement's turning to the use of increased fees and charges may be viewed as a realistic strategy made necessary by the reduction in tax funds through the 1980s.

However, it represented more than this. Instead, leading practitioners, university educators, and other leisure-service authorities at this time urged the recreation, park, and leisure-service field to adopt an aggressive entrepreneurial stance. Rather than respond passively to emergencies and fiscal cutbacks, the need was to be "proactive" risk-takers, thinking creatively and working toward a preferred future. Increasingly, emphasis was placed on new approaches to strategic planning, as shown in Table 3.1, which contrasts newer and older approaches to planning.

More and more leisure-service managers have adopted strategic planning approaches designed to accomplish the following functions:

Establish the organization's mission, goals, and program of internal and external activities.

Allocate human and financial resources and links with other agencies to accomplish these activities.

Assess whether goals and objectives are being met.

Systematically evaluate programs, staff, and resources, and provide a basis for establishing new priorities, policies, and projects.

Seen in this light, strategic planning is essential for organizations striving to flourish in a rapidly changing environment. The process itself requires a fundamental change both in the structure and the operational philosophy and style of organizations.

TABLE 3.1   Traditional and Strategic Planning Contrasts

Traditional	Strategic
1. Emphasis on stability and efficiency	Dynamic and change-oriented; willing to risk failure
2. Creates blueprint for future decisions	Vision of future guides today's decisions
3. Reactive	Proactive
4. Inaction in face of ambiguity	Action-oriented, even in face of ambiguity
5. Internal focus	External focus
6. Relies on tried and tested	Emphasizes innovation and creativity
7. Fixed, lock-step process	Ongoing, changing process
8. Facts and quantitative measurement emphasized	Less tangible and qualitative factors emphasized

Source: Adapted from Smith, Bucklin Associates, *The Complete Guide to Nonprofit Management* (New York: John Wiley and Sons, 1994): p. 3.

Public recreation and park departments, along with many national youth-serving organizations and numerous cultural groups, adopted a vigorous marketing approach that had evolved in the American business world over the preceding period. Making use of target marketing, environmental scans, sophisticated pricing, and promotional methods, they packaged leisure services in ways calculated to stimulate public demand and lead to an ever-growing appetite for their programs.

In adopting this marketing emphasis, leisure-service managers were following a popular national trend. Respected professionals like doctors and lawyers frankly advertise their services and in some cases operate as part of regional or national chains. Churches and cultural institutions all market their products and services today. Hospitals often house subsidiary industries, such as food or laundry services, while television evangelists not only provide entertainment directly to huge audiences but in some cases establish resorts or theme parks based on religious themes.

As later chapters will show, cities themselves have adopted vigorous marketing approaches—advertising lavishly, promoting their images and tourist appeals with subsidized tours of travel agents, building huge convention and exposition centers, developing new sports stadiums to attract professional teams—as part of a powerful new entrepreneurial strategy (see page 342).

Viewing the Public as "Customers."   Linked to this new marketing emphasis, managers in all types of leisure-service agencies were increasingly urged to regard the public at large, or members of their organizations (as in the case of military recreation), as *customers*. This designation was consistent with the trend toward regarding the overall recreation, park, and leisure-service field as an industry.

The American Association for Leisure and Recreation, a national body representing thousands of leisure professionals who work in educational settings, adopted a new identity in the mid-1980s in its use of the term *recreation industry* to describe the leisure-service field. Similarly, *Trends,* a publication of the National Recreation and Park Association and the federal government's National Park Service, has concluded that public recreation and park administrators are inseparable from their commercial counterparts:

> Managed recreation is a profession that provides services to consumers of all demographic stripes and shades. Under this designation, a public park superintendent is in the same business as a resort owner, as are a theme park operator and the fitness director of a YMCA . . . . There are many changes overtaking the industry . . . . [and it is becoming] more competitive, more complex, and more in need of a high degree of professionalism to manage these changes.[14]

Recreation directors in public agencies, military morale and welfare units, hospitals, nursing homes, and employee-service programs are now urged to adopt an "entrepreneurship" approach, along with their openly commercial counterparts in profit-seeking businesses. They are regarded as part of the total spectrum of business-sponsored entertainment and play, including major motion-picture and music recording companies, professional sports teams and stadiums, theme parks and cruise-ship owners, television networks, magazine publishers, and toy and sports-equipment manufacturers.

If all members of the public were equally able to pay for the use of this variegated leisure system, the accommodation that has been made would be entirely appropriate. However, the reality is that great numbers of Americans—over 35 million in the early 1990s—are living below the poverty line. Millions of others, including the elderly, the physically and mentally disabled, at-risk children and youth in urban ghettos, and other special populations, are clearly unable to pay more than the most minimal costs of leisure involvement. Within a dominant marketing and revenue-seeking orientation, it is likely that the poor and those with other disabilities will have limited access to positive recreational opportunities, and will seek less socially desirable forms of play.

Trends in the Mid- and Late 1990s

As the twentieth century drew to a close, several important social and economic trends affecting recreation and leisure were evident.

These included the following: (1) a wave of continued cutbacks in government operations, particularly in programs involving social services and the environment; (2) heightened conservative pressures that evidenced themselves in policies affecting public support of the arts, criminal justice and penal policies, welfare and health care; and (3) continued resistance by those supporting more liberal social policies accompanied by, at century's end, evidence of strong economic recovery for many states and the nation as a whole.

Cutbacks in Support for Social Programs and the Arts

Fiscal reductions that slashed public recreation and park budgets during the 1970s and 1980s were part of government cost-cutting that affected many other areas of social service, including welfare, health care, disability-related programs, and the environment.

This overall policy reached a peak in the mid-1990s, as the 1994 Congressional election stamped the public's approval on the majority party's "Contract with America." Budget proposals submitted in 1995 contained such elements as Medicare and Medicaid cuts, reduced federal programs for families with dependent children, declining cash payments for farmers or the student loan program, increased fees in national parks and lowered environmental regulations—linked to overall tax reductions and heightened tax-credit eligibility serving the well-to-do.

Newspaper headlines in major publications at this time illustrated the impact of governmental budget cuts:

Fiscal Crisis May Hurt Health Care: Los Angeles Makes Choices It Doesn't Really Want to Face

Public Hospitals Around Country Cut Basic Service; Some Face Elimination

Many States Fail to Fulfill Mandates on Child Welfare; One Neglected Child "Climbed into a Trash Can and Asked to Be Thrown Away"

Decline Is Seen in Legal Help for City's Poor

Administration Plans to Cut "Safe City" Youth Programs

Santa Monica Tries to Curb Charity to Homeless

Safety Net Cut, Charities Turn to the Public

In Colorado, a Move to Tax Nonprofits; Social Programs Could Be in Peril

Fighting Poverty Programs: Hartford Faces Vote to Bar New Nonprofit Services

Debating High Costs of Special Needs; State Board of Regents Is Reviewing the Expense of Educating Handicapped Children at Upstate School[15]

Numerous other examples may be cited of reductions in federal and state support for environmental programs: "Panel Votes Almost $1 Billion Cut for Environmental Protection Agency," "Wildlife Refuge System Faces Uneasy Future," and "Report Says New York Cuts Environmental Enforcement." Numerous other reports document reductions in grants to support the areas, such as civic orchestras and opera companies, theater and dance, and other cultural programs.

Conservative Trend in Social Policy

While the cuts just described reflect a determination to reduce the scope of government generally, they also were linked to a powerful public reaction to what were viewed as the excesses of the 1960s and 1970s. Increasingly, politicians who argued for strong conservative legislative agendas found support at election time.

Criminal Justice System

In 1998, it was reported that crime statistics had declined for the sixth straight year, with the biggest drop in the northeastern states and in big cities. The U.S. Justice Department and Federal Bureau of Investigation reported that:

> Violent crimes declined by 5 percent, led by 9 percent decreases in murders and robberies. There were smaller decreases in the categories of aggravated assault, down 3 percent, and rape, down 1 percent . . . . Murders in the Northeastern states declined 13 percent . . . .[16]

Strikingly, however, although the crime rate has steadily fallen, the nation's prison population has continued to grow over the same period of time. In August, 1998, Fox Butterfield reported:

> the Justice Department said the number of Americans in local jails and in state and federal prisons rose to 1,725,842 in 1997, up from 1.1 million in 1990. During that period, the incarceration rate in state and federal prisons rose to 445 per 100,000 Americans in 1997, up from 292 per 100,000 in 1990.[17]

Some critics suggest that growing prison statistics are due to a prevailing "lock'-em-up" mentality in Washington and state houses, encouraged by politicians seeking popular support. Increasingly, judges are being urged to "throw the book" at criminals, and harsh drug offender laws account for great numbers of individuals being imprisoned for relatively trivial infractions.

Beyond the rapidly climbing imprisonment rate, the actual management of prison populations has become steadily more vindictive, with sharply reduced efforts to provide rehabilitation or vocational education services. J. Michael Quinlan, former director of the Federal Bureau of Prisons, has commented that the most important ingredient in managing safe and secure prisons is preventing idleness by keeping inmates productively occupied through work, education, drug treatment, or structured recreation. Instead, a harsher policy has prevailed in many states. Butterfield writes:

> This spring Alabama restored the chain gang, once a symbol of Southern racism and brutality. In Mississippi, prisoners now wear striped uniforms with the word "convict" branded on the back. Ten states are considering caning. Others have abolished television privileges, weight-lifting equipment, and computers. In last year's crime bill, Congress eliminated Pell grants, which had provided federal subsidies to prisoners taking college courses.[18]

Other states have turned back to chain gangs; some, like Maryland, are pioneering in the use of electric "stun belts" to keep prisoners in line. Other states are now charging prisoners for visits to prison hospitals. In 1997, two decades after the Supreme Court reinstated the death penalty, states were executing prisoners at a steadily accelerating rate. Expanding from their traditional Southern base and with states such as Connecticut, New Jersey, and Ohio considering the death penalty, executions are now at a forty-year high.

Apart from the humanitarian issues involved in the overall hardening of public attitudes and policies, a practical effect of the growth of prison populations and the construction of huge, new, expensive prisons has been that funding for other vital services is significantly reduced. In 1995 for the first time, California spent more on its prison system than on its two major university systems. Throughout the state, there has been a major decline in public services, heavily due to California's tough new "three strikes and you're out" law, which compelled the building of fifteen new prisons in the late 1990s, at a cost of $4.5 billion.[19]

The direct implication of such changing policies for recreation and leisure services is that with greater emphasis on punishment and reduced support for rehabilitation and crime-prevention programs, recreation services for at-risk youth receive less funding.

Affirmative Action and Other Race-Connected Issues

A second major area illustrating the pronounced conservative trend in the United States in the mid- and late 1990s involved policies having to do with racial and other ethnic minorities.

In 1996, California voters approved Proposition 209, which banned state use of racial quotas and preferences. In this state and in Texas, which passed similar legislation banning affirmative action in colleges and universities, African American, Indian, and Hispanic admission and enrollments dropped sharply in the elite university centers and in medical, law, and business schools.

While substantial evidence showed that racial-minority students admitted under affirmative action guidelines had performed successfully in their studies and in their later careers, the new policy had the effect of severely reducing the opportunity for many African American, Hispanic, and other racial-minority individuals to enter the mainstream of national life.

Other examples of the trend away from programs designed to meet the needs of racial and ethnic minorities were found in campaigns against bilingual education or remedial education in public four-year colleges that, while debatable, were generally intended to assist students from impoverished socioeconomic backgrounds. One of the chief groups to suffer from budget cuts in the mid-1900s was Native Americans living on reservations, when the Bureau of Indian Affairs was forced to lay off thousands of employees responsible for a wide range of services to tribes—including welfare, law enforcement, education, and management of natural resources.[20]

Similarly, stronger efforts to limit immigration from poorer to third-world nations and to deny educational opportunity for children of illegal immigrants, as approved in California's Proposition 187, illustrated conservative thrusts in public life at this time. Growing numbers of immigrants were forcibly returned to their countries of origin because of minor infractions committed many years before, without the possibility of judicial appeal. As another example of strong conservative pressures at this time, the 1980s and 1990s saw powerful attacks on the National Endowment on the Arts and the Public Broadcasting

System. These recipients of public funding support were viewed as too liberal, or as offensive to more conservative political or religious groups.[21]

Challenges to the Leisure-Service Movement

In general, most recreation, park, and leisure-service agencies are concerned with promoting socially progressive values and encouraging a sense of community and civic responsibility in the constituents they serve. In the early days of the playground movement, recreation leaders sought to encourage respect for those of different backgrounds within a framework of human dignity and personal worth. Shared, democratic decision making and volunteer leadership in program planning and ongoing operations characterized the philosophical framework within which most public and nonprofit recreation, park, and leisure-service organizations functioned.

The pronounced trend toward more conservative social policies of the 1990s therefore represented a challenge for many leisure-service organizations. It was accompanied by a growing tendency for millions of Americans to withdraw from participation in varied community-based programs serving the public at large.

Privatization and Withdrawal from Public Life

With greater prosperity for many groups in society and continuing poverty and economic insecurity for others, a distinct separation between upper and lower socioeconomic classes has become increasingly evident in U.S. society. Economists agree that this gap is far more pronounced than in other western, industrialized nations, and that it is illustrated in the marked decline of the middle class.

Today, growing numbers of wealthy families are relying on private leisure resources and opportunities, rather than the shared cultural or play experiences that they might have enjoyed in the past. Often, when they do take part in public recreation and park programs, it involves the use of fitness centers, golf course or tennis centers, day camps, or adult classes that require substantial fees or charges and that tend to restrict participation by poorer groups. Rather than use public playgrounds today, the children in such families typically take private classes in gymnastics or sports skills, or attend commercially sponsored play centers.

Millions of Americans today live in gated communities, with their own tennis courts, swimming pools, fitness centers, and marinas, or in so-called "Edge Cities" (see page 353), with generous resources for play. As an extreme example of this trend, in March 1999 the 18,000 residents of the Leisure World retirement community in Laguna Hills, California, voted to transform their association into a city, with its own City Council responsible for providing community services. Following a state certification process that took more than a year, the citizens of the new Laguna Woods, who average 77 years of age, will continue to live behind gated barriers, although a number of city businesses will be able to operate outside the walls of the retirement community.[22]

As television, video games, and other forms of electronic entertainment contribute to the appeal of safe, home-based leisure, privatism in play accelerates. Harvard social scientist Robert Putnam documented the pronounced trend for Americans to withdraw from PTAs, church clubs, and other social groups in community life in an influential 1995 article, "Bowling Alone."[23]

Changing Social Values

Many of the shifts in American life that have just been described may be linked to a trend away from idealism and toward a hard-edged materialistic stance. This may be illustrated in the attitudes of the nation's youth, as shown in a study released in 1997 by the University of California at Los Angeles and the American Council on Education that compared the attitudes of 9 million freshmen—male and female—on 1500 campuses who responded to questionnaires about their life goals and values from 1967 to 1996. The survey, repeated year after year, revealed the following changes:

> In 1967, 82 percent of entering students said it was "essential" or "very important" to "develop a meaningful philosophy of life"—making that the top goal of college freshmen. Today, that objective ranks sixth, endorsed by only 42 percent of students.
>
> Conversely, in 1967, less than half of freshmen said that to be "very well off financially" was "essential" or "very important." Today it is their top goal, endorsed by 74 percent.[24]

Still other changes showed that there was a sharp decline in the number of students who felt it was important to keep up to date with political affairs and in the percentage who felt that capital punishment should be abolished. In general, the survey through the years documented the growing conservatism, self-centered concerns, and materialistic views of a cross-section of the nation's college youth.

Outlook for the Future

While this chapter has described a number of negative trends during the past three decades, it also has emphasized the widespread involvement of millions of Americans of all ages and backgrounds in recreation and leisure pursuits. In the final years of the 1990s, a number of other, positive trends became apparent.

First, after a number of years of financial stringency, the United States was experiencing a period of healthy economic growth. Many states and cities were successfully balancing their budgets and in 1997 the federal government's Congressional Budget Office announced that the nation's budget would be balanced in the following year—with a substantial budget surplus to be generated in the years following 2001.

Given this optimistic economic outlook, a growing number of states and cities were expanding their land acquisition and recreation resource development efforts.

In December 1996, the National Recreation and Park Association announced that state and local bond initiatives had overwhelmingly approved over $4 billion in bond issues for open space and land and water conservation in cities, suburbs, and rural areas. As a single example, Dade County, Florida, approved a $200 million park and recreation bond issue by a two-to-one margin.

Tourism too was flourishing around the nation. In California, a state that had been battered by earthquakes, fires, urban riots, and recessions, amusement parks and attractions from San Diego to San Francisco were racking up record numbers of visitors. City after city was undertaking major projects to redevelop waterfront and other rundown or abandoned industrial areas, to provide space for civic attractions, housing, and shopping.

The National Endowment for the Arts and the Public Broadcasting System had survived legislative attempts to terminate their funding and, with growing public support, were optimistically engaged in new projects to enrich the nation's culture.

In many urban centers, volunteer community organizations were taking fuller responsibility for "adopting" parks and other recreation facilities, and in some cases actually managing them under contract. Volunteerism in general was thriving in American society, with a report by Independent Sector, a group that studies and represents nonprofit organizations, indicating that 93 million volunteers contributed a stunning 20.3 billion hours of their time annually in varied service projects.[25]

Increasingly, recreation, park, and leisure-service practitioners and educators were accepting the challenge of developing benefits-based programs to meet significant public needs. In 1998, Bev Driver, one of the key figures in this growing movement, expressed the important need to articulate the benefits of recreation outside the field itself:

> The public, other public agencies, related social service professionals, those responsible for the provision of leisure services in the private sector, and legislators at all levels of government must understand and appreciate the benefits of parks and recreation to the same extent that they understand the social benefits of education and medical services.[26]

As one example of this growing trend, many public recreation and park agencies began to assign high priority to serving at-risk youth and documenting the positive outcomes of new social programs.

Finally, two important studies reveal the state of mind of Americans at century's end. A national, state-by-state survey found that, despite negative beliefs to the contrary, 87 percent of Americans reported that they were in a good state of physical and mental health—a positive forecast in terms of readiness for active participation in recreation pursuits.[27] Similarly, a 1998 study by the Pew Research Center for the People and the Press reported that at the end of 1997 almost 50 percent of Americans surveyed reported that they were "highly contented" with their lives—a far higher percentage than in past studies.[28]

Given these positive developments, it seems clear that recreation and leisure will continue to play important roles in the day-by-day lives of Americans in the years that lie ahead. To complete this overview of the broad field of recreation, parks, and leisure services, Chapter 4 describes the varied organizations that comprise the modern leisure-service system. The next several chapters outline a number of the major trends and issues that face practitioners in this field today and the demographic, social, and economic factors that influence them.

Summary

The final two decades of the twentieth century were a time of significant change that affected the role of recreation and leisure in American society. Widely publicized research concluded that work hours had lengthened considerably for the population at large, although some studies challenged these findings. However, it was undisputed that the pace and stress of work *had* risen sharply for many employees, and that leisure itself represented a new source of time pressure and crowded schedules for the public.

Fiscal cutbacks linked to the rising cost of government resulted in many public recreation and park departments imposing new fees and charges and adopting a strong marketing orientation. Communities able to impose such charges were able to expand and diversify their programs and services, while others—particularly inner-city neighborhoods with primarily minority-group populations—suffered from marked deterioration of their facilities and skeletonized programs. Socially oriented recreation and park programs, such as those receiving federal support in the 1960s and 1970s, declined, and growing privatization and reliance on commercially provided programs threatened the well-being of public leisure services.

Accompanying this trend, there was a significant retreat from the era of the counterculture, with the nation accepting more conservative values and social policies. At the same time, in the final years of the 1990s, the economy boomed, many recreation and park agencies acquired new open spaces and facilities, and there was a widely shared feeling of well-being and confidence in the future throughout most of the United States.

Key Concepts

1. In the 1980s, Harris polls and other sources of economic statistics claimed that American work hours had increased sharply, with a resultant decline of leisure, as reported in a popular text by Juliet Schor.
2. However, other time-diary studies of systematic samples of employees by John Robinson of the University of Maryland found the reverse to be true, with many individuals gaining additional free time. For certain groups in society, work pressures clearly have grown, based on increased job demands, changing family patterns, and responsibilities and employment trends, as shown in later chapters.
3. Beginning in the 1970s and accelerating in the 1980s, taxpayer resistance to rising government budgets resulted in severe cutbacks in public spending in many states. As a result, numerous public recreation and park agencies were forced to reduce staffs and both programming and maintenance budgets.
4. In response, the aggressive marketing and revenue-seeking approach adopted by many departments led to the new conceptualization of leisure

as an "industry" and regarding participants as "customers"—a trend questioned by many recreation professionals with a strong social-service orientation.

5. The growing gap in American society between the upper and lower socioeconomic classes that became increasingly evident during the 1990s was reflected in the "apartheid" contrast between many thriving recreation and park agencies in wealthy communities and those in poorer settings.

6. The conservative trend in American values at this time was linked to repressive criminal justice policies, a retreat from concern with racially based affirmative action, mounting threats to the environment, and similar shifts. At the same time, many recreation and leisure-service professionals began to fight vigorously for positive, "benefits-based" programs and more socially oriented services.

7. At the very end of the 1990s, high levels of employment, a steadily rising stock market, a building boom, and a general atmosphere of public optimism in the future represented a sharp turnaround from the preceding years and a positive forecast for the oncoming twenty-first century.

Endnotes

1. Samuelson, R. 1995. *The Good Life and Its Discontents.* New York: Times Books, p. 3.
2. DeGrazia, S. 1952. *Of Time, Work and Leisure.* New York: Twentieth Century Fund, pp. 131–135.
3. Harris, L. 1987. *Inside America.* New York: Vintage, Random House, p. 20.
4. Schor, J. 1991. *The Overworked American: The Unexpected Decline of Leisure.* New York: Basic Books.
5. Schor, J. 1992. Are We Really That Lazy? *Newsweek* (February 17): 42–43.
6. Samuelson, R. 1989. Rediscovering the Rat Race. *Newsweek* (May 15): 57.
7. Sobel, R. 1992. Working in America. Book Review, *Philadelphia Inquirer* (February 23): K–1.
8. See Robinson, J. 1991. How Americans Use Time. *The Futurist* (September-October): 23–27.
9. Rybcznski, W. 1991. *Waiting for the Weekend.* New York: Viking.
10. Crompton, J., and B. McGregor. 1994. Trends in the Financing and Staffing of Local Government Park and Recreation Services, 1964/65–1990/91. *Journal of Park and Recreation Administration* (21/1): 19.
11. Kraus, R. 1980. *New Directions in Urban Parks and Recreation: A Trends Analysis Report.* Philadelphia: Temple University and Heritage Conservation and Recreation Service, p. 6.
12. Foley, J., and V. Ward. 1993. Recreation, the Riots, and a Healthy L.A. *Parks and Recreation* (March): 68.
13. Cohen, A. 1997. Competing Interests. *Athletic Business* (October): 33.
14. Zenger, J. 1987. Leadership: Management's Better Half. *Trends:* 4:3.
15. Headlines drawn chiefly from front-page articles in *New York Times* in 1995 and 1996.
16. Cushman, J. 1998. Serious Crime in U.S. Fell in 1997 for a 6th Year. *New York Times* (May 18): A–15.
17. Butterfield, F. 1998. "Defying Gravity," Inmate Population Climbs. *New York Times* (January 19): A–10.
18. Butterfield, F. 1995. Idle Hands Within the Devil's Own Playground. *New York Times* (July 16): E–3.
19. Miller, M. 1998. Explaining California's "Mississippification." *U.S. News and World Report* (May 18): 32.
20. Indian Bureau Sees "Devastation" in Its Budget. 1995. Washington, DC: *Associated Press* (September 9).
21. To illustrate, federal funding for the National Endowment for the Arts declined from $188.1 million in 1980 to $86.9 million in 1996. See *Statistical Abstract of the United States,* 1998: 270.

22. Terry, D. 1999. In This Brand-New City, No Shortage of Elders. *New York Times* (March 4): A–14.

23. Stengel, R. 1996. Bowling Together. *Time Magazine* (July 22): 35.

24. Hornblower, M. 1997. Learning to Earn. *Time Magazine* (February 24): 34.

25. Gerson, M. 1997. Do Do-Gooders Do Much Good? *U.S. News and World Report* (April 28): 26–36.

26. Driver, B. 1998. The Benefits Are Endless . . . But Why? *Parks and Recreation* (February): 26–27.

27. Brody, J. 1995. Gloomy Reports to the Contrary, 87% of Americans Feel Healthy. *New York Times* (March 29): C–10.

28. Boldt, D. 1998. A Happy Revolution is Sweeping the '90s. *Philadelphia Inquirer* (February 14): A–31.

4 The Leisure-Service System Today

In the last decades of the twentieth century, leisure service agencies [are] challenged to develop a more flexible and client-oriented comprehensive delivery system to better respond to the dynamic context of community life. There is ample evidence that our communities are changing; indeed, they are more diverse in ethnicity, culture, and lifestyle than ever before. Community life, represented by the diverse and changing composition of individuals and families, results in an ongoing barrage of shifting values, interests, beliefs, and lifestyle preferences. Agencies must monitor carefully and respond to these changes if they are to provide relevant services and programs to their constituents.[1]

Earlier chapters in this book dealt with leisure as a phenomenon of growing importance in national and community life. It is clear that, while it may be viewed from a purely personal perspective, leisure also has significant economic, health-related, and social implications in contemporary culture and has become the responsibility of thousands of different agencies throughout the nation. Taken all together, the emergence of this network of leisure-service organizations and the realization of leisure's importance in national life have given rise to a new but rapidly growing profession. This chapter examines the leisure-service system, its varied specialized objectives, and its practitioners.

It also makes clear that many of the traditional functions of different types of leisure-service organizations—and the relationships among them—are changing rapidly as a consequence of the trend toward fuller degrees of cooperative partnerships among program sponsors, along with the growing practice of privatization in various areas of public service.

Agencies Comprising the Leisure-Service System

There are eight major types of organizations within the overall leisure-service system, based on distinctly different missions or program emphases, patterns of sponsorship, and funding sources:

1. Public or governmental agencies
2. Nonprofit or voluntary organizations
3. Commercial, profit-oriented businesses
4. Therapeutic recreation service
5. Private-membership associations
6. Campus recreation sponsors in schools and colleges
7. Armed forces morale, welfare, and recreation units
8. Employee recreation and fitness programs

Beyond these major categories of program sponsors, the leisure system may also be understood in terms of clusters of agencies that deal with common concerns, such as travel and tourism, sports management, arts programming, or environmental protection. In addition, there are numerous organizations that do not provide programs as such, but that sponsor research, advocacy, public relations, or the promotion of higher standards of professional performance.

Public Leisure-Service Agencies

This category includes numerous governmental departments and other agencies that are primarily supported by public taxes, although they may also gain revenue from fees or charges, grants, contracts, and contributions. They operate on federal, state, and local levels of government.

On the federal level, leisure-service agencies include the National Park Service in the Department of the Interior, the Forest Service in the Department of Agriculture, the Bureau of Land Management, the Fish and Wildlife Service, the U.S. Army Corps of Engineers, and the Tennessee Valley Authority. Numerous other offices or bureaus have functions related to environment, commerce, tourism, and the needs of special populations.

Among the major land-managing agencies, the National Park Service and the Forest Service have sharply differing functions. The Park Service has two chief responsibilities, conservation and outdoor recreation, as shown in the following mission statement:

> The National Park Service is dedicated to conserving unimpaired the natural and cultural resources and values of the National Park System for the enjoyment, education, and inspiration of this and future generations. The Service is also responsible for managing a great variety of national and international programs designed to help extend the benefits of natural and cultural resource conservation and outdoor recreation throughout this country and the world.[2]

In contrast, the Forest Service is committed to serving a variety of needs, including outdoor recreation, cattle grazing, timber cutting, watershed and wildlife purposes, under the Multiple-Use Sustained-Yield Act of 1960. In Canada, the federal government has a broader range of leisure-related responsibilities, including major programs operated under the Fitness and Amateur Sport Branch that sponsor and assist sports organizations and competitions, promote applied research in sport and fitness, set standards, develop leadership, and provide special assistance to disadvantaged and disabled groups.[3]

In the United States, all fifty states have departments, bureaus, or administrative units responsible for parks, conservation, and outdoor recreation, as well as other offices concerned with tourism, cultural programs, and the needs of special populations. Typically, states maintain hospitals, special schools, and correctional institutions that include recreation as a basic service. In addition, state agencies serve as a liaison between the federal and local governments within several areas of leisure-service programming, such as services for the elderly or disabled. State universities also have a major responsibility for preparing professional workers in the leisure-service field.

The most important type of public leisure-service agency in terms of meeting the everyday needs of most Americans consists of recreation and park departments sponsored by local government, either on the township or municipal level, or by counties or special park districts. Specialized leisure programs are offered by the public schools, departments of human services, libraries, and other educational, cultural, or social-service departments linked to local government.

Public local recreation and parks agencies have three major areas of responsibility: (1) *operating facilities for public use*, such as parks, playgrounds, indoor recreation centers, outdoor sports facilities, swimming pools, nature centers, art centers, senior centers, and such other specialized units as skating rinks, ski centers, marinas, and riding stables; (2) *providing recreation programs under leadership*, involving instruction, supervision, and organizational direction of such programs as after-school and summer playground and day-camp activities, adult classes, sports leagues, performing arts workshops, and a host of other activities; and (3) *promoting and stimulating recreation in the community at large*, by assisting other agencies, training leadership, coordinating volunteer efforts, providing facilities for use by other groups, and working closely with other environmental, educational, and social-service organizations.

Beyond the obvious purpose of providing fun and creative challenge for community residents, the specific goals of local park and recreation departments are to improve the overall quality of life for residents, promote mental and physical fitness, help curb juvenile delinquency and other negative pursuits, strengthen family and neighborhood unity, assist persons with disabilities, sponsor and promote programs in the arts, and protect and improve the natural environment (see page 18).

To achieve these purposes, local public programs may include a host of sports leagues, day camps, cultural and civic events and celebrations, special activities for the elderly or for disabled persons, and cooperative relationships with many community organizations. In some cases, municipal or county recreation and park departments may offer a range of classes that introduce members of the public to varied leisure activities and give them the opportunity to practice them on increasingly more advanced levels of skill and satisfaction. For example, the Montgomery County, Maryland, Department of Recreation offers hundreds of classes in local recreation centers or on a countywide basis, in such areas as children's fitness, arts and crafts, dance, youth and adult fitness, music, and other such varied interests as:

growing government funding, many nonprofit organizations *are* meeting such needs.[5] For example, at this time Catholic Charities USA, a network of about 1400 social-service agencies, received about $1.3 billion, or two-thirds of its revenues, from federal, state, and local governments. Similarly, the Salvation Army draws about 17 percent of its income from government.

In a striking example of how individual churches have entered the human-service field, the African Methodist Episcopal Church in Queens, New York, with 9000 members and a towering new $23 million cathedral, operates an extensive government-funded social-service network, including:

> . . . a city-funded walk-in clinic and federal Head Start classrooms . . . . a city-sponsored prenatal-counseling program for teen mothers, a state-sponsored housing and community-renewal program . . . a city-assisted mental health center and state Stop Driving While Intoxicated program . . . and numerous other anti-poverty services, including recreation.[6]

Numerous youth-serving organizations—such as the Girl Scouts of the USA, with 2.6 million girls on five levels; the Boys and Girls Clubs of America, also with 2.6 million youth served in 1850 club facilities; the Boy Scouts of America, with a total of over 5 million youth and adult members; or other major associations, such as the Young Men's Christian Association or the Police Athletic League—combine a host of social services with such recreational activities as sports, camping, the arts, conservation education, or citizenship and community-service volunteer programs.

The nonprofit volunteer organization field also includes thousands of membership groups devoted to promoting interest or sponsoring instruction, competition, or program standards in a huge range of recreational pursuits. In some cases, such organizations represent the spontaneous interest of members in a given activity, such as a sports or hobby pursuit. In other cases, as in bowling, hunting, fishing, or riflery, a major part of their funding and program planning is drawn from manufacturers of equipment or operators of commercial facilities serving participants—as part of a total public relations effort.

A key point with respect to the funding of nonprofit organizations is that, although they are charitable in nature and meet significant social needs, they often collect substantial revenues through fees for membership or participation. As a consequence, some nonprofit leisure-service organizations have been challenged by lawsuits in recent years, claiming that they are in competition with commercial businesses and should have their tax-exempt status withdrawn.

Commercial Recreation

The largest and most extensive form of organized leisure-service sponsorship today, in terms of the variety of programs offered and the sheer scope of participation and revenues earned, is provided by commercial recreation. Many thousands of leisure-service businesses large and small offer fitness and health-related activities, travel and tourism, and opportunities for participation in such pursuits as bowling, racquetball, horseback riding, and a host of other pastimes. In the broadest sense, all forms of commercially sponsored entertainment and hospitality, including admission to for-profit theater and concerts and the operation of nightclubs and bars, are part of this field.

The services offered by commercial recreation business may include instruction, the rental of equipment or use of special facilities, the provision of entertainment, hospitality, and social contacts, and other kinds of leisure-related opportunity. In some cases, recreation is the sole element that is offered to the public; in others, it is part of a complex of offerings. In some huge shopping malls that have been built in recent years, recreation is a major attraction that helps to draw great numbers of people to the overall facility. For example, the West Edmonton Mall, in Alberta, Canada, is the world's largest shopping complex. This sprawling indoor facility is crammed with 836 stores, 110 restaurants, 20 movie theaters, and a large hotel. An appealing destination for tourists in its own right, the mall attracts as many as a hundred thousand visitors a day, about 40 percent from the United States. Its recreation facilities include a mammoth amusement park (entry free of charge) with forty-seven rides; a miniature golf course; a $5 million skating rink; a huge water park with a surf pool an artificial lake, submarines that take tourists on underseas adventures, and a replica of Columbus's ship, the *Santa Maria*.

Similarly, the Mall of America, the largest shopping mall in the United States, in Bloomington, Minnesota, has numerous recreation attractions, including a huge amusement park, Camp Snoopy. Such enterprises demonstrate the degree to which leisure has become part of the commercial structure of the nation, both as a highly profitable business in its own right, and as a "threshold" attraction that draws customers to other businesses.

As later chapters will show, the expansion of commercial recreation business has been greatly stimulated by a host of technological innovations within every type of leisure activity. Crossley and Jamieson cite the importance of high-speed, relatively inexpensive air travel for the expanding travel and tourism industry. They continue:

> Electronic innovations generated a huge home entertainment industry of television, stereo equipment, video recorders, and computers. Synthetic materials improved the performance and durability of ski equipment, golf clubs, skateboards, and sports balls of all types.
>
> Theme parks and water-play parks capitalized on a variety of innovations. Service innovations such as time-sharing [of vacation resort properties] have also had significant impact. Undoubtedly, the future holds a continuing variety of new facilities, products, and services [influenced by technology].[7]

A marked distinction separates commercial recreation businesses from public and nonprofit agencies in that they are conducted primarily for the purpose of making a financial profit and do not require public support or approval to initiate new enterprises or services. However, if they are to maintain a favorable level of popular approval and involvement, they must be sensitive to the public's reaction to their policies or programs.

As an example, the Disney Company has come under heavy attack by conservative or right-wing religious factions because of its relatively liberal hiring policies or sponsorship of "gay-oriented" events (see page 198). Similarly, Time Warner, the huge entertainment and mass media conglomerate, was pressured by harsh attacks in the mid-1990s for its acquisition of a company producing so-called "gangsta rap," with excessive violent and sexist content. Commercial recreation sponsors must be alert to the views of groups concerned with gender, racial, religious, or environmental issues, along with other factors linked to safety, public taste, or the most important concern, *profitability* of a given venture.

Therapeutic Recreation Service

A fourth important component of the organized leisure-service field involves therapeutic recreation service. Historically, this field was known either as "hospital recreation" or as "recreation for the ill and handicapped," and tended to provide recreation as a morale-related service for individuals with physical or mental disabilities or illnesses, in residential treatment settings. In time, it broadened its scope to include those with a broader range of disabilities and to embrace the purpose of equipping individuals with disabilities to live independently in community settings.

Today, recreation provided as part of treatment service is often closely linked to other treatment functions. Within the "clinical" or "prescriptive" approach to therapeutic recreation, patients are carefully evaluated and treatment plans are developed to achieve specific objectives linked to the physical, emotional, social, or cognitive skills that are needed for recovery or rehabilitation.

Underlying all applications of therapeutic recreation service is the principle that it represents a form of psychosocial habilitation or rehabilitation. Practitioners must be prepared to deal with such factors as the individual's self-perception (often marked by poor self-esteem, excessive dependency, or "learned helplessness") as well as negative environmental factors.

In a recent discussion of the Leisure Ability model of therapeutic recreation, Stumbo and Peterson point out that it is one of the most widely used theoretical models in this field. Based on such elements as internal locus of control, motivation, and freedom of choice, the Leisure Ability Model defines three components of service:

> . . . treatment, leisure education, and recreation participation . . . . The overall intended outcome of therapeutic recreation services, as defined by [this model], is a satisfying, independent, and freely chosen leisure lifestyle.[9]

The role of therapeutic recreation in helping persons who are disabled gain or regain skills of independent living related to self-care and maintenance, travel, shopping, attending public events, and developing satisfying leisure pursuits and social lives is related to the field's second important function: assisting disabled persons who live in the community setting. Here, so-called special recreation programs are provided by community organizations like Special Olympics, the Easter Seal Society, and other groups that serve specific populations such as those with physical, mental, or visual disability, or that provide activities for different categories of disabled persons. In general, their goal is to promote mainstreaming of such persons, having them participate in nonsegregated community recreation programs wherever possible.

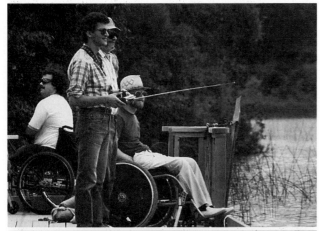

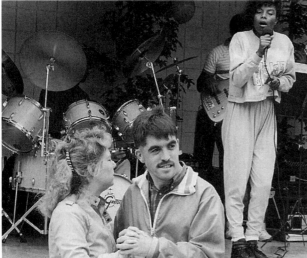

Persons with developmental, emotional or physical disabilities today are served by varied community agencies, often along with nondisabled persons. Here, individuals in wheelchairs enjoy fishing (Oakland County, Michigan Parks and Recreation), take part in student dance (Long Beach, California), take ski vacations sponsored by South East Consortium for Special Services, New York, and learn gardening skills (San Francisco RCH, Inc.).

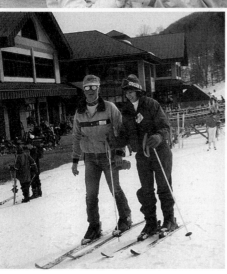

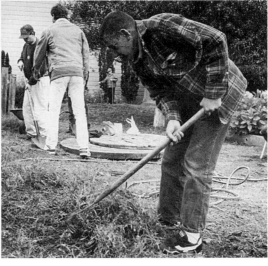

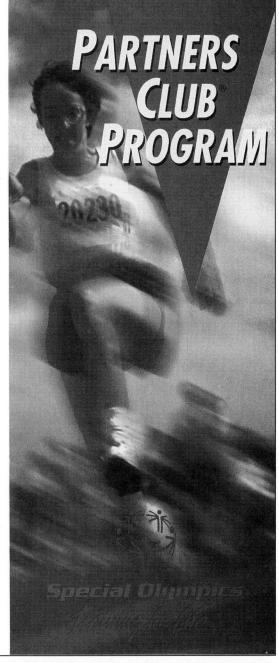

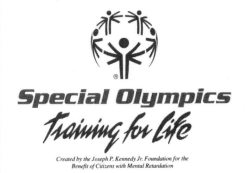

For more information
about Partners Club®,
call your local
Special Olympics office.

Special Olympics
Training for Life

Created by the Joseph P. Kennedy Jr. Foundation for the
Benefit of Citizens with Mental Retardation

Materials Provided By
Special Olympics International
1325 G. Street, NW, Suite 500
Washington, DC 20005-3104
(202) 628-3630

FIGURE 4.1 Social integration of persons with disabilities is promoted by the "Partners" program of Special Olympics, which joins diabled and nondisabled individuals in training and competition, in cooperation with hundreds of other community organizations.

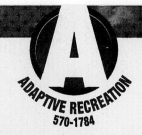

Citywide recreation activities and classes for individuals with disabilities. For any information on programs, contact Adaptive Recreation at 570-1784, unless otherwise noted.

NEW YOUTH PROGRAMS & ACTIVITIES

Beginning Line Dance. Ages 11-15. All you boot scooting' boogiers come and learn the Tush Push, the Elvira and everybody's favorite, Black Velvet. Come on out and have a good time! Classes meet M, beginning June 15, for eight weeks. Classes held from 6-7 p.m. and are designed for youth with developmental disabilities. Instructor: Benavidez. Fee is **$16**/person.

SUMMER SIZZLERS
Ages 9-14

Adaptive Recreation is offering activities geared especially for youth ages 9-14 who have developmental disabilities. Limited transportation is available. Pre-registration for all events is mandatory. Call Adaptive at 570-1784 for information.

Reptile Safari. Can reptiles wink or blink their eyes? Can you crawl out of your skin, change colors on a whim, bury yourself in the mud or slither across hot sand? Discover who can. Must provide own transportation. Date TBA, 9:30 a.m.-Noon. Fee is **$15**/person.

Walt Disney's Mulan. Join friends for an excursion to the El Capitan Theatre to see a presentation of Disney's newest release. Fee includes show, transportation and supervision. Fee is **$15**/person. Call Adaptive for details.

RETURNING ACTIVITIES

Adaptive Recreation in Special Environments (ARISE). Ages 9 and up. This after-school program for people with disabilities includes arts, music, dance, sports, special events and excursions. M-F, 2-5 p.m. at Stearns Champions Park. Summer hours: M-F, 1-5 p.m. For information, call Adaptive.

Bowling. All ages. For details, call Java Lanes at 597-5558.

Dining Out Program. Ages 18 and up. Dinner program for young adults with developmental disabilities. Participants pay own meal costs. 1st and 3rd W of mo., 6:30-9:30 p.m. For reservations, call 570-1687 after 2 p.m., M-F.

Indoor Sports and Games for Disabled Senior Adults. 2nd & 4th Sa of mo., 1:30-6:30 p.m. at Stearns Champions Park.

Lip Reading. Sponsored by Long Beach City College. Th, 10 a.m.-Noon at the Senior Center. For more, call 570-3500.

Mommy and Me Aquatics. Five-week course introduces kids with disabilities, ages 5-8, to water safety and beginning swimming. One-hour, twice weekly. Call Special Olympics at 421-2882 for details.

Movie Night Out. Young adults with developmental disabilities ages 18 and up. Evenings out to the theatre in small groups. Must pay your own ticket and snack costs. 2nd W of mo., 6-10 p.m.

Quad Rugby. Offered in cooperation with Long Beach Memorial Rehabilitation Hospital. For information, call 933-9043 or Adaptive.

Residential Camp for Developmentally Disabled. Ages 16 and up. Summer camp is **$250** and runs June 8-12.

Sailing for the Physically Challenged. Beg. & Int. Rigging modification, cockpit adaptation and techniques for those with physical disabilities. Contact Duncan Milne at (714) 722-5371 for details. Class free to all qualified disabled persons.

Square Dance Class. Ages 15 and up. An 8-week program (Mar. 30-June 1 & June 15-Aug. 31) for people with developmental disabilities. M, 7-9 p.m. Fee is **$16** at Stearns Champions Community Center. Call Adaptive for more information.

Sign Language Introduction. Th, 5:30-7:30 p.m. Call Adaptive for dates.

Special Events Nite. Ages 18 and up. Monthly activities such as plays, baseball games and ice skating. Call Adaptive.

Did You Know About?
Pick-Up Basketball. Take part in pick-up basketball games for people with physical disabilites. Games are free and at Stearns Champions Park. All are welcome. Call Adaptive for details.

Other Services And Activities

California Pools of Hope, Inc. Therapeutic swimming for all ages. Facilities include wheelchair ramps, stairs and lifts. People with arthritis meet Tu/Th from 9-10 a.m. and a low-impact aerobics class is conducted W/F from 9-10 a.m. General pool hours are Tu-F, 9 a.m.-4 p.m. and Sa, 9 a.m.-2 p.m. For more information, call 537-2224.

Citizens' Advisory Commission on Disabilities (CACOD). Meets the 2nd Th of mo. at Noon at City Hall. For information, call Dolores Barrows at 570-6304.

Community Advisory Committee for the Handicapped (CAC). A support group for parents who have special education students in the Long Beach Unified School District. Call 987-8000.

Deaf Telephone Communication Center (TTY). Information and referral services available by calling 436-6706.

Energy Rebate Program. Disabled residents receive tax breaks on utility fees. For details, call these centers: Central Facilities, North Facilities, West Facilities, Senior Center and Houghton Park. See pg. 28 for facility phone numbers.

Girl & Boy Scouts. 1-3 p.m. 1st Sa of mo. at Stearns Champions Park.

Long Beach Alcohol and Drug Abuse Rehabilitation Program. An outpatient program that provides confidential treatment and prevention of alcoholism and other drug problems. For information, call 570-4100.

Long Beach Early Intervention Council. Made up of parents and service agencies that represent infants and toddlers with special needs. For info, call the council at 985-8481.

Special Olympics Practice. Includes swimming and seasonal team sports on Tu/Th, 6:45-8:30 p.m. Call 421-2882 for registration.

Stroke Association of Southern California. Support groups and education. For information, call 985-9971.

FIGURE 4.2 The range of varied program activities for disabled persons of all ages is shown in this "Adaptive Recreation" listing from Long Beach, California. Numerous other educational and social-service agencies are involved in sponsoring social, sports, and outdoor recreation pastimes.

Some therapeutic recreation organizations, such as RCH, Inc., in San Francisco, provide a wide range of services, including vocational, counseling, educational, transportation, and other forms of assistance, for all age groups and those with different disabilities. Through the years, many thousands of clients of RCH, Inc., have been successfully integrated into community life.

As an example of programming in sports for persons with disabilities, the National Wheelchair Athletic Association in Colorado Springs, Colorado, is a multisport organization begun in 1956. Serving individuals with varied disabilities, including post-polio, spinal cord injury, spina bifida, amputations, and other conditions, NWAA involves thousands of participants who compete annually in regional, national, and international tournaments, including Victory Games, Pan American Games, World Games, and Paralympics. Competition offered for both men and women includes archery, track and field, basketball, quad rugby, rugby, shooting, swimming, table tennis, tennis, and weight lifting.

Although they have long been regarded as separate fields, today there is steady movement toward merging the two areas of service, therapeutic recreation with emphasis on treatment goals and special recreation in community settings.

Private Membership Organizations

The fifth category of leisure-service organizations consists of associations, societies, or clubs that provide recreation for their members, rather than for the community at large.

Country clubs have served upper- and middle-class Americans for many years, specializing in such pursuits as golf, tennis, yachting, and social events for member families. In addition, many private-membership clubs are based on other outdoor recreation interests, such as hunting and fishing, skiing, family camping, riding, and similar pastimes. Usually, such clubs own their own land and are not as restrictive in terms of their membership policies as private athletic or social clubs have tended to be. Many such clubs have been places where the wealthy and powerful members enjoy relaxation, sociability, and deal-making. However, in recent years, such clubs have been on the decline. For example, one of the most famous and exclusive of such clubs, New York's Downtown Athletic Club, formerly had a total membership of 4000 successful businesspeople and professionals and a long waiting list. Today this club's membership is dwindling and its financial affairs are in disarray; in the late 1990s, it owed New York City over $3 million in back taxes. Like it, almost all of the private clubs throughout the United States are in difficulty for a variety of reasons. When Congress withdrew the club-dues tax deduction, companies limited the number of executives they would assist with membership costs. Beyond that, the "stuffy," exclusive, old-boy network atmosphere of such private membership clubs is no longer appealing for young people in a more democratic, fitness-oriented, and socially liberal and diverse era.

Some private membership organizations are structured nationally or regionally, to promote participation and influence public attitudes within a given area of leisure activity. For example, in the field of outdoor recreation and conservation, membership organizations such as the Sierra Club, Appalachian Mountain Club, and the Audubon Society may maintain networks of facilities, sponsor tours and training programs, and at the same time promote environmental causes and lobby for needed legislation.

A unique type of private-membership organization involves the provision of recreation programs for people based on residence. Many wealthy families live in resort communities or have vacation homes in developments that provide skiing, sailing, or other forms of outdoor play, making use of facilities that are restricted to property owners. However, such private-membership leisure opportunities are not necessarily limited to the affluent. In one giant development, Starrett City, in Brooklyn, New York, middle-income tenants drawn from various ethnic populations—approximately half of Hispanic, African American, and Asian backgrounds—enjoy a variety of sports, aquatic, fitness, and club activities that are limited to families in residence.

Campus Recreation: Programming in Schools and Colleges

A sixth major group of sponsors of organized recreation programs is commonly referred to as *campus recreation*—services provided for students, and often faculty and staff members, in colleges and universities.

In a broad sense, this type of leisure-service sponsor also should include public school systems, which often provide after-school or evening sports, social and cocurricular programs for their students, as well as adult classes or continuing education activities for the community at large. However, the primary emphasis of campus recreation is on the programs provided in college and university settings.

Such activities may be sponsored under various administrative structures—either through an athletic department (for sports and outdoor recreation activities) or under the supervision of a dean of students or division of student life. Campus recreation covers a wide range of activities and purposes, ranging from networks of fraternities and special-interest or social clubs, to intramural and intercollegiate sports, cultural programs that include concerts, theater, dance, and other performing groups or spectator events, outings, publications, and volunteer service projects.

Often leisure activities are housed in college unions or campus recreation centers. For example, at San Diego State University in California, the

> Associated Students Organization sponsors a remarkable range of films, concerts, recreation and athletic programs, legal services and other activities. This multi-million dollar corporation, funded by annual student fees . . . operates the Aztec Center, the college's student union building. In addition, it runs a highly successful travel service, intramurals and sports clubs, special events, leisure skills classes, lectures, movies, concerts, an open-air theater, a large aquatics center, a campus radio station, a child-care center, a black students council, a general store, a campus information booth, and many other services and activities. Within this spectrum, the bulk of the leisure activities on the San Diego campus are operated directly by the Recreation Activities Board, a unit within the overall Associated Students Organization.[9]

free clinics

Local Outdoor Recreation Opportunities
Wednesday, March 19 @ 7pm in the ARC
Come and learn all about the many incredible opportunities for outdoor recreation in beautiful Southern Illinois. Learn favorite spots from fishing to ghost towns.

Bike Maintenance Clinic
Thursday, March 20 @ 7pm in the ARC
Do not miss your chance to learn some secrets from a local expert about how to keep your bike in perfect running condition. This is a great prep for the Mountain Biking trip to Kinkaid Lake.

Introduction to Rock Climbing
Wednesday, March 26 @ 7pm at the Climbing Wall in the Student Rec. Center
Face your fears, and come on in and learn all about the basics of rock climbing from our friendly staff. Try on a harness, tie some knots, and climb like a monkey!

All you ever wanted to know about BACKPACKING, but were afraid to ask.
Wednesday, April 9 @ 7pm in the ARC
Hike on in and learn about backpacking basics such as pack sizing, food planning, and route selection. This is a primer to our Ozark Trail trip April 11-13. Plus, you get to try out our new Osprey backpacks and receive a $1 off coupon for backpack rental.

Crazy Campus Canoeing
Wednesday, April 16 from 4 - 6pm at the Lake-on-the-Campus Boat Dock
Come and learn some basic water safety and canoe paddling strokes.

Low Impact Camping
Wednesday, April 23 @ 7pm in the ARC
Learn the basics of the "Leave No Trace" ethic. This clinic will be taught by a certified outdoor leader, so come and absorb some important knowledge if you love the outdoors.

Mountain Biking @ Kinkaid Lake
Saturday, March 22
Challenge yourself on the beautiful trails at Kinkaid Lake. Forget those Mountain Dew commercials; this is real mountain biking through some of the most amazing scenery around. Bring your own bike, helmet, and bandaids! Transportation and trip leaders provided. Mandatory pre-trip meeting is Tuesday, March 18 @ 7pm in the ARC.
S=$5 M=$7 U=$9 C=$9

april

NEW! All Women's Rock Climbing Trip to Giant City
Saturday, April 5
If you've never tried rock climbing before, but have always wanted to, here is your chance! Join us for an all women climbing trip that is fun and challenging. Basic climbing techniques and safety will be covered. Please, no testosterone allowed! Transportation, gear, and female trip leaders included. Mandatory pre-trip meeting is Tuesday, April 1 @ 7pm in the ARC.
S=$12 M=$14 U=$16 C=$16

Backpacking the Ozark Trail, Mark Twain National Forest
Friday, April 11 - Sunday, April 13
Take some time to get away. Spend a weekend with us on the Current River section of the awe-inspiring Ozark Trail. Hike along the river and experience the panoramic mountain top views. Mileage will be kept to a moderate 5-7 per day, so there will be plenty of time for relaxation. Transportation, gear, and trip leaders are included. Mandatory pre-trip meeting is Tuesday, April 8 @ 7pm in the ARC.
S=$25 M=$27 U=$30 C=$30

Current River Canoe Trip
Friday, April 18 - Sunday, April 20
Take a weekend away from classes and work and join us for this float down one of Missouri's most beautiful and popular canoeing areas. Come prepared to have fun and relax on the Current River. No experience is necessary and price includes transportation, all gear, and trip leaders. Mandatory pre-trip meeting is Tuesday, April 15 @ 7pm in the ARC.
S=$20, M=$22 U=$25 C=$25

Earth Day Celebration! Full Moon Night Hike @ Giant City State Park
Tuesday, April 22 @ 8pm in the ARC
Come and celebrate what mother earth has given us and relax on a beautiful night hike. Must preregister by Monday, April 21 at the Information Desk.
Transportation and trip leader included.
S=$1 M=$2 U=$4 C=$4

Rock Climbing @ Cedar Bluff / Camping @ Ferne Cliff
Saturday, April 26 - Sunday, April 27
This two day climbing trip is sure to be an incredible experience. On the first day, learn basic climbing philosophy, safety, and technique on some beginner climbs. The second day we will try some more challenging routes and advanced techniques. No experience is necessary, and price includes all transportation, gear, and trip leaders. Mandatory pre-trip meeting is Monday, April 21 @ 7pm in the ARC.
S=$20 M=$22 U=$24 C=$24

Outdoor Adventure Programs is dedicated to providing outdoor experiences for all individuals. We will try to accommodate, as much as possible, all of our programs to the needs of those with disabilities.

FIGURE 4.3 Outdoor recreation trips and clinics offered by the Office of Intramural-Recreational Sports at Southern Illinois University, in Carbondale.

Sport Clubs

Interested in a new sporting experience, then try...

Aikido	Outdoor Adventure
Badminton	Racquetball
Ballroom Dancing	Rodeo
Baseball	Roller Hockey
Bike Racing	Rugby (Men's & Women's)
Boxing	Sailing
Canoe & Kayak	Soccer (Men's & Women's)
Cricket	Table Tennis
Equestrian	Triathlon
Fencing	Ultimate Frisbee
Footbag	Volleyball (Men's & Women's)
Karate	Water Polo
Kendo	Water Skiing
Lacrosse	Weightlifting
Martial Arts	Wrestling

        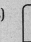

For more information, call (618) 453-1256.

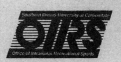

Southern Illinois University at Carbondale

OIRS

Office of Intramural Recreational Sports

Sport Club List Flyer.pm

FIGURE 4.4 Varied sports and other club activities serve men and women students at Southern Illinois University.

The goals of colleges and universities in providing or assisting such services are in part to fulfill the responsibility of *in loco parentis*—that is, to oversee the lives of young men and women entrusted to their care by attempting to control negative or destructive forms of play and by providing positive alternative leisure opportunities. In addition, the image and reputation of institutions may be enhanced by student activities that help to build public awareness and assist in the recruitment and retention of students. Various student programs contribute to the learnings stressed by the formal curriculum, including programs in the arts, humanities, sciences, and social sciences, as well as in career-related subject fields.

Beyond these functions, campus recreation services are often linked administratively with such university functions as student orientation programs, ongoing relationships with students' families, the supervision of Greek-letter fraternities and sororities, campus life during vacation periods, student community service and multicultural activities, residence-hall programs, and student conduct codes and judicial affairs.

In many institutions, recreation is not singled out as a separate, identifiable branch of university services, but is interwoven with other administrative functions. With the pronounced trend in the late 1990s to reverse the "hands-off" policies of the 1960s and 1970s, when most universities abdicated responsibility for supervising students' lives, today they feel a growing need to provide varied forms of enriching campus programs and experiences (see page 112).

Armed Forces Recreation

A seventh major type of organized recreation sponsor involves the nation's military forces and consists of programs and facilities operated by the Morale, Welfare and Recreation (MWR) Program within the Department of Defense. In the 1980s this program served approximately nine million people, including active-duty, reserve, and retired military personnel, civilian personnel, and dependents. Operating on virtually all 923 Department of Defense installations in the United States and 363 bases in twenty-nine foreign countries, the Morale, Welfare and Recreation program at this time had a total budget of approximately $3 billion, much of it derived from self-generated revenues, and employed 215,000 people, including 8700 military personnel, 8900 civilian employees on government-funded salaries, and almost 200,000 employees on nonappropriate salaries.[10]

Recognizing that the MWR program contributes significantly to the quality of life in the military community, the Department of Defense is mandated to conduct a varied program of activities that:

- Maintain a high level of esprit de corps, enhance job proficiency, contribute to military effectiveness, aid in recruitment and retention by making military service an attractive career, and aid service personnel in the transition from civilian to military life.
- Promote and maintain the physical, mental, and social well-being of military members, their families, and other eligible members of the military community.
- Encourage constructive use of off-duty leisure time with opportunities for acquiring new talents and skills that contribute to the military and civilian community.

■ Provide community support programs and activities for military families, particularly when the service member is on an unaccompanied tour or involved in armed conflict.

Within each of the major branches of service, the MWR program typically covers a broad range of physical, social, cultural, and entertainment pursuits. For example, the Special Service program of the U.S. Air Force provides such activities and facilities as: (1) sports, including self-directed, competitive, instructional, and spectator events; (2) motion pictures; (3) service clubs and entertainment, including parties and special events, dramatic and musical activities; (4) crafts and hobbies; (5) family activities, particularly for children and youth; (6) special-interest groups, such as aero, automotive, motorcycle, and power-boating clubs, and hiking, skydiving, and rod and gun clubs; (7) rest centers and recreation areas; (8) open messes; and (9) libraries.

Special efforts are made throughout the armed services to compensate for the stress and boredom of military life and to overcome problems of drug and alcohol abuse that have affected many servicemen and women. Consistently, studies have shown that armed forces recreation programs have contributed to the morale of military personnel and their dependents and are an important factor in the retention and reenlistment of men and women within the Department of Defense.

During the mid-1990s, as part of an overall reduction in the military forces in the United States, there was a sizable cutback in the number of armed forces personnel and military bases. Despite this trend, armed forces recreation planners have continued to initiate numerous innovative programs, often in partnership with other community groups.

For example, the Marine Corps Air Station at Cherry Point, North Carolina, has entered into an "open gate" relationship with regional residents, improving community relations and providing needed revenue for the MWR program. The Navy Seabee Base in Gulfport, Mississippi, cosponsored the 1996 USA Junior Boxing Championship, in cooperation with U.S. Amateur Boxing, Inc. The Kirtland Air Force Base in Albuquerque, New Mexico, initiated successful family-center programs, and other military bases around the country promoted the *Start Smart* Sports Development program for children. Still other military recreation units have developed cosponsorship arrangements with the Boys and Girls Clubs of America, and with the Young Men's Christian Association, illustrating a widespread trend toward partnerships described later in this chapter.[11]

Employee Services and Recreation

The eighth important segment of the leisure-service system consists of programs sponsored by companies for their employees and often their families. In the latter half of the nineteenth century, such programs began when the severe work ethic and "sweatshop" conditions of many factories were replaced by a new concern for worker well-being and the quality of life in American communities. Labor-management friction in the first decades of the twentieth century, often leading to strikes and violent confrontations, also compelled many company owners to provide improved employee benefits and services in an effort to prevent unionization of their employees.

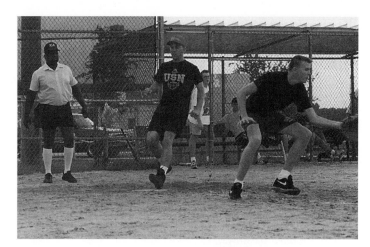

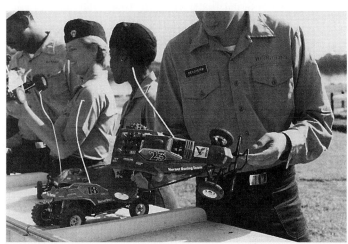

Military recreation includes varied sports, hobbies, social activities, and outdoor recreation pursuits, as shown in Orlando, Florida, Naval Training Center MWR program. Even on active duty, participants enjoy volleyball on deck of aircraft carrier during the Gulf War.

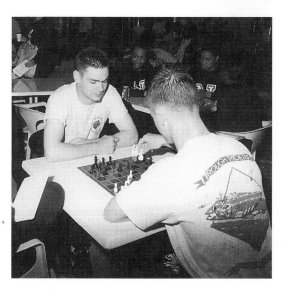

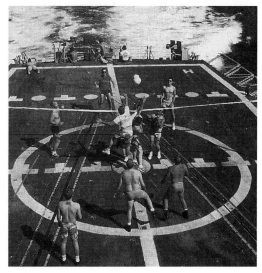

Many industrial concerns, insurance companies, banks, and other concerns therefore began recreation programs or sponsored sports teams to promote the loyalty of their employees, create a favorable image and sense of fellowship and high morale, and promote job performance. Employee recreation—which was generally regarded as an integral part of personnel management—varied in its administrative sponsorship. Some companies took complete responsibility for organized recreation programs, providing facilities and leadership, sometimes with an advisory council of employees. Others provided facilities and a degree of financial support, with employees taking responsibility for planning and conducting programs. Some corporations built large gymnasiums, meeting rooms, and recreation centers; activity programs included varied sports, classes and clubs in hobby interests and areas of personal development, family activities, parties, picnics, and a wide range of other pastimes.

In the 1980s and early 1990s, the range of employee services broadened to include clinics and support groups dealing with health needs, stress management, drug and alcohol abuse; some companies provided a greater diversity of services, such as discount buying clubs and chartered travel programs. By the mid-1980s, the National Employee Services and Recreation Association (NESRA) had almost 3000 member companies that offered such human resources programs as employee assistance, health and fitness activities, sports, travel, education, and pre-retirement planning. Michael Murphy summed up NESRA's basic philosophy:

> that employee services, recreation, and fitness programs make good business sense. That a work environment which satisfies its users' physical and psychological needs is conducive to greater productivity. That happy and healthy employees result in reduced absenteeism and turnover, and higher workforce morale. That the time for a humanized workplace is now.[12]

Other Components in the Leisure-Service System

Beyond the eight major types of recreation sponsors just described, the leisure-service system may also be seen as an assembly of organizations that focus on specific areas of public interest, or that regulate, promote, and set standards for or improve performance in the delivery of programs and services.

For example, the field of sports management includes a host of different types of sponsors, such as schools and colleges, sports leagues sponsored by youth-serving organizations or religious groups, sports for persons with disabilities, stadium and professional team owners, sports equipment manufacturers and others that represent the full range of public, nonprofit, commercial, and therapeutic agencies.

Similarly, there are numerous organizations that represent different elements in the travel and tourism field, such as travel agents, cruise ship or resort operators, theme park owners, and similar bodies. While members of such groups obviously compete against each other in fighting for a larger market share of business, they also recognize their common interests and cooperate on important joint efforts.

While other groups of sponsoring organizations concerned with therapeutic and special recreation service, performing arts or museum management, or outdoor recreation and environmental issues may have different agendas or needs, they also have typically formed national societies or trade associations. They tend to have the following key functions:

1. Promoting popular interest and involvement in their field of activity. This is done through public relations and advertising, publishing newsletters and magazines, sponsoring major events and developing links to social causes.
2. Funding or conducting research dealing both with pragmatic concerns such as marketing studies or risk-management methods, and with the outcomes and benefits of their fields of leisure interest.
3. Carrying out lobbying or promoting legislation to achieve varied forms of government assistance to support their own policies and projects.
4. Training leadership on different professional levels and setting standards for professional performance in fields as diverse as sports officiating, scuba diving, or ballroom dance instruction, linked with instructional guides and programs for people entering their fields on different age levels.
5. Establishing levels of participation or rules for organizations in areas such as sports, including different types of leagues, along with policies and penalties for infractions of regulations on player eligibility, practice periods and game schedules, recruitment of athletes and the role of sports agents, transfer from institutions in amateur sport and free-agentry in professional sport, or linkages with business sponsors and television contracts.

While most such organizations and associations do not directly sponsor ongoing programs, other than expositions, conferences, or in some cases, major tournaments, they obviously play a key role in the operation of the overall leisure-service system. As such, they have been part of three late twentieth-century trends that affect all recreation, park, and leisure-service organizations: *partnerships, privatization,* and *professional development.* These three important Ps are discussed in the concluding sections of this chapter.

Partnerships Among Leisure-Service Organizations

Although many recreation, park and leisure-service agencies may compete vigorously among themselves, the more significant trend during the 1990s has been in the direction of partnerships. Sometimes called *synergy*—a term implying that when two or more groups join in cooperative efforts they achieve successes beyond what any of them might achieve independently—partnerships have taken varied forms in recent years.

As a key example of partnerships in the leisure-service field, Crompton and Richardson point out that many state and local government departments of commerce or tourism work closely with private entrepreneurs in the joint promotion of tourism. Publicly owned parks, seashores, historic monuments, gardens, marinas, zoos, and historic mansions attract tourists, who also patronize commercial cruises, tours, theme parks, and other attractions.

Public and private agencies may also cooperate in carrying out festivals or other events that encourage tourist visits.[13]

Many private companies assist by funding sports programs for children, youth, or special populations, locally or as part of nationwide programs. A useful example is Hershey's National Track and Field Youth Program, which is designed to introduce children between the ages of 9 and 14 to physical fitness through track and field events, and which is run in cooperation with the National Recreation and Park Association, the President's Council on Physical Fitness and Sport, and many local public recreation and park agencies. Timber and utility companies cooperate with park authorities in making their lands and water-based recreation sites available for camping, boating, and other forms of outdoor recreation.

As an example of partnerships involving military recreation, the community of Radcliff, Kentucky, has joined with its neighbor, Fort Knox, to sponsor extensive convention programs and other leisure activities serving the public on the fort's base—thus providing needed revenues for the military Morale, Welfare and Recreation operation and Radcliff with an ideally situated facility that it could not build on its own.

In the area of special recreation, many nonprofit organizations serving persons with disabilities have joined with public, college, private, and other agencies to sponsor joint services. In many cases, several communities have combined their special recreation programs to form associations that offer adapted activities for different groups in various locations, while sharing funding and leadership responsibilities. The Maine-Niles Association of Special Recreation in Illinois is one such body; another is the Southeast Consortium for Special Services in Westchester County, New York, which serves nine towns, cities, and villages with the bulk of its funding from the State Office of Mental Retardation and Developmental Disabilities.

Another growing example of partnerships within the sports field has seen city after city contribute millions of dollars to assist private football or baseball club owners in building elaborate new stadiums. Such controversial arrangements—at a time when many municipalities have been under severe financial constraints—are obviously intended to help cities lure professional franchises to them, both for the added income they would bring and to enrich the communities' images.

Many other examples of different types of partnerships among leisure-service organizations may be cited. For example, the Fairfax County, Virginia, Park Authority has developed linkages between eight of its recreation centers and major employment and office-building complexes around the county. Through intensive marketing efforts with companies and cooperative planning, the Park Authority has been able to involve hundreds of employees in its specially formed noontime aerobics classes, water fitness programs, racquetball leagues, and other programs.

Within the overall field of parks management, many public agencies under financial pressure in recent years have found partnerships a useful means of gaining support. Vaske, Donnelly, and LaPage write:

> Unwilling to see parks and natural areas closed to their owners (the public) during periods of budget austerity, managers have for years been building an impressive catalogue of partnerships with public and private entities. Today, those partnerships

represent not only significant cost savings to taxpayers, but have greatly expanded the quality of public service.[14]

In general, there are a number of important benefits that businesses gain by forming partnerships with public or nonprofit leisure-service organizations. These include the goal of improving a company's corporate profile with financial institutions, shareholders, or the public at large; increasing awareness of the company and its products or services; benefits to the company's personnel in terms of skills development and morale, when staff members are assigned to community-linked functions; and finally being able to call upon municipal government or other agencies for assistance when needed.

Privatization Approaches

The term *privatization* tends to have two meanings in the leisure-service field: (1) the growing trend for many families or social groups to seek their leisure outlets within private settings, rather than within public facilities and programs; and (2) the practice of assigning responsibility for public functions to private organizations, usually on a contractual business.

Today, many communities contract with such private, profit-oriented organizations to provide health services; construct and maintain roads and highways; provide utilities, trash pickup, building maintenance, and food services in city-owned structures; and similar functions.

Over the past fifteen years, within the growing penal system, many public authorities have turned to both profit- and nonprofit groups to provide medical care, food services, and other functions in prisons and jails. In a number of cases, profit-oriented companies have assumed contracts to provide total management for correctional centers and low-security jails, with mixed results in terms of substandard medical care and reports of widespread brutality in privately run institutions.[15]

The rationale for the growth of privatization through subcontracting of government responsibility is simple: It is often more efficient and cost-effective than having the work done by public employees. Private companies are not subject to Civil Service regulations and, in many cases, union pressures. In programs that expand and contract according to seasonal or climatic factors, they can be highly flexible in hiring and discharging practices and are not subject to bidding procedures in terms of buying or renting materials and equipment.

Beyond this, there has been an accelerating trend toward reducing the scope of government operations. As Chapter 3 pointed out, this has stemmed in part from the conviction that government operations tend to be wasteful and inefficient, linked to the powerful drive toward reducing taxes of the past two decades. It also is related to the libertarian position that government—particularly the federal government—has become so large and powerful that it poses a threat to the rights and freedoms of ordinary citizens.

Examples in Parks and Recreation

The funding of private groups or special recreation associations to meet the needs of persons with disabilities, described earlier, is an example of privatization.

More typical is the growing practice of subcontracting with profit-oriented companies, some of which have chains throughout the country, to run golf courses, tennis complexes, or other municipally owned leisure facilities.

Many communities today contract with private companies to carry out other functions, such as landscaping, tree-trimming, maintenance, and security services. In other settings, city and county governments develop Design/Build/Operate (D/B/O) arrangements with private architectural and construction firms, in establishing new facilities—thus tapping public capital and the expertise and economies of the private sector. In a limited number of cases, particularly in California, communities have contracted with private companies run by their former employees to operate public playground, day camp, and recreation center programs.

At another level, a growing number of schools today are contracting with private, nonprofit organizations to run their afterschool programs, which were formerly conducted by school or recreation department personnel. For example, the afterschool program of Roosevelt High School, a huge old structure in the Borough of the Bronx, in New York City, is now managed by Phipps Houses, a low- and middle-income housing developer operating with the help of a foundation grant. In an effort to combat the school's high dropout rate, in an area marked by poverty and varied social problems, and to promote more interest in school activities, the Phipps Houses program includes such features as a "hip-hop" music and dance revue, break dancing, karate, fashion modeling, "double-Dutch" rope jumping, and similar club activities reflecting popular teen culture.[16]

Operation of a Major Park.   In a striking example of privatization, in February 1998, a private group officially took control of Central Park in New York City—possibly the most famous park in the United States and a landmark in the history of parks and recreation. Under the deal, the Central Park Conservancy, which had played an important role in raising funds and helping the park recover from severe deterioration during the 1980s and early 1990s, took over

> . . . control of the park's daily operations, with the city ultimately giving it up to $4 million a year based on how much private money [the Conservancy] raises. The city, however, will continue to handle larger decisions about the park, deciding, for instance, when and where to hold concerts and how to deploy police officers there.[17]

Although the Parks Council, New York's advocacy group for the parks, supported the decision to privatize Central Park, some citizens and community groups expressed concern about whether the city's growing reliance on private money would hurt parks in poorer neighborhoods. Others suggested that the move was clearly intended to escape the demands of labor unions representing the city's employees, and that the Conservancy was overly concerned with maintaining the park's beauty and historical treasures, but gave little priority to city residents who wanted to use it for sports and other forms of active recreation.

Implications of Privatization

Privatization may be seen as having both positive and negative outcomes. While it may represent a more economical and efficient way of carrying out managerial and programming functions, when agency tasks are subcontracted to private groups, the likelihood is that more affluent neighborhoods or communities are likely to benefit chiefly. Since organizations like the Central Park Conservancy depend heavily on private or foundation funding to supplement public grants—this approach is unlikely to be successful in poorer community settings.

When for-profit organizations take over responsibility for managing golf or tennis facilities on a contractual basis, they typically raise fees for participation—again biasing the service in favor of more affluent residents. In some cases, when such arrangements have not proved sufficiently profitable, the commercial contracting firm has withdrawn from the arrangement, and it has become necessary to seek new managing groups. One of the arguments supporting publicly operated recreation and parks that was cited years ago by George Butler was that such arrangements represented *permanent* commitments—which obviously is not the case in privatization agreements.[18]

In terms of the other type of privatization described in Chapter 3, the tendency of many wealthier families to withdraw to the use of private facilities, the danger here is that widespread community support for the public operation of varied recreation and park programs is threatened.

Professionalism in the Leisure-Service Field

As earlier chapters have shown, the provision of recreation, park, and leisure services has become increasingly complex and sophisticated in an era of economic pressures and rapid social change. As a consequence, there has been a continuing effort to develop a higher level of professionalism in the overall leisure-service field and within its specialized delivery systems.

Although people have been employed for thousands of years in providing recreational experiences—as entertainers, fencing and dancing masters, zookeepers, gardeners, sports coaches, and in hundreds of other leisure-related roles—the emergence of professionalism in this field has essentially been a twentieth-century phenomenon.

What did it mean to be professional, and why did those working in the recreation, park, and leisure-service field seek this designation—apart from the higher degree of status that it implied? A position paper of the Society of Park and Recreation educators defined *profession* as follows:

A profession is a vocation whose practice is founded upon an understanding of the theoretical structure of some department of learning or science and upon the abilities accompanying such understanding. This understanding and these abilities are applied to the vital practical affairs of man . . . . The profession . . . considers its first ethical imperative to be altruistic service to the client.[19]

Expanding this definition, H. Douglas Sessoms has identified the following elements as important criteria of professionalism in contemporary society:

1. Professions align themselves with a social concern, the ameliorating of some social ill, and they frequently result from a major social movement.
2. Professions establish their body of knowledge, a set of concepts and procedures generally known to those within the profession.
3. Specified programs of education and training, generally involving internships, are needed in order for one to learn the necessary concepts and practices of the profession.
4. To assure that programs of professional preparation are reliable, that individuals have the prerequisite skills and understandings to practice, programs of accreditation and certification are created.
5. Those within the profession create organizations to serve it. These organizations often establish codes of ethics, norms of practice that are enforced by the profession.[20]

Through the final decades of the twentieth century, recreation, park, and leisure-service educators and practitioners have made significant progress in meeting these criteria. A growing body of published research has identified the unique functions and competencies attached to leadership, particularly in public recreation and park agencies and in therapeutic recreation service. Journals related to leisure concepts, administrative strategies and methods, and other theoretical and practical concerns add to this body of knowledge each year.

Trends in Professional Preparation

Professional authority based on formal academic training has been achieved through the expansion of a higher education system of college and university curricula ranging from two-year community college programs to institutions that offer the doctorate in this field. The relatively few such curricula that were established in the post–World War II years expanded rapidly during the late 1960s and 1970s, to the point that there were an estimated 500 degree-granting programs throughout the United States and Canada. Many of these were poorly staffed or represented minor curriculum options within a larger department of health, physical education, and recreation.

During the 1980s and 1990s, professional preparation in recreation, parks, and leisure studies was consolidated and strengthened, as a number of marginal college programs discontinued their offerings, while others developed fuller and more specialized staffs and degree requirements. Many shifted their focus from a broad approach to recreation leadership, programming or management, or park operations, to sharply defined emphases on such fields as sports management, therapeutic recreation, or tourism and hospitality management.

Accreditation

A key factor in the field's advancement has been its recognition and approval as an appropriate area of professional study by the Council of Postsecondary Accreditation (COPA) in the mid-1980s. This means that parks, recreation, and leisure studies are now validated as a legitimate field of academic specialization: Today, approximately one hundred colleges and universities have met the requirements of the Council on Accreditation (a joint function of the National Recreation and Park Association and the American Association for Leisure and Recreation).

Credentialing in Leisure Services

The National Recreation and Park Association's National Certification Board began in 1990 to conduct a Certified Leisure Professional Examination, to serve as the basis for identifying individuals as qualified practitioners in the field. In addition, forty-three states and the National Therapeutic Recreation Society conduct NRPA-recognized certification programs. A number of other specialized professional societies, such as the National Employee Services and Recreation Association (NESRA) maintain certification requirements, usually based on a combination of professional education and experience.

While curriculum accreditation and personnel certification procedures have upgraded professionalism in the leisure-service field, the reality is that they do not control the admission or continuing employment of many recreation and park workers. Table 4.1 presents current employment statistics within this overall field and in related fields. In several cases, recreation personnel are lumped together indiscriminately with other specialists, making it difficult to determine how many are recreational practitioners and how many are in related fields. In addition to these job categories, there are substantial numbers of therapeutic recreation specialists, workers in museums, zoos, membership organizations, and similar agencies, who are part of the total leisure-service field. Beyond these groups, there are also many individuals working in areas of the commercial recreation field, including such marginal or specialized fields as gambling casinos or sports betting, or pornography and the

TABLE 4.1 Estimated Employment in Leisure-Related Fields

All government park and recreation agencies (1995)	387,000
Writers, artists, entertainers, and athletes (1997)	2,234,000
Natural resources management (1995)	421,000
Instructors and coaches, sports and physical training (1996)	303,000
Amusement and recreation attendants (1996)	288,000
Social, recreation, and religious workers (1997)	1,357,000

Source: Statistical Abstract of the United States (1998): pp. 331, 417, 420.

Note: A number of these categories are overlapping or include recreation employees as part of a larger group. They do not include statistics of armed forces recreation workers, those employed in after-school or campus recreation, or therapeutic recreation personnel, estimated as approximately 30,000 in the late 1980s. Also, they do not include those employed in the manufacture or sale of recreation-related equipment, or the construction and maintenance of leisure facilities.

related "sex trades," who are not usually thought of as recreation professionals but who clearly are involved in satisfying leisure demands of many Americans.

Clearly, there are at least several hundred thousand individuals who have recreation programming or resource management as a primary job responsibility in the United States today—as well as several million workers who hold support roles in terms of planning, promotion, safety and security, environmental functions, or other management tasks.

A relatively small segment of this overall group consists of individuals who should be classified as professionals, in terms of their specialized job functions, academic training, certification status, and other criteria. Chiefly, these are managerial personnel in recreation and park departments, recreation therapists or supervisors, members of armed forces MWR units, school and college program managers, and specialists in employee recreation programs. A substantial number of government recreation workers must meet Civil Service requirements, usually based on a combination of education and professional experience, or, if they work in health-care settings, must satisfy state personnel requirements. Finally, a substantial number of recreation professionals employed in voluntary agencies such as the YMCA, YWCA, or YM-YWHA, Boy and Girl Scouts, Boys and Girls Clubs, and similar national federations must meet hiring requirements and take part in training and continuing education programs established by these groups.

Employment Trends

A number of studies in the 1980s and 1990s identified recreation as a field in which employment would continue to grow, although some of them focused primarily on low-paid jobs as technicians or program aides, rather than on higher-level management positions.

Ethnic/Racial and Gender Factors

Within this overall growth, employment patterns will be influenced by demographic factors linked to ethnicity and gender. Studies during the 1960s and 1970s indicated that members of racial and ethnic minorities were increasingly being hired in the recreation and parks field, but that relatively few had reached the upper levels of public or voluntary agency administration. During the late 1970s and 1980s, this pattern changed as numerous large cities throughout the country appointed African American and Hispanic American professionals to executive-level positions as directors of public park and recreation departments. This trend has also been evident in federal agencies such as the National Park Service and the Forest Service and in many state recreation, park, and conservation departments.

A somewhat similar situation is evident with respect to the role of women as leisure-service professionals in the United States. Henderson, Bialeschki, and Sessoms point out that in the early years of the playground and recreation movement, most program leadership was provided primarily by women, and men were not the majority staff members until the 1930s.[21] Particularly with the merger of the park and recreation movements, however, men took over the bulk of management positions—especially those entailing facilities development and maintenance responsibilities. Women were relegated to direct program leadership positions for the most part, often working with preschool groups, the elderly, or girls' and women's programs. This situation began to change in the 1970s, as women moved increasingly into a range of supervisory and management roles. A professional profile survey of women employed in the recreation and park profession revealed in the late 1980s that a substantial percentage of women were employed on administrative levels, and that they were generally positive about their career development.

However, Henderson, Bialeschki, and Sessoms report that pay inequity still exists through much of the leisure-service field, and that men continue to dominate executive levels of employment—particularly within the private or commercial sector. And, in 1992, Henderson stressed that women continue to face the glass ceiling that hinders their advancement in recreation and parks careers, just as in other areas of employment. In many job settings, women are subject to sexual harassment, and the problem may also be exacerbated by other demographic factors such as ethnicity and disability.[22]

Role of Professional Societies

As in other fields of professional service that have developed higher education curricula and standards for admission to practice over time, recreation, parks, and leisure services continue to make steady progress. In large measure, this is due to the work of such organizations as the National Recreation and Park Association and its specialized components, such as the American Park and Recreation Society, the National Therapeutic Recreation Society, and the Society of Park and Recreation Educators. Other professional societies include the American Therapeutic Recreation Association, the Armed Forces Recreation Society, the American Association for Leisure and Recreation, the National Employee Services and Recreation Association, the National Intramural and Recreational Sports Association, and dozens of other organizations and trade associations concerned with promoting specialized branches of commercial recreation.

NRPA in particular has been effective in promoting public awareness of the leisure-service field, pressing for sound legislation related to urban needs, open space and other environmental concerns, and juvenile delinquency, and drawing attention to the needs of the aging and other special populations and similar recreation-related issues. It has constantly stimulated research and publication and has been instrumental in establishing numerous special schools and workshops across the United States that provide in-service education for practitioners.

In Canada, the Canadian Parks/Recreation Association has expressed a broad vision of its own role—along with the efforts of provincial professional societies—in improving community life and utilizing the following strengths:

> Our diverse, multitalented membership being active in virtually every community in the nation.
>
> Our communication abilities to mobilize this corps of committed Canadians around important issues.
>
> Our traditional interests in lifestyle, the environment, and our heritage being discovered and revitalized by new movements that need our support.
>
> Our ability to motivate and support grassroots community initiatives.
>
> Our growing credibility as an organization capable of producing innovative and cost-effective national programs accessible to all citizens.[23]

Typically, CP/RA achieves its varied goals by appearing before legislative committees and elected officials, sponsoring national and provincial programs of education and environmental action, offering clinics and symposiums, and generally providing leadership to a host of national and local organizations within various sectors of the overall leisure-service field.

Professional Identity and Role

Despite the evidences of professional growth that have been described throughout this chapter, it is probable that many members of the public are not yet familiar with the field of leisure services as a profession.

While they undoubtedly recognize the specific occupations in which practitioners work—recreation therapist, fitness director, ice arena manager, park naturalist, or park and open-space planner—the likelihood is that they do not appreciate the common identity among these different job specializations. The unifying element that potentially unites the eight major sectors within the field, as well as activity interest clusters and specialized organizations, is a shared concern with leisure and its contribution to the quality of life in contemporary communities.

As this text has shown, the important contributions made by recreation, parks, and leisure-service organizations include the promotion of physical and mental health, intergroup understanding, economic and environmental well-being. However, it is becoming increasingly difficult for leisure-service professionals to make hard choices among conflicting needs and priorities.

Should recreation and leisure be viewed primarily from an entrepreneurial or a human service perspective?

How will changing population trends influence the provision of recreation opportunities in the years ahead? What trends with respect to meeting the needs of racial, gender, or disabled minority groups are likely to challenge leisure-service providers?

How are choices to be made between different types of outdoor recreation uses, in terms of their impact on the natural environment or their economic benefits for surrounding communities?

What is the long-range impact of the growing popularity and acceptance of forms of leisure that flaunt accepted moral codes of behavior and are potentially destructive to participants?

Can leisure-service practitioners and educators unite in the effort to educate the public in the creative and constructive values and uses of free time—and is it their responsibility to do so?

Such questions, along with their implications for managerial philosophy and operational strategies, are discussed in the following chapters of this text. They are placed ^within the context of predicted changes that lie ahead, in the oncoming decades of the twenty-first century, with respect to demographic, social, economic, and environmental conditions.

Summary

This chapter describes the eight major types of organizations providing leisure services in the United States today, as well as other clusters of program sponsors in such activity areas as sports management or travel and tourism. It discusses the role of societies or trade associations that promote different types of recreational pursuits.

It then examines three major trends in the field today, dealing with privatization, partnerships, and professional development, concluding with a brief discussion of the public's awareness and understanding of leisure services as a career field and professional discipline.

Key Concepts

1. In analyzing the overall leisure-service system, it is essential to recognize that there are eight distinct types of organizations that are characterized by their sponsorship patterns, funding sources, goals and objectives, and program emphases.

2. Of these eight types, the one type of sponsor that has a primary responsibility for meeting overall public needs, as well as providing a range of indoor and outdoor facilities and resources, is the public, tax-supported agency on local, state, and federal levels.

3. Nonprofit leisure-service organizations tend to meet more specialized needs in terms of age groups served or more sharply focused program emphases. Usually, they are not regarded as recreation agencies, but may be considered "educational," "social-service," "religious," or "youth-serving" organizations. However, recreation is often a major part of their ongoing responsibilities.

4. Commercial recreation businesses offer the greatest range of program offerings and respond to more advanced public interests, often with expensive, technologically based programs and facilities. They also are the most sophisticated and effective, in terms of promoting their offerings and shaping public leisure values and involvement.

5. Therapeutic recreation has essentially two thrusts: treatment-based or "clinical" service in residential or other medically directed treatment or rehabilitation centers and community-based special recreation programs designed to meet broader, ongoing recreation needs.

6. A key trend that tends to unify and strengthen the leisure-service field today consists of partnerships through which different types of agencies share their resources and collaborate in joint programs and projects.

7. Privatization in the recreation and park field has two kinds of emphases: withdrawal of wealthier community residents to private groups, programs, and facilities and the assignment of government functions to private nonprofit or commercial subcontracting groups.

8. Professional development applies chiefly to several hundred thousand individuals who have levels of training, responsibility, and expertise related to meeting leisure

needs, rather than the several million men and women working in "support" or "related" roles in the leisure-service field. Elements promoting professionalization include specialized higher education, credentialing and certification of personnel, and the work of specialized professional associations and societies.

Endnotes

1. Murphy, J.F., and R.F. Dahl. 1991. The Right to Leisure Expression. *Parks and Recreation* (September): 106.

2. *Informational Brochure.* 1996. Washington, DC: The National Park Service.

3. Searle, M.S., and R.E. Brayley. 1993. *Leisure Services in Canada: An Introduction.* State College, PA: Venture Publishing, Chapter 5.

4. *Guide to Recreation and Leisure Service.* Fall 1992. Rockville, MD: Montgomery County, MD, Department of Recreation.

5. Arenson, D., 1995. Gingrich's Vision of Welfare Ignores Reality, Charities Say. *New York Times* (June 4), pp. 1, 16.

6. Cohen, A. 1997. Feeding the Flock. *Time Magazine* (August 25): 46–48.

7. Crossley, J.C., and L.M. Jamieson. 1993. *Introduction to Commercial and Entrepreneurial Recreation.* Champaign, IL: Sagamore, pp. 23.

8. Stumbo, N., and C. Peterson, 1998. The Leisure Ability Model. *Therapeutic Recreation Journal* (2nd Q.): 82–95.

9. See *Breakaway: Recreational Guide to San Diego State University.* (n.d.). San Diego, CA.

10. Lankford, S., and D. DeGraaf. 1992. Strengths, Weaknesses, Opportunities and Threaters in Morale, Welfare and Recreation Organizations: Challenges of the 1980s. *Journal of Park and Recreation Administration* (Spring): 31–45.

11. See several articles in *Parks and Recreation* describing trends in military recreation, December 1996 and December 1997.

12. Murphy, M. 1984. The History of Employee Services and Recreation. *Parks and Recreation* (August): 38.

13. Crompton, J., and S. Richardson. 1986. The Tourism Connection: Where Public and Private Leisure Services Merge. *Parks and Recreation* (October): 38.

14. Vaske, J., M. Donnelly, and W.F. LaPage. 1995. Partnerships for the 21st Century: A Return to Democracy. *Journal of Park and Recreation Administration* (Winter), 13(4): 1.

15. McGraw, D. 1997. Abuse, Private Jails, and Videotape. *U.S. News and World Report* (September 1): 36. *See also* Ward, J. 1998. The Pros and Cons of Long-Term Privatization. *American City and County* (May): 54–60.

16. Archibold, R.C. 1999. In School. *New York Times* (March 24), p. A–25.

17. Martin, D. 1998. Private Group Signs Central Park Deal to Be Its Manager. *New York Times* (February 12): A–1.

18. Butler, G.D. 1967. *Introduction to Community Recreation.* New York: McGraw-Hill.

19. *Education for Leisure.* Proceeding of the 1975 Dallas-SPRE Institute. Arlington, VA: National Recreation and Park Association, p. 18.

20. Sessoms, H.D. 1990. The Professionalization of Parks and Recreation: A Necessity? In *Recreation and Leisure: Issues in an Era of Change,* eds. T.L. Goodale and P.A. Witt. State College, PA: Venture Publishing, p. 248.

21. Henderson, K., M.D. Bialeschki, and H.D. Sessoms, 1990. Occupational Segregation. Women and the Leisure Services. *Journal of Physical Education, Recreation and Dance* (October): 49–52.

22. Henderson, K. 1992. Being Female in the Park and Recreation Profession in the 1990s: Issues and Challenges. *Journal of Park and Recreation Administration,* 10/2: 18.

23. *Descriptive Brochure.* 1996. Ottawa, Ontario, Canada: Canadian Parks/Recreation Association.

5 Forecasting the Future: Trends and Issues

The century to come, and the centuries to follow, will be complex, fast-paced, and turbulent. Human beings everywhere have learned to live with, even thrive on, explosive increases in the volume of knowledge, the capacities of technology, the potential for travel, the electronic immediacy of once distant culture. Change has become almost addictive, a jolt to energy and creativity.

. . . to make the dreamed-for future work, people everywhere are going to have to know much more about, and demand much more from, themselves. . . . To embrace the future fully, one must give to it the very best of oneself. For the future to be bright, it must be lit by the lamp of learning, the true Olympic torch.[1]

In a rapidly changing society at the brink of a new millennium, for any field of public service or economic activity it is essential to look ahead and to determine—to the extent that it is possible to do so—the trends, issues, and challenges that lie ahead.

The rate of change over the past several decades has been immense, in terms of population growth, the improvement of medical care and the extension of life expectancy, technological advancement, and the growth of cities. What changes can we look forward to in the future, and how will these affect our lifestyles, our social values, and our patterns of leisure and recreational participation? Predicting the future is always uncertain, and yet it is possible to define a number of oncoming trends with reasonable assurance by extending current population shifts and economic and technological developments.

This chapter begins this process by reviewing the methods that may be used to forecast the future and then summarizing a number of the major predictions that have been made for the years ahead, both in terms of overall society and then with respect to specific leisure-related trends and issues. It then presents the findings of a recent survey of recreation, park, and leisure-service educators, in which they were asked to rate the importance of eighteen demographic, social, economic, and environmental trends and their implications for the future.

Forecasting Methods Applicable to Leisure

Obviously, it is never possible to predict the future with absolute certainty, or stock analysts and individual investors would be far wealthier than they are today, and many errors of economic policy or political strategy might have been avoided.

Nevertheless, it is possible to predict many future events and trends with a reasonable degree of success—particularly in terms of short- rather than long-range forecasts. Indeed, the field of "futurology," while not a fully accepted social science, makes extensive use of other social or behavioral sciences, including economics, social psychology, political science, and other disciplines.

How is this done? The simplest approach is to examine past and current trends—particularly those that can be quantified and analyzed statistically—and to develop straight-line projections based on them. Often such projections are expressed not as precise forecasts of future happenings, but rather within margins of statistical probability, or on a contingency basis, assuming that other factors prevail. Cummings and Busser argue that mere extensions

> ... or projections of past trends into the future do not constitute forecasts by themselves. Projections are simply mechanical functions, while forecasts require judgment. Quality forecasting estimates are derived through objective and systematic questioning and do not depend solely on subjective hunches, biases, guesses, and blindspots of the forecasters.[2]

The overall process of making predictions about the future, then, includes both gathering as much significant information as possible about past and current events, cycles, or conditions and applying individual or group judgment about future circumstances in order to arrive at forecasts.

Sometimes this is a group process, in which a number of individuals regarded as experts in a given field are asked to give their judgments in a series of polling episodes over time. Their views are refined, reshaped, and blended in order to arrive at shared predictions. Known as the *Delphi method*, named after the ancient Greek oracle on the island of Delphos, this approach is sometimes used in planning studies. As a variant of it, authorities in a given discipline may simply develop a set of probable forecasts and, through discussion groups or weighted scoring approaches, reach agreement on predictions.

As this chapter will show, the kinds of future predictions that are made may range from sweeping forecasts of population change or technological innovation to narrower and more detailed statements of social trends or environmental gains and losses. A number of the kinds of predictions that have been presented in recent years are now presented.

Examples of Forecasts

In 1990, the United Way of America's Strategic Institute, working with its volunteer Environmental Scan Committee, identified more than one hundred specific trends in contemporary society and grouped them into nine major "change-drivers." These forces included the steady maturation of American society in terms of aging and social and political changes; increasing diversity moving the nation from a "mass" to a "mosaic" society; redefinition of individual and societal roles, with a blurring of the differences between public and private-sector functions; continued growth of an information-based economy; the increased globalization of business and economic activity; personal and environmental health becoming key areas of public concern; a major restructuring of global economic patterns and American businesses; redefinition of traditional concepts of family and home; and, finally, a rebirth of social activism.

In 1992, writing in the *Journal of Park and Recreation Administration,* Daniel McLean and Ruth Russell discussed a number of other projected trends that social scientists believe lie ahead. These include such elements as a stronger "greening movement" based on continuing environmental decline; increased economic dislocation and social malaise for many families; the emergence of new leadership, based on "powershifts" involving the knowledgeable, the news media, and the innovator. McLean and Russell write:

> Anticipatory democracy will be more prevalent at all levels. There will be a decentralization of power in all organizations with a disappearance of large sectors of middle management. Visionary leaders will be the leaders of the future—those who can share and empower others in their vision. [There will be a] social revolution different from any experienced before. . . . promoted by humans who have evolved into opportunity creators—people who imagine, create, and implement opportunities for better futures.[3]

A collaborative study by the Canadian Park/Recreation Association and the Rethink Group, a research and planning organization, identified a number of "macro" trends that were expected to influence Canadian society in the decades ahead. These included the following:

1. *"Adultism": The Altered Family.* This will involve a shift from a youth-oriented to an adult-oriented society with an increasingly older population. By the year 2016, we will see a fixed working-age cohort at about 60 percent of the population, with the percentage of children declining as the percentage of elderly persons increases.

   Single-person households will decline to 30 percent by 2011, with projections that the percentage of working women will rise to 75 percent by the early 2000s [with growing] need for day-care programs and services for latchkey children.

2. *Structural Economic Change.* We are witnessing a shift from one complex of production technologies to another with the combination of computer and telecommunications advances speeding the transition from an industrial to a post-industrial economy. Society will become increasingly divided into "technocrats" and "technopeasants." For many, there will be temporary dislocation and unemployment; older "technopeasants" will face early forced retirement.

3. *Electronic Entertainment "Cocoons."* Homes are steadily evolving into the information age, with television, VCRs, computers, and word processors, videogames, and CD-ROMs offering communication and entertainment. Electronic systems will link the home with the community in terms of shopping, banks and other businesses, and entertainment options. Families will increasingly rely on the safety and comfort of their homes for recreation; virtual reality will make it possible to explore a host of new experiences.[4]

Other major trends identified in this Canadian futurist report include the following: mounting intercultural and intergroup problems, budget cutbacks and the shrinking leisure dollar in public agencies, and the decline of established agencies, with an emphasis on moving away from centralized authoritarian structures toward community-based leadership.

Numerous other predictions made over the last several years emphasize the growing role of technology and its impact on such diverse fields as energy production and use, environment, farming and food, medicine, space exploration, transportation, and manufacturing. There is widespread agreement that globalization is inevitable, in terms of worldwide trends in commerce, travel and cultural exchange, and that the twenty-first century will represent an "information" age, in which the gathering and exchange of knowledge will replace industry and manufacturing as key elements of national economies.

Many futurists are highly optimistic about the future, with some authorities predicting a "macroindustrial era"—a new age of abundance and prosperity. Within this oncoming period of turbocharged economic and technological growth, it is expected that there will be general improvement in the human condition on a global scale marked by increased ability to control and direct the course both of nature and of human societies.[5] Whether such projections are likely to prove true is uncertain. A recent analysis of predictions made in the late 1960s in *The Futurist* showed a scorecard of both "hits" and "misses" in such areas as medical, economic, urban, leisure, science and technology, and communications processes.[6]

Forecasting in the Leisure-Service Field

Apart from such general areas of forecasting, a number of reports have been developed that project trends and future needs within the organized recreation and park field itself.

NRPA/National Symposium Committee Report

Early in the 1990s, the National Symposium Committee held a national conference to identify critical future needs in recreation, parks, and leisure services. Its report, published by the National Recreation and Park Association, contained statements both of future trends and of priorities for the leisure-service field in meeting the changes lying ahead. Examples of the conference's conclusions follow:

Park and recreation professionals must be able and willing to identify, analyze, promote, and respond to change in society.

There is a strong trend toward greater participation in the decision-making process by citizens and employees; new leadership techniques will be required of park and recreation professionals to facilitate consensus building.

Multicultural diversity will continue to grow rapidly; parks and recreation must find ways to celebrate the variety of cultures within the community.

The wellness movement will continue to grow, and parks, recreation, and leisure services must facilitate and identify directly with this movement.

Success will depend on an organization's ability to build cooperative relationships and establish networks and coalitions with other organizations.

It is essential to improve the image of the profession, both externally and internally, so that the relationship between park and recreation programs and values and contemporary social needs is clearly apparent.

Tourism has emerged as one of the world's growth industries and an increasingly important part of leisure expression; parks and recreation must be involved in mutually beneficial partnerships with tourism.

Environment will increasingly become a focus on international concern; the park and recreation profession should play a leadership role in shaping environmental policy.

The park and recreation profession must develop and articulate clearly defined mission statements, goals, and objectives of the field.[7]

In a similar conference, the Illinois Park and Recreation Society held a "Gateway to the Future" planning meeting that summed up its visions for the early years of the twenty-first century. In its report, it argued that park and recreation agencies needed to become:

The champion of the wellness imperative for all citizens and communities—recognized as the key preventive service in the health field;

A catalyst and advocate for the environmental movements—stewards of our natural environments, leaders in environmental education, committed to ecologically sound operations and services;

Programming and facilities that are accessible to all—increasingly responding to challenged, disadvantaged, and "at-risk" individuals, "families" and neighborhoods—providing the cultural and social connections that build harmony;

Excellence in government management—demonstrating responsiveness, optimal use of all available resources, generating creative revenue alternatives to invest in quality services; and

Leaders in the public sector movement toward partnerships and strategic alliances that help achieve the full potential of our leisure, learning, health, police, and social service enterprises.[8]

Clearly, such conference conclusions represent forceful statements of the roles that recreation, park, and leisure-service agencies must play if they are to flourish and to make an important contribution to community and national life.

Trends and Issues: Views of Leisure-Service Educators

To probe beyond such general forecasts and recommendations, a survey was conducted in the fall of 1998 to determine the views of leisure-service educators with respect to trends, issues, and challenges facing the field at the beginning of the twenty-first century.

Eighteen demographic, social, and economic trends were drawn from the literature that were believed to have significant implications for the recreation, park, and leisure-service field. A panel of 195 current college and university department chairpersons and other faculty members active in the Society of Park and Recreation Educators was asked to rate the importance of these trends and issues for recreation, park, and leisure services.

The findings of the first section of the study are presented in Table 5.1. A summary of survey findings with respect to a second group of items representing issues and challenges for the field is presented in Chapter 14, and fuller details of the overall study are given in Appendix A.

TABLE 5.1   Predicted Trends Affecting Leisure in Twenty-First Century. Leisure-Service Educators Survey (September 1998).

Trend	Weighted Score
1. Age-related population shifts (growing number of elderly persons, changing birthrate, etc.)	494
2. Impact of high-tech equipment (computers, E-mail, Internet, etc., on leisure pursuits and business/professional practices, etc.)	443
3. Increasing racial and ethnic diversity in American society	442
4. Economic trends, with growing numbers of wealthy and poor populations and decline in middle-class numbers	419
5. Impact of deinstitutionalization and managed health care (reduced services, shorter treatment stays, on therapeutic recreation)	403
5. Influence of mass media of entertainment (movies, television, video games, "rap" music, etc.) on children and youth	403
7. Increased recognition of leisure as health-related field (fitness benefits, mental health, avoiding negative behaviors)	392
8. Continued breakdown in family structures and values	374
8. Reduced scope of government functions, shift toward privatization	374
10. Efforts to roll back environmental programs and permit fuller commercial exploitation of wildlands	367
11. Changing gender-related values; views toward alternative lifestyles	358
12. Trend toward telecommuting, with home worksites using computers	349
12. Growing conservatism in social policy, welfare cutbacks, harsher penal codes, attacks on affirmative action and immigration	349
14. Company mergers and downsizing, causing more double job-holding, increased job pressures, and reduced leisure time for many	342
15. Changing view of leisure, from earlier view of its moral/religious meaning to its identity as "commodity" or "industry"	331
16. Residential living shifts away from older central cities and rural towns toward suburbs, "edge" cities, "sun belt" states	314
17. Documented decline of public participation in community organizations	313
18. Greater concern about opportunities for persons with disabilities	306

Note: Items are listed in rank order of importance, based on survey findings, with 1 being the highest and 18 the lowest. Three sets of items were tied, and share ranks 5, 8, and 12. Number of survey respondents: 107.

Preliminary Review of Survey Findings

As indicated, selection of the trends listed in the survey was based on a systematic examination of articles in professional journals, newspapers, and news magazines in the mid- and late-1990s and other sources dealing with demographic, social, and economic trends. Items also reflect research papers presented at national conferences and editorials and policy recommendations found in professional society newsletters in the United States and Canada.

Each of the eighteen trends is now briefly reviewed and is then discussed in fuller detail in the following chapters of this text. It should be understood that while survey respondents gave fuller weight to some trends than others, as shown in the ranking, *all* of the trends were judged to be significant.

Trend 1: Age-Related Population Shifts

This was judged to be the most important trend affecting leisure needs, behaviors, and service policies. Clearly, each age-group in the population, from children and adolescents through later maturity and the elderly, has unique leisure needs and interests.

The surge of children and youth moving through the nation's schools and colleges clearly presents a challenge for educational administrators—but also for leisure service programmers and managers. Similarly, the growing number of elderly persons with varying degrees of health, economic security, and capability for independent living—coupled with greater self-awareness and political "clout"—will make older men and women an immense force to be reckoned with in the years ahead.

Beyond the needs of individual age groups, the steady increase in the overall populations of the United States and Canada through changing birth and death rates and continuing immigration will represent a major concern for leisure-service agencies.

Will it be possible to provide a basic floor of recreational facilities and programs for *all* citizens—what might be called an "opportunity spectrum"—or will some groups receive lavish leisure services while others are recreation-poor?

With a steadily increasing population, will it be possible to maintain and protect the nation's natural resources and wilderness areas and revive the crowded and rundown slum areas that so many socially and economically disadvantaged live in?

Can recreation be made a more effective tool in overcoming various forms of deviant or antisocial leisure behavior, particularly among at-risk youth and young adults? Such questions pose serious concerns for professionals in this field at the brink of the twenty-first century.

Trend 2: Impact of High-Tech Equipment on Leisure Pursuits and Business or Professional Practices

All futurist surveys agree that one of the most important changes in the years ahead will be the continuing development and proliferation of advanced technological devices and practices in all areas of community life, from health to business and communications to leisure.

Clearly, the impact of home computers, the Internet, video games, CD/ROMs, and a host of new kinds of equipment in sports, outdoor recreation, and entertainment has already affected leisure behavior significantly. With a substantial portion of home computer use involving varied forms of play and entertainment, and with much social contact today involving high-tech equipment, what will the long-range effect of this trend be on other forms of play or leisure involvements?

Will increased reliance on physically passive kinds of recreational equipment cut into active sports and outdoor recreation, and will this have a negative effect on children and youth?

Similarly, will reliance on television and other home-based leisure pursuits continue to promote the electronic entertainment "cocoons" discussed in the Canadian futurist report—and in further withdrawal from public social involvement?

Computers have already entered heavily into the planning and management of public and other recreation and park agencies, with a stronger emphasis on sophisticated marketing, pricing, and promotional methods? What new uses will high-tech equipment evolve in the delivery of leisure services?

Trend 3: Increasing Racial and Ethnic Diversity in American Society

All demographic and census studies show that the population of the United States has become increasingly multiracial and multiethnic over the past several decades, with minority populations becoming the majority in a number of leading cities. African Americans, Hispanic Americans, and, to a lesser degree, Asian Americans are increasing in numbers due to differing birth rates and to immigration impacts.

The history of racial and ethnic discrimination and its impact on recreation, parks, and leisure practices in the United States has been discussed in earlier chapters. Today, although public policy and social attitudes of the public at large has made immeasurable gains in terms of reducing prejudice and providing fuller educational and economic opportunity for minority groups, there continues to be a stubborn residue of prejudice and distrust on both sides of the national majority/minority divide.

Recreation and leisure have provided impressive forms of opportunity for blacks and Latinos in particular—through their success in professional sports and popular forms of entertainment. Beyond these gains, how can the organized recreation system be more effective in serving minority groups, particularly those who comprise a disproportionate segment of socially and economically disadvantaged persons?

Can leisure services meet the dual need to provide programming that is keyed to the unique cultural needs and interests of racial and ethnic minorities, and at the same time provide equal opportunities for the disadvantaged by helping them enter the mainstream of community life more fully?

In what ways can leisure services contribute to reducing lingering racial tensions and discrimination and promoting respect for all groups in society? For a unique and largely separate population, Native American tribes living on reservations, can outdoor recreation and tourism in particular provide an important new channel for economic progress?

Trend 4: Economic Trends, with a Growing
Rich/Poor Dichotomy

As Chapter 6 will show, although the United States is one of the wealthiest nations in the world, it also has one of the most pronounced contrasts between its rich and poor populations.

Through the 1980s and 1990s, economic studies show that the numbers of wealthy and poor citizens increased, while those in the middle-income income brackets declined markedly. In part, this was the result of major waves of downsizing, and the firing of millions of manufacturing and middle-management personnel by large corporations—in many cases individuals who have been unable to find new positions at comparable salary levels. This trend has contributed to a major sense of insecurity for many persons, to increased work-related pressures, and to more double-job-holding individuals and families.

Its importance for leisure also stems from the fact that so many recreational opportunities today come at a significant cost. As earlier chapters have shown, most public and nonprofit leisure-service agencies have moved vigorously into an entrepreneurial, marketing programming strategy. While many new forms of recreational activities have been devised and new programs and services provide the public with outstanding leisure opportunities, they rely heavily on substantial fees and charges for participation. The economic trend of the past two decades makes it increasingly difficult for many middle- and lower-class families to enjoy a full range of recreational activities.

Can public and nonprofit leisure-service agencies in particular justify themselves if they bar substantial population groups from participation on economic terms?

What methods can be used to provide adequate opportunities to the economically disadvantaged, or to assist recreation, park, and leisure-service agencies in poorer communities or neighborhoods to sponsor more varied programs?

Is the trend toward increasingly elaborate and expensive leisure pursuits, as described in Chapter 12, inevitable, or is the urge toward a simpler, more organic, "do-it-yourself" lifestyle that some have expressed a potential solution to this problem?

Trend 5 (Tie): Impact of Deinstitutionalization and
Managed Health Care

While increased concern about those with mental and physical disabilities has led to greater efforts to provide needed special recreation programs in community settings, other trends in recent years have diminished support for therapeutic recreation service in clinical settings.

Deinstitutionalization represented a massive effort during the 1960s and 1970s to reduce the numbers of individuals with mental illness or severe mental retardation who were confined to huge, custodial state hospitals or special schools by moving them out into the community. This was done partly for humanitarian reasons—with the conviction that many of these individuals had been unjustifiably confined and should be able to enter community life—and partly for economic purposes, to close down or cut back the large, expensive institutions that had housed them.

Unfortunately, however, the funds needed to provide special-care services, group housing arrangements, and other forms of support were never adequately provided, and great numbers of people who are seriously mentally ill and unable to cope live today as homeless persons in the community or with the most meager kinds of living arrangements. Today, a growing number of mentally ill persons—particularly those with substance-abuse problems—are confined not in hospitals, but in jails. Often, they receive no treatment and are preyed on by hardened criminals in such settings.[9]

The effect on therapeutic recreation has been that many treatment settings where practitioners functioned in the past are now closed, and community-based services are often almost nonexistent. Similarly, the impact of managed-care treatment plans has been to sharply reduce costs, cutting down on patient stays and eliminating many forms of adjunctive therapies—again undercutting the provision of therapeutic recreation as a treatment service.

What will be the long-range effect of this trend on the therapeutic recreation profession, which has traditionally dedicated itself to a range of services in clinical settings?

Can special recreation in the community incorporate a fuller level of prescriptive and adapted approaches to serve individuals with more severe levels of disability, and will adequate financial support be provided for such services?

Trend 5 (Tie): Influence of Mass Media of Entertainment on Children and Youth

The long-standing concerns about the impact of television, movies, video games, and rap and rock music on children and youth are reviewed in Chapter 11, which describes the widely held beliefs that in their most extreme forms these entertainment media contribute to violence, racial prejudice, drug involvement, and sexual abuse among many young people.

With new evidence that the Internet has become a channel for other types of negative play—including sexual predation practiced against the young and the easy entry of pornography into the home—many parents and civic groups are seeking solutions in the form of V-chips, stronger policing of the media, and similar policies.

The shocking slaughter of twelve students and a teacher and the wounding of numerous other students at Columbine High School in Littleton, Colorado, in April 1999 focused the nation's attention on the impact of violent "point-and-shoot" video games on many young people. The two disturbed students who used high-tech weaponry and homemade bombs to carry out this massacre had been fascinated by such violent games as *Doom* and *Quake*—in which players stalk their opponents through dungeon-like settings, firing steadily at human targets. Beyond this, one young assailant was revealed to have maintained a Web site on America Online, in which he displayed Nazi-like prejudice and racial antagonism and a fascination with violent attacks that served to forecast the Columbine School massacre.

Apart from a higher level of moral concern and social responsibility on the part of commercial vendors (rap groups, album makers, video-game producers and the like), which seems like an improbable development, how can the leisure-service industry counter such negative attractions?

Can a concerted effort to teach and promote leisure values and can honest discussions of varied forms of play and their impacts within youth-serving organizations contribute to more discriminating tastes and behaviors? Many youth-serving groups have been known for years as "character-building" organizations. Should it be their function to advocate for better levels of youth entertainment, to serve on community coalitions to restrict or limit destructive products or programs—within Constitutional restraints protecting free speech? Should this problem be part of their overall professional responsibility?

Trend 7: Increased Recognition of Leisure as Health-Related Field

This represents one of the most solidly documented areas of contribution of recreation and leisure in modern society. Numerous studies have shown the value of physical forms of play to personal health, and in a broader sense the value of varied forms of activity to total wellness.

Recognizing that obviously aerobic exercises, strenuous sports, and outdoor hobbies promote physical well-being and help prevent major forms of disease, it has also been demonstrated that people engage in such pursuits most consistently and with fullest commitment when they are part of a recreational or social context, rather than a grim, "exercise for health's sake" rationale.

Clearly, this area of organized recreation's contribution to public life needs to be pursued vigorously in the years ahead, with more diversified and purposeful programming and stronger public relations efforts to familiarize the public with the total wellness impact of leisure involvement.

In addition to such efforts, can public, nonprofit, employee-service, military, and other leisure-service agencies successfully make the case that leisure lifestyles that avoid tobacco, alcohol, drugs, and stress—or, more positively, offer healthy, outgoing, social pursuits—can promote health at any age? While this is widely known within the leisure-service field itself, how can it become a matter of common knowledge?

Trend 8 (Tie): Decline of Family Structure and Values

There is widespread agreement that since the 1960s the structure and stability of families in modern society have been seriously weakened, as evidenced by the high rate of divorce, the growing numbers of children born out of wedlock, the incidence of physical abuse among family members, and similar problems.

As Chapter 6 shows, while the cozy picture of the happy family of the 1950s, as depicted in familiar situation comedies, is often a romantic fiction, the reality is that stable and secure families are essential if children are to grow up in responsible, self-fulfilling ways. Increasingly, leisure-service agencies have focused their efforts on providing family-centered programs and helping to build positive family values and relationships.

What are the realistic prospects for the family of the future? What role do recreation and leisure play in building strong families and avoiding the pathologies that often trouble both urban and rural neighborhoods today? While it is generally assumed that social problems are less severe for youth in upper-class suburban or small-town neighborhoods, the

Littleton, Colorado, tragedy showed that no social class is immune from the dangers of youth violence. There, and in a number of other communities through the late 1990s, one of the root causes of the sudden attacks—apart from the easy availability of semiautomatic guns—seemed to be the failure of parents to maintain close emotional ties with their children, or even to be concerned about their systematic preparations for the slaughter that was to come.

Beyond such questions, there are new issues to be decided. What constitutes a family —in an era in which there are great numbers of single-family households and in which same-sex couples are increasingly seeking to adopt children or to be recognized as legitimate married couples and responsible family units? As a community service that helps to build cohesive family structures, such issues need to be faced by leisure-service agencies.

Trend 8 (Tie): Reduced Scope of Government Functions and Shift Toward Privatization

As shown earlier, more and more government units today have been abandoning traditional functions and turning to subcontracting a wide range of functions. At the same time, the distinction between different types of leisure-service agencies has become increasingly uncertain. With many types of nonprofit or cultural organizations adopting marketing strategies, there has been growing pressure to withdraw their charitable tax-exemption status.

Private-membership organizations have become more and more public, in that their past policies of racial, social, or gender exclusion have come under attack and been weakened by state legislation or court decisions. Within this context, is it possible to say definitively exactly what functions *should* be governmental, when nonprofit community organizations run parks, neighborhood groups sponsor youth sports leagues, and city councils contribute millions of dollars to the construction of privately owned stadiums and arenas?

What are the long-term implications of growing numbers of well-to-do families withdrawing from the use of public leisure programs and facilities, and relying on private or commercial recreation services?

Beyond such general questions, does government have a legitimate responsibility for supporting the arts, meeting the needs of disabled populations and the elderly, promoting intercultural understanding, and similar functions that we have come to accept in recent years?

Trend 10: Efforts to Reverse Environmental Recovery Programs and Permit Fuller Commercial Use of Wildlands

While major progress has been made since the 1960s in overcoming varied forms of environmental pollution, recovering the health of rivers and lakes, restoring wildlife habitats, and protecting endangered species, this continues to be a controversial issue in national life.

Constantly, there are efforts to open up formerly protected parks and wilderness areas to commercial use through roads, mining, oil drilling, lumbering, or the introduction of facilities to serve outdoor recreationists and tourists. With the need for jobs as a constant refrain voiced by local residents and their representatives in state legislatures or Congress, it is often outside groups of conservationists who mobilize to resist such pressures. Within this context, recreation and park professionals may be torn between different groups of outdoor enthusiasts and troubled by the inability to maintain effective environmental controls or maintenance operations with inadequate funding.

As Chapter 13 will demonstrate, new successes have been achieved in placing huge new tracts of wildlands and open space under protection on a permanent basis. What role do recreation and park agencies have in this process? Are they able to demonstrate that outdoor recreation represents a continuing source of employment and income in many settings through ecotourism and the sustained use of natural environments, rather than the short-term exploitation by lumbering or mining that may then have long-term destructive effects?

Trend 11: Changing Gender-Related Values and Views Toward Alternative Sexual Lifestyles

For a number of years, there has been steady pressure by feminist groups and their allies for fuller opportunity and equality of opportunity for participation in leisure activities such as sports, in which they had traditionally been harshly restricted.

The fact that respondents to the survey did not rate this trend as a high-priority concern may indicate that many believe this battle has been won, with women achieving much higher rates of participation in sports and outdoor recreation and gaining access to other areas of community recreation from which they had formerly been restricted. However, while significant progress has been made, many would argue that the struggle for full equality in the recreation, park, and leisure-service field will continue, to ensure full equality in both participation and career roles. Certainly, many organizations serving women and girls receive far less support than their male counterparts. In those athletic or other organizations that have merged male and female memberships, the argument has been made that the priorities of women and girls are given less support.

Beyond such feminist concerns, there is growing awareness of the special needs of men and boys, who have traditionally been subjected to a limiting set of expectations regarding appropriate "masculine" behaviors. In addition to policy questions regarding gender issues, there is the broader question of sex as a factor in the leisure behavior of Americans. Here, the traditional morality of past generations has been replaced by a widely accepted code involving fuller freedom for both sexes. At the same time, a substantial group of citizens—often linked to more conservative religious denominations—opposes such freedom.

This split in contemporary values is illustrated in terms of public attitudes with respect to homosexuality. While lesbians and gays are generally much more widely accepted than in the past, resistance to their lifestyles continues to be evidenced on many fronts: religious, political, and in a growing wave of violence against homosexuals during the late 1990s. What are the policy questions facing recreation, park, and leisure-service agencies in this area?

Trend 12 (Tie): Trend Toward Telecommuting, with Home Worksites

While this shift has been relatively limited thus far, many futurists predict that it will become far more widespread in the years ahead. As Chapter 14 shows, an increasing number of companies have relocated to distant or rural sites, making use of computers to conduct their business.

What will working at home mean for employees who adopt this new workstyle? While it will make their lives more flexible and reduce commuting and travel time, it may also mean that work is no longer carried out in a face-to-face, social environment. In effect, will it add to social isolation for many employees? As a positive possibility, will it mean that men and women who telecommute, using home worksites, will be all the more eager to take part in organized leisure activities away from their homes? If so, what kinds of programs and activity schedules will meet their needs?

Trend 12 (Tie): Growing Conservatism in Social Policy

The trend of the late 1980s and 1990s, as shown in Chapter 3, has been markedly in the direction of reducing social services for all ages, cutting back on welfare support for families, imposing harsher sentencing and penal policies, and mounting legislative efforts to eliminate affirmative action regulations in business, education, or government.

This pronounced conservative shift can be seen as a reaction to the counterculture of the 1960s and 1970s, an expression of religious fundamentalism and distrust of government, or simply part of an ongoing cycle in public attitudes and values. Its relevance for recreation, parks, and leisure services, as shown earlier, is that the basic principles underlying these programs involve commitment to improving the lives of people and strengthening communities and natural environments. A major thrust of many leisure-service professionals has been not simply to meet the needs and interests of the public for play or entertainment as an amenity, but to meet significant social needs.

While it is difficult to predict whether there will be a swing away from the conservative trend just described, the clear mandate for recreation, park, and leisure-service professionals will be for them to serve as proactive advocates for meeting the needs of disadvantaged persons, those with disabilities or other groups with special needs. Both within their own programs and in collaboration with other community groups, will leisure-service practitioners be able to meet this challenge?

Trend 14: Impact of Company Changes That Increase Work Pressures and Reduce Leisure Time

As the discussion of Trend 4 (see page 99) points out, many corporations have reduced their workforces, merging and downsizing for greater stockholder profit, using "outsourcing" methods to slash full-time employee rolls, and throwing many individuals into the labor market. Forced often to take two poorly paid jobs with greater work pressures, such individuals are clearly in need of the restoring and refreshing values of creative, self-directed play. Yet, in many cases, as surveys have shown, they have significantly less free time than in the past to enjoy individual or family recreation.

Again, it is not possible to predict whether this trend will continue, and whether work hours will be extended and leisure hours diminished. In some cases, unions have begun to militate and even strike against excessive overtime hours. In any case, leisure-service managers will need to consider the need to provide the kinds of programs that will be restorative for employees experiencing severe work stresses and free-time shortages. Flexible program scheduling and supportive group-centered services—such as those offered by many company personnel units—may be helpful in meeting such needs.

Trend 15: Changing View of Leisure from Moral or Religious Meaning to Identity as an Industry

As shown earlier, at the inception of the recreation movement, playgrounds, parks, and recreation centers were justified for their contribution to community life, and play itself was often referred to in moral or religious terms. Moving sharply from this idealistic concept of recreation and play, today it is common practice to regard all forms of leisure involvement or sponsorship as a type of commodity or industry—with participants regularly referred to as "customers."

In part, this practice emerged from the growing reliance on fees and charges and the accepted emphasis on marketing services for financial support during the 1980s and 1990s. It also came from the strong thrust toward "reinventing government" that many civic leaders adopted at this time, which preached that all government agencies needed to be run on a "bottom-line," businesslike basis.

Recognizing the necessity for all leisure-service organizations to operate as efficiently as possible, streamlining their services and seeking funding support in innovative ways, it is also essential that leaders in this field stress that it is more than an industry. Like medicine, law, social work, or education—all of which have significant economic needs and priorities—it is also a field of important human-service values. The issue that will constantly confront recreation, park, and leisure-service managers in the decades ahead will be the need to reconcile economic priorities and financial pressures with the commitment to providing significant social programs and serving populations that cannot pay fees and charges for participation.

Trend 16: Shift Toward Suburbs, "Edge" Cities, and Sun Belt States

The internal migration of millions of families over the past several decades, both away from the central cities into suburbs or more prosperous small towns and from rural areas to metropolitan regions, brought about sharp social and economic contrasts between residents in both types of areas. A second important trend has been the continuing shift from wintry regions to such states as Arizona, Florida, Texas, or California.

While there have been some reversals of these trends, with many older persons deciding to retire in the north, or with wealthier individuals returning to cities to enjoy their cultural advantages and conveniences, the overall patterns of migration seem likely to continue. What are their implications for the leisure-service field?

Clearly, for cities and towns in northern, wintry regions, one of the strategies has been to maximize the leisure opportunities offered by their climates—in terms of winter sports and pastimes—such as those explored by many so-called "Winter Cities." For others, the severe disparity of living conditions and recreational services between impacted inner-city neighborhoods and wealthier surrounding communities, there appear to be few solutions at present.

In some states, efforts have been made to equalize educational services and standards between wealthier and poorer school districts by adjusting tax rates and state funding allocations to strengthen the weaker districts. Such efforts have met with strong political resistance, and it is questionable whether any regional approach to sharing recreation and park funding resources among rich and poor communities would receive public approval.

Trend 17: Reported Decline of Public Participation in Community Organizations

This trend is a controversial one, based as it is primarily on an article by Harvard University professor Robert Putnam that reported a sharp decline in public participation in a host of community organizations throughout the United States. Putnam documented this shift with varied statistics from parent-teacher organizations, adult bowling leagues and other sports groups, membership clubs, and organized social and service groups. He speculated as to the causes, ranging from increased reliance on home-based entertainment to fear of crime to the gradual loss of a sense of civic involvement and "community" among many Americans.

At the same time, there is widespread evidence that volunteerism is flourishing—not only in terms of individual efforts in social-service settings, but also through organized groups that work for community betterment and provide funding support and billions of man- and woman-hours of contributed time each year.

The relatively low rating given by survey respondents to this trend suggests that they do *not* regard it as a matter of real concern. Certainly, many public recreation and park agencies are able to recruit substantial numbers of residents as advisory council members or program volunteers, and such youth-serving groups as Boy and Girl Scouts or Little League are generally heavily assisted by adult leaders and coaches. At the same time, the trend reported by Putnam and the specific examples of organizations that have suffered major membership losses need to be carefully studied. Why has this shift occurred, and what are its implications for other recreation, park, and leisure-service organizations?

Trend 18: Greater Concern About Opportunities for Persons with Disabilities

This trend, which one might have expected to receive a higher rating, ranked lowest of all eighteen items in the survey. One might draw several inferences from this, the first being that the leisure-service educators responding felt that sufficient support is now being given to programs for persons with disabilities, in both segregated and integrated settings. Certainly, due both to recent legislation and to increased public interest, special recreation services and adapted physical facilities for play are now found in most community and nonprofit recreation organizations.

One might also speculate that, since the majority of leisure-service educators are generalists, with therapeutic recreation service constituting a separate, highly specialized professional concern, they would tend to assign it a lower priority than other issues.

At the time of the passage of the Americans with Disabilities Act in 1990, it was estimated that there were approximately 43 million citizens of all ages with disabilities that were significant enough to limit them seriously in some aspect of life activity—education, work, family life, leisure, or civic involvement. Canadian reports indicate a similar proportion of persons with disabilities. The recognition that leisure represents an important aspect of life satisfaction and self-fulfillment for such persons (many of whom cannot work or find other rewarding outlets in life) *must* increasingly pose a challenge to recreation, park, and leisure-service professionals in all types of agencies.

What policies might be effective in arousing fuller public and professional concern and support for programs designed to bring persons with disabilities more fully into the mainstream of community life?

Implications of Survey Findings

Each of the trends just reviewed represents an important concern, both in terms of understanding the present and future roles of leisure in American society and the kinds of choices facing practitioners and decision makers in the leisure-service system, today and tomorrow.

They are therefore discussed more fully in the eight chapters that follow, as part of a broad analysis of expected changes in American society that will have a significant impact on leisure involvement and recreation and park programs.

Summary

From an overview of the recreation, park, and leisure-service system, this chapter turns to forecasting future trends and issues that will affect the leisure-service field. It summarizes a number of major predictions offered by futurologists with respect to such trends as increased globalization, the emergency of an information-based society, the impact of technology and electronic data processing, shifts in family values and structures, and changes in work and leisure patterns. It then presents a number of the key findings of professional recreation and park study groups or forecasting bodies, with respect to professional challenges or priorities in the twenty-first century.

The chapter concludes with a summary of the findings of a 1998 survey of leisure-service educators that sought to measure the perceived importance of a number of social, demographic, and economic trends for recreation and park agencies and practitioners.

Key Concepts

1. One of the most important influences in the decades ahead will involve the overall growth pattern of the nation, along with the specific increases among such population groups as adolescents and young adults, or the elderly.

2. Advancing technology, both in terms of the kinds of leisure pursuits it will provide and its use in the management of recreation and leisure agencies, will constitute another major influence.

3. Concerns related to two major types of "minorities"—racial or ethnic subgroups who will soon comprise a majority and gender-related groups that have been discriminated against the past—will also provide an important challenge for leisure-service planners in the future.

4. The growing dichotomy between rich and poor, with a decline in the middle socio-economic classes in the United States, will pose both an ethical and a practical problem for leisure-service managers, given the growing reliance on fees and charges to support many programs.

5. Therapeutic recreation services, while not recognized as one of the highest priorities in this study, do represent an area of growing need, particularly because of trends in health care that have resulted in greater numbers of persons with disabilities living in the community.

6. Issues related to supporting family structures, resisting the influence of mass media entertainment forms that promote negative forms of play, and problems of at-risk youth will present critical challenges to leisure services in the years ahead.

7. There is a need to promote public awareness of leisure as a health-related field and to balance the marketing emphasis with continuing concern about recreation's social role and contribution.

8. Environmental concerns must be part of the leisure service field's mission, along with the need to adapt to changing work patterns and the trend toward privatization of public functions.

Endnotes

1. Henry W. 1992. Ready or Not, Here It Comes. *Time Magazine* (Fall, special issue): 32.

2. Cummings, L., and J. Busser. 1994. Forecasting in Recreation and Park Management: Need, Substance, and Reasonableness. *Journal of Park and Recreation Administration* (Spring): 36.

3. McLean, D.D., and R.V. Russell. 1992. Future Visions for Public Parks and Recreation Agencies. *Journal of Park and Recreation Administration* (10/10: 48–49.

4. Macro Trends Prescribe Canada's New National Vision for Recreation and Parks. 1993. *Leisure Watch* (2/3): 1–4.

5. Zey, M. 1997. The Macroindustrial Era: A New Age of Abundance and Prosperity. *The Futurist* (March/April): 9–14.

6. Cornish, E. 1997. Futurist Forecasts 30 Years Later. *The Futurist* (January/February): 45–49.

7. Mobley, T., and R. Toalson, eds. 1992. *Parks and Recreation in the 21st Century.* Arlington, VA: National Symposium Committee and NRPA.

8. From the Leading Edge: Innovative View of the Future. 1993. Presentation at NRPA Congress, San Jose, CA (October).

9. Goodman, W. 1999. Confining the Mentally Ill, Not in Hospitals but in Jails. *New York Times* (March 11): B–13.

6 People I: Demographic Trends Affecting Leisure

As the New Year begins, the nation's population is estimated to be just under 269 million, an increase of 2.4 million in the last year, the Census Bureau reported. The growth rate of 0.9 percent in 1997 was the same in 1996 and is the projected rate for 1998. The figure reflects a flattening of the growth rate in the United States, which since 1990 has been 8.1 percent. Census Bureau analysts report that the stabilization of the growth rate can be attributed partly to the declining number of births. . . . The news is encouraging to some, like those in Zero Population Growth, a nonprofit group that advocates the slowing of population growth worldwide.[1]

American marriage and family life have changed dramatically in the past three decades. The "traditional" family of the 1950s and 1960s . . . has been reshaped by high rates of teenage and nonmarital childbearing, sharp increases in the divorce rate, postponed marriage and childbearing, smaller families, single-parent families, stepfamilies, and dual-earner marriages. Many scholars call this diverse array of family types the "postmodern family."[2]

We now turn to a more detailed analysis of several key demographic factors that influence life in the United States today and that will have a growing effect on leisure in the years ahead.

They include the following: (1) population trends, including changes in the United States resulting from immigration, shifting birthrate, and life-expectancy rates; (2) the needs of different age groups in American society, linked to new patterns of family life; and (3) the growing rich/poor polarization of socioeconomic groups in the United States, with a resultant decline of the middle classes. Each factor is explored, both in terms of current trends and future prospects.

Importance of Demographic Analysis

Clearly, it is not possible to forecast future changes in terms of leisure needs and behaviors without developing realistic projections with respect to population growth, including such elements as birthrate, immigration, and life expectancy. For example, Robert Ditton cites one segment of the outdoor recreation field—fisheries management:

> In addition to decreased rates of population growth, changes will occur in population characteristics: The population is aging, minority populations are increasing, and traditional, married-couple family households are decreasing.
>
> Generalizations are difficult since these trends vary by state, but as the composition of the population varies, more people are less likely to participate in recreational fishing (based on previous study results on participation by age cohort, gender, race, and ethnic group), and more anglers will participate less frequently. . . . Managers can either intervene now or take no action and let changing population trends dictate their futures.[3]

Within every area of public leisure involvement, ranging from television-watching to boating or visiting gambling casinos, changing population patterns affect both the demand for recreational opportunities and the specific needs and interests that must be served.

Patterns of Population Growth

For centuries, population growth was regarded as desirable. In an era in which the life span was short, with high rates of infant and childhood mortality and with vast wilderness and prairie areas on the North American continent to be settled, European immigration was encouraged and rising census reports were viewed optimistically. However, by the mid- and late-1990s, population growth began to be seen as a danger, both on a global scale and within the United States itself.

In a recent book, *Juggernaut Growth on a Finite Planet,* Lindsey warns that uncontrolled population growth has been devastating to human societies at every level. He argues that:

> Poor nations endure famine and destruction of their resources. Emerging nations struggle with the problems of industrialization. Affluent countries face joblessness, failing social structures, growing disparities between the rich and poor, ethnic conflict, and environmental degradation. We are all rapidly descending into troubles of our own making.[4]

While it might be countered that many of these difficulties stem from misguided social and economic policies rather than population growth alone, there is no question that many of our most severe ecological problems are the direct effect of steadily increasing population numbers and their impact on surrounding environments. For example, planners for the Chesapeake Bay region on the eastern seaboard recognize that dense residential settlement, with increasing sediment and nutrient pollution stemming from overbuilding and road construction, has been the root cause of great environmental stress on the bay and its tributaries.

At another level, the impact of surging population totals was illustrated in the mid- and late-1990s, when a huge wave of children of Baby Boomer families reached its peak, bursting school enrollments in many cities and school districts. Education Secretary Richard Riley issued a report showing that the 1996–1997 school year represented the midpoint of a twenty-year trend of rising enrollments. With the projection that by 2006 schools would be educating 54.6 million children, almost 3 million more than in the mid-1990s, many schools were facing alarming overcrowding, substandard, and often dangerous conditions.[5]

The professional literature in recreation, parks, and leisure studies has reflected these concerns. Edginton, Jordan, DeGraaf, and Edginton, for example, wrote in 1995:

> The world population, expanding at an alarming rate, will dramatically impact society—including leisure patterns and opportunities—for decades to come. As of 1990, the Canadian population stood at 27 million with more than 75 percent of Canadians living within two hours of the Canada–United States border. . . . Population in the United States, estimated in 1990 to be 250 million people [is projected to reach approximately 268.3 million people by 2000].[6]

In actual fact, the U.S. Census Bureau reported that the nation's population reached 270.5 million in August 1998. However, other reports show that, surprisingly, the rate of population growth has sharply declined as part of a major worldwide trend.

Reports of Declining Birth and Population Growth Rates

In November 1997, demographer Ben Wattenberg reported that, far from facing "global chaos as the planet's population grows exponentially," instead there has been a worldwide decline in fertility rates around the world. Strikingly, this trend has been underway since the 1980s.

> European birthrates of the 1980s, already at record-breaking lows, fell another 20 percent in the 90s, to about 1.4 per woman. . . . Italy, a Catholic country, has a fertility rate of 1.2 children per woman, the world's lowest rate—and the lowest national rate ever recorded (absent famines, plagues, wars, or economic catastrophes). In the United States, birthrates have been below replacement for 25 straight years . . .[7]

Wattenberg points out that the population explosion—in which the world's total population increased from 1 billion to 2.5 billion from 1750 to 1950 and to 6 billion over the last half-century—has largely been a consequence of rising life expectancy. Factors leading to lower rates are heavily based on the shift to urbanization in industrialized countries. With the move away from rural living, where children are needed to help with farm work, to cities where the need is for fewer mouths to feed, families simply want and plan for fewer children. Other factors include more education and new aspirations for women, legal abortion and more effective contraceptive methods, later marriage and a higher divorce rate, greater acceptance of homosexuality, and—finally—vastly lower infant mortality rates.

While population growth is likely to continue in undeveloped nations, demographers predict that birthrates will remain low in industrialized societies, with the new danger that countries like Italy, Sweden, and France, among others, will soon find themselves with poorly balanced societies, with huge numbers of elderly citizens and not enough young people working to support them with essential services.

Ultimately, the world population is projected to stabilize around 2200 at about 11 billion. For the near future in the United States, the most significant population forecasts show that today's dramatically higher numbers of children and youth will be moving into colleges and then the adult work force over the next decade or two and that the elderly population will continue to represent a increasingly higher proportion of the population. Beyond that, a major element in population growth will continue to consist of immigrants from other countries—particularly developing nations, which tend to have higher birthrates.

Influence of Age Groups on Leisure

A key factor that affects leisure values and behavior in American society is one's age or, stated more broadly, one's place in the life cycle, extending from infancy and childhood through later maturity and aging. At each stage of development, there are specific tasks that must be mastered as part of healthy physical, emotional, social, and intellectual growth. This chapter outlines the role played by leisure in this process and the challenges that face individuals today in a rapidly changing society. A concluding section of the chapter examines recreation's contribution to family life and the impact of disability on Americans of all ages.

First, it should be recognized that there have been major changes in the ways that different stages of the life cycle have been perceived in recent year, with accepted forms of behavior at each stage. Gail Sheehy comments that there has been a revolution in the life cycle within the space of one short generation. Puberty, she writes, arrives earlier by several years than it did at the turn of the century. Adolescence is now prolonged for many individuals well into their twenties, as they continue to attend college and graduate school and, in increasing numbers, live at home. She continues:

> True adulthood doesn't begin until 20. Most baby boomers, born after World War II, do not feel fully "grown up" until they are in their forties. . . . Unlike members of the previous generation, who almost universally had their children launched by that stage of life, many late-baby couples or stepfamily parents [have adolescent children as they move into the middle years]. . . . The territory of the fifties, sixties, and beyond is changing so radically that it now opens up whole new stages of life . . .[8]

Despite such changes, for all persons the human life cycle represents a similar process of development in which varied biological, psychological, and other tasks or milestones are chronologically encountered. Osgood and Howe write:

> Life is portrayed as a progressive unfolding of crises and resolution. Certain psychological tasks must be completed before the individual may move on to other

stages. . . . The psychologic crisis of ego development, which confronts the individual at various life stages, influences personal values; motivations for behavior; the meanings, significance, and satisfactions derived from various activities (including leisure activities); and patterns of life involvement.[9]

Leisure Availability in the Life Cycle

There are marked differences in the amount of leisure available to people throughout the life cycle. To illustrate, during the mid-1960s, the Southern California Research Council carried out a study of the amounts and uses of leisure for almost thirteen million residents in its region, based on extensive surveys of all age groups and social classes. Documenting leisure patterns at each life stage, it found that the bulk of time in infancy was spent in self-care or maintenance activity, such as rest, sleep, and eating. In early childhood, play and beginning study activities occur. In later childhood and adolescence, school, self-care, and recreation pursuits dominate time use, with children assuming some chores at home, and adolescents increasingly taking on outside work activities as well. For adults, discretionary time amounted to between 25 and 50 hours a week. For the young and the old, it rose to between 50 and 70 hours weekly, with leisure increasing dramatically for retired persons.

Leisure, Play, and Recreation in Childhood

Childhood is a period generally regarded as extending from infancy or the toddler stage through the age of approximately 12, although the onset of puberty or adolescence may actually occur well before or after that age. It is a time for physical and psychomotor growth and for dealing with such tasks as gaining a sense of self and relating to others; learning responsibility and self-discipline; and developing social, cognitive, and communicative skills.

Apart from study and self-maintenance responsibilities and occasional chores, play fills a major portion of the child's time. It is a phenomenon that appears among various living species and in all human societies, as shown in Chapter 1. A leading psychoanalyst, Bruno Bettelheim, stressed play's importance in the emotional development of children:

> . . . children use play to work through and master quite complex psychological difficulties of the past and present. So valuable is play in this connection that play therapy has become the main avenue for helping young children with their emotional difficulties; it is a "royal road" to the child's conscious and unconscious inner world.[10]

Beyond these values, play contributes to the child's physical and intellectual development, ability to deal with others, perseverance, and confidence. In a detailed review of the values of play experience that have been documented by research, Lynn Barnett emphasized its contribution to the child's cognitive growth, including divergent thinking and problem-solving skills.[11]

As we examine leisure and play in the lives of children today, it is important to recognize the real problems that face many youngsters in contemporary society. For example, while many children grow up in happy and financially secure homes and communities, too many others experience stress from parental abuse or neglect, family breakup, or neighborhood poverty and pathology.

The period of the 1980s represented a "terrible decade for children," according to a report issued in 1991 by the nonprofit Center for the Study of Social Policy. Nationally, there were substantial increases in the percentage of children living in poverty, juveniles who were incarcerated, out-of-wedlock births, violent deaths of teenagers, and the percentage of babies with low birth weights, which often leads to physical and mental impairment.

Beyond such changes, it is apparent that many children have lost their "innocence" in terms of having a harsher and crueler understanding of the adult world. Based on hundreds of interviews with elementary school children, researcher Marie Winn comments: "their testimony about marijuana, sex, and pornographic movies on cable television would have deeply shocked parents a decade or two ago. The reticence and shyness once associated with childhood have clearly gone the way of curtsies and pinafores."[12]

Linked to such changes, Winn writes, are profound changes in adult conceptions of childhood itself. In the past, most parents felt obliged to shelter their children from life's ugliness; today, many appear to accept the belief that children must be exposed early to adult experience in order to survive in an increasingly uncontrollable world. Neil Postman, author of *The Disappearance of Childhood,* agrees, commenting that with the new technologies, including both cable television and the Internet, there are fewer and fewer secrets in medical, sexual, or political matters. Children become "adult" at a very early age.

Role of Parents

Recognizing that children's play can be a positive force in the child's development, it is helpful to examine the role of parents in children's leisure lives. Barnett and Chick write:

> The most salient force in the young child's environment is the presence and influence of parental models. Play behavior is a dimension of experience and exploration available to most children, but it has been shown that the richness and frequency of play arise from a set of optimal conditions that include the behaviors of parents for identification and modeling. Parents have been shown to exert a strong directing influence on their children's imaginative and cognitive play styles, and, in a more subtle manner, parental attributes and personality traits produce correlates with children's tendency toward playfulness.[13]

It is clear that parents play a critical role in helping children develop constructive leisure values and habits of participation. In many situations, however, parents may fail to show interest or may provide a negative model, as in the case of families where parents have problems related to drugs or alcohol or sexual promiscuity. Other problems may be linked to the lack of community resources for healthful recreational pursuits.

On the other hand, some parents who are social "strivers" may attempt to use children's play to compensate for their own lack of success or prestige by having the child become a successful athlete or performer—or may do so to help the youngster embark on a hopefully lucrative career. This may take the course of enrolling children in a relentless schedule of music or ballet classes, figure skating, or other pursuits at an extremely early age. One parent describes how she and her competitive, highly status-conscious friends sought to have their children enter the "fast lane" in infancy:

> we compress their time and pack it with play dates, lessons of all kinds and enriching experiences like camping and skiing . . . It begins in the first year of life, when infants are enrolled in special gyms . . . [at a] "children's fitness center," where the babies crawled around a padded obstacle course . . . one of the babies started walking at eight months, which caused a stir. "See that!" the mothers whispered to their charges. "Look at Megan, you can do what she does. You just have to be more assertive!"[14]

In contrast with such efforts, other programs to provide children with organized play activities vary greatly in quality and scope. While team sports like soccer or Little League Baseball serve millions of elementary-age children, most youngsters of this age lack adequate physical education programs in their schools and do not meet important fitness standards. Currently, only seventeen states have mandatory physical education classes and only a third of all schoolchildren take such classes daily. In many communities, the traditional practice of children playing outdoors after school has largely disappeared. In many homes, they watch television instead; if they live in impacted urban neighborhoods, they are warned to stay indoors where they will be safe.

As evidence of this trend, in the late 1990s a number of public school systems, such as schools in Atlanta, Georgia, eliminated recess periods and instead placed heavier and heavier emphasis on academic homework.

Reflecting the impact of socioeconomic status, millions of children in disadvantaged communities lack neighborhood resources for constructive play. At the same time, wealthier children are wooed as a key target audience by major airlines, cruise ships, hotel chains, and theme parks. To promote family travel, airlines publish children's magazines and activity books and offer lounges and other special attractions for children. Many companies today are creating new kids' products, such as computer technology designed for children, specially packaged children's frozen meals, an array of cosmetics and toiletries for boys and girls, and an estimated $17 billion worth of entertainment-based licensed products featuring such stars as TeleTubbies and Rugrats.

A key example of how commercial interests and lack of meaningful parental concern threaten the healthy development of America's children in their leisure may be found in television programming. Studies by the A. C. Neilsen Company have shown that the average child in the 2-to-11-year-old age group watches television for over 27 hours a week. While there are a few excellent children's television programs, these have declined in number and are inaccessible in some sections of the country. On the other hand, television programs, rap music, and video games with high levels of violence and other objectionable content are widely available everywhere.

In the late 1990s, it was reported that the number of juveniles arrested for violent crimes had risen sharply across the United States. Boys and girls as young as 10 were using steroids to enhance athletic performance, with growing evidence of other social problems in this age group. At the same time, a 1999 research report by the Urban Institute concluded that the vast majority of American families were thriving and providing a positive environment for raising children.[15]

In considering the role of children's play, it is important to recognize the work of youth groups such as the Boy Scouts and Girl Scouts, Boys and Girls Clubs, 4-H Clubs, the leading sports leagues, church-sponsored groups, Police Athletic Leagues, Junior Achievement, and a host of other special-interest groups that serve millions of boys and girls with positive and constructive youth programs. These organizations often provide a valuable cross section of outdoor recreation activity and camping, along with arts and creative pursuits, homemaking skills, and leadership training.

Adolescents and Leisure

The adolescent or teenage period in the human life cycle extends from the onset of puberty, roughly between ages 11 and 14, to the late teen years, when individuals begin to be perceived as young adults. Adolescence is a time when young people must develop a healthy and realistic sense of self and of their sexual identity. They must master the academic challenges in school and college that equip them to function effectively as adults in community life and the related task of choosing career options and preparing for future employment.

Increasingly, Beth Kivel writes, there is evidence that leisure provides an important context for young people in terms of developing meaningful individual or personal identity, and in terms of their social roles and group relationships.[16]

In past centuries, adolescence was not recognized as a separate period of life. Instead, children often assumed adult responsibilities at an early age. However, they began to assume a separate identity in the early twentieth century, as the years of schooling were prolonged and entrance into the work force was postponed. Wartella and Mazzarella point out that teenagers became recognized as a group needing public policy action and intervention at this time, with growing concern about how they spent their time: "concern with children's leisure was part of a list of child-related interests among Progressive reformers. . . . [As high school attendance became the predominant pattern] children became the focus of scientific studies. . . ."[17]

Surveys of major cities documented the ways in which adolescents were spending their time—particularly in such forms of commercial recreation as movies, public dances, poolrooms, and vaudeville and burlesque theaters. By the end of the 1920s, the American public came to realize that adolescents were developing an autonomous and highly commercialized peer-oriented leisure culture.

Particularly after World War II, mass cultural forms such as movies, television, popular movies, and distinctive styles of dress all captured teenage audiences and served to set them apart in American society. The mass media helped to create a separate teen culture, marked by its own customs and tastes and resistant to the traditional values of adult American society. In time, the generations were so physically segregated by the factors of suburban living, forced school attendance, and after-school work and play that the young spent

> the greater portion of their day in a world dominated by peers, so the mass media ideologically segregated them; youthful language, style of dress, goals, and behavior became more and more foreign to adults—as well as more and more commercialized. . . . [T]eenagers, by erecting barriers of fashion and custom around adolescence, had walled off a secret and potentially antagonistic area of American culture.[18]

This trend was made more vivid and threatening by the youth rebellion of the 1960s and 1970s, when growing numbers of high school and college students resisted parental authority and became increasingly involved in potentially self-destructive leisure pursuits. A 1989 report by the national Parent's Resource Institute for Drug Education, Inc. (PRIDE) reported that alcohol and drug abuse were serious problems in both low-income housing projects and affluent suburbs. Strikingly, both forms of substance abuse were consistently higher for white students than for black—a refutation of popular beliefs. In 1990, a study by the Search Institute for the Lutheran Brotherhood reported that 5 percent of American children commonly attend drinking parties as early as the sixth grade, and as many as 61 percent do so regularly as high school seniors. The study also reported that numerous children lacked adult supervision, watched television extensively, had parents with alcohol and drug problems, and had been physically or sexually abused by adults. A major panel report in 1990 concluded that because of problems related to substance abuse, unplanned pregnancies, venereal disease, and emotional problems, many modern teenagers were "unlikely to attain the high levels of educational achievement required for success in the twenty-first century."

As late as 1998, research reports indicated that teenagers' social problems were continuing to grow, with a dramatic rise in the number of juveniles arrested for violent crimes between the mid-1980s and mid-1990s. The patterns of adolescents constituting a separate social group through the 1990s was documented by a recent book, *A Tribe Apart*, based on an in-depth study of eight suburban Virginia adolescents, which confirmed that they spent much of their time unsupervised and isolated from the adult world. The power of the adolescent "tribe," Hersch writes, is more than simply a group of peers. Instead:

> It becomes in isolation a society with its own values, ethics, rules, worldview, rites of passage, worries, joys, and momentum. It becomes teacher, adviser, entertainer, challenger, nurturer, inspirer, and sometimes destroyer.[19]

Within this complex society, as the Littleton, Colorado, school massacre (see page 100) illustrated, many adolescents today attach themselves to varied cliques—"jocks," "nerds," "Goths," "preps," or even "trenchcoat Mafias." Reflecting a hierarchy of social acceptance or rejection, such cliques often are based on socioeconomic status and racial or ethnic identification. For many unpopular or "different" students, social isolation and alienation become inevitable. Clearly, recreation leaders in public and nonprofit leisure-service agencies should be sensitive to such groupings and should seek to overcome their negative effects.

Studies of Adolescent Values and Behaviors

A number of systematic studies have sought to identify and analyze adolescent views of leisure and their own free-time involvements. Douglas Kleiber, Reed Larson, and Mihaly Csikszentmihalyi, for example, studied several thousand accounts of adolescents' reporting on various dimensions of leisure during their daily lives. Based on these reports, they grouped the activities of teens into three major categories: (1) *productive*, such as classwork, studying, jobs, or other productive tasks; (2) *maintenance*, including eating, personal care, transportation, chores and errands, and rest and napping; and (3) *leisure*, including socializing, sports and games, television watching, nonschool reading, arts and hobbies, and other freetime pursuits.

Within the third category of involvement, the researchers identified two basic kinds of leisure. The first, which they called "relaxed leisure," involved such free-time activities as socializing, watching television, reading, and listening to music—pursuits that provided pleasure without making high personal demands of participants. The second form of leisure they called "transitional." It includes activities that require a degree of effort and demand, such as sports and games, crafts, and hobbies. These more structured pastimes, they concluded, serve adolescents as preparation for more serious adult roles. At a stage in their development when young people are often bored and disinterested in responsibilities placed on them by adults,

> these transitional activities would appear to provide a bridge. They offer the experience of freedom and intrinsic motivation within highly structured systems of participation, systems that require discipline and engage an adolescent in a world of symbols and knowledge outside the self [and lay] a groundwork for experiencing enjoyment in more obligatory adult activities.[20]

Later research examined the issues of boredom, time pressures and stress, and imposed social control of free-time activities, as they affect adolescent leisure behavior. For example, Shaw, Caldwell, and Kleiber studied teenage students in a working class town in Ontario, Canada, and found that about half of the students experienced time pressures and being "rushed" to do their work. About 30 percent of subjects reported problems of boredom, and over half reported the lack of choice and control by others in sports or social activities.[21]

Sanford Dornbusch, Director of the Stanford University Center for the Study Families, Children and Youth, points out that, while peer influence among adolescents is powerful, there is no single, dominant peer culture or value system in America: "Instead . . . researchers have found multiple peer cultures that support the diversity of adolescent values and behavior. . . . Indeed, the variation in values among adolescents was as great as the variation between adults and youths."[22]

Teenagers as Commercial "Targets"

Adolescents in the mid-1990s represented a huge market for business, spending an estimated $83 billion a year on their personal needs. They have been and are a prime target for the marketing of travel opportunities, fast foods, rock music concerts, and other forms of entertainment, cars, clothes, and a host of other leisure-oriented products and services. They congregate by the thousands at spring breaks at Florida or Texas beachside resorts, and flock through shopping malls, attending video-game arcades and movie theaters or simply "cruising."

On the other hand, particularly in disadvantaged urban neighborhoods, lacking financial resources or the opportunity for organized, constructive recreation, many teenagers simply "hang out," committing vandalism and break-ins, randomly assaulting strangers driving or walking through their neighborhoods, or engaging in other casual forms of delinquency. When asked why and how such incidents occur, teenagers often complain that they have "nothing to do"—that life is boring, and that they just want to "chill out" with their friends. James Calloway points out that a significant number of today's youth are overstimulated by the mass media, spiritually empty, and emotionally isolated from needed support systems: "[They] show less emotion, devalue life and are lonely, fearful and anxious. They seek life-threatening adventures and events which excite and stir their human spirit. Lesser challenges will not do."[23]

For all adolescents, the issue of passive versus active uses of leisure represents a serious problem in terms of fitness and other health-related needs. According to American Medical Association studies, children and teenagers who watch four hours or more of television a day are significantly fatter than those who watch for two hours or less. It has been confirmed that childhood obesity sets the stage for overweight adulthood, with accompanying risk for high blood pressure, diabetes, and heart disease. Yet, as in elementary schools, high school physical education is being widely cut back. Illinois is the only state with required daily physical education for all four high school years, and in many programs, real aerobic exercise is almost totally lacking.

Conflicting Reports of Adolescent Life

Despite the negative views of teenage behavior and social problems cited earlier, there is evidence that the picture is not totally gloomy. Writing in *U.S. News and World Report,* David Whitman points out that on many measures today's adolescents are better off than their parents were a quarter century ago:

> They are less likely to smoke, drink, or do drugs, less likely to die at an early age, . . . and more likely to finish high school and college. And they do every bit as well as their parents' generation, if not somewhat better, on aptitude and achievement tests.[24]

A 1998 poll conducted by *The New York Times* and CBS News concluded that today's teenagers are worldly, shaped by a culture that has dropped many of its inhibitions and sophisticated in ways that contrast sharply with earlier generations. Goodstein and Connolly write:

They carry beepers, prefer permanent tattoos to body piercing, and are just about as likely to take lessons in shooting guns as they are to play a musical instrument. Four in ten personally know someone who is gay or lesbian, and six in ten say distributing condoms in school is a good idea.[25]

Yet, the same poll reports that late-1990s adolescents trust their government, admire their parents, and believe in God; strong majorities say they never drink alcohol and never smoke cigarettes or marijuana. Despite the reality that today's older teens are more concerned about making money and less about having a meaningful philosophy of life than their peers were in 1970s, increasing numbers of high school students are now doing community-service volunteerism work in their free time. At the same time, when asked what problems confront youth today, they cite threats that their earlier counterparts did not face: hard drugs, AIDS, school violence—shown in horrific examples of youth killing fellow students and teachers in the late 1990s—and peer pressure. On the positive side, Gallup polls show that nine out of ten teenagers report that they are close to their parents, are personally happy, and are optimistic about their future.

Increasingly, varied youth-serving organizations are seeking to acculturate youth to desirable social values, expose them to varied environments and positive growth experiences, and use challenging pursuits as a way of diverting their aggressive or hostile drives. In poorer settings, recreation often serves as a "threshold" activity that helps to bring neighborhood youth through the doors of the agency, where they may then be involved in academic tutoring and counseling, drug and alcohol prevention and treatment programs, job training and career counseling services, and other types of assistance designed to overcome the effects of the constricting ghetto environment.

Leisure During the Adult Years

The adult age bracket is a broad one, ranging from the late teens or early twenties to the so-called mid-life years, which are generally considered to extend to the sixties. The eighteen-year "baby boom" of 1946–1964, when birth rates peaked at 25.3 births per 1000 population, swelled the numbers of adults in the United States who are now in the age bracket from their late thirties to early fifties. In contrast, during the eleven-year period after 1964, the rate fell to a low of 14.6 births per 1000 of so-called "Generation X-ers." In 1997, there were 77 million American "baby boomers," compared to only 44 million "Xers," in their twenties and thirties.

For the latter group, economic prospects have been sharply less favorable than for their older brothers and sisters. William Finnegan points out that the economic prospects for most young people have been deteriorating for a generation:

Entry-level wages for male high school graduates, for instance, fell 28 percent from 1973 to 1997, in real dollar terms . . . Home ownership among younger families has also fallen sharply. . . . The great American middle class is by any measure, shrinking, and more and more young people are being shunted into the ranks of the working poor.[26]

Developmental Tasks

Authorities identify a number of the key developmental tasks or challenges that confront those entering the period of early adulthood. These tasks, Osgood and Howe suggest, are:

> related to the psychological need to establish intimacy. The urge to merge generally culminates in marriage, settling down, buying a home, and starting a family . . . as primary developmental tasks of young adulthood. Much of the leisure in this late phase of young adulthood is centered around the marriage, carving out the roles of the wife and husband.[27]

Beyond such needs, young adults also face the task of developing economic independence, assuming civic and community roles, and in the broadest sense continuing to develop as fully rounded persons. For young men and women who attend college, much leisure involvement centers around campus pursuits, such as dormitory parties and friendships, participating in intramural sports or attending sports events, going to dances, listening to music, membership in sororities and fraternities, and other social, political, and literary activities.

As Chapter 4 points out, many colleges and universities are taking a more proactive role today in supervising the lives of their students than was the case in the years following the counterculture revolution. Campus authorities are striving to reduce student drinking and are offering liquor-free social programs. Sexual harassment and fraternity activities are issues of concern, and fuller orientation programs are offered to help young students make the transition to university life. Counseling services and varied cultural and public service activities are part of this newer thrust toward a more structured campus environment. Ethan Bronner writes:

> Three decades after American college students defiantly threw off the vestiges of curfews, dress codes, and dormitory house mothers, a revolution is under way in undergraduate life . . . colleges are offering and students are often demanding greater supervision of their lives.[28]

For young adults who do not attend college, commercially sponsored agencies such as health spas or racquetball clubs, singles bars or clubs, rock concerts, and other forms of entertainment provide sociality. In addition, churches and synagogues, employee recreation programs, and public recreation and park departments also provide opportunities for sports and social recreation. Many of the pursuits that young people engage in at this stage of life represent a continuation of interests first developed during childhood and adolescence. For example, McGuire, Dottavio, and O'Leary found that 70 percent of all outdoor recreation activities enjoyed by older adults were first engaged in before the age of 21.[29] Similarly, Scott and Willits confirmed strong continuity from adolescence through the adult years in five major types of leisure activities, including socializing and intellectual pursuits, involvement in formal organizations, and artistic or creative pursuits.[30]

For many young adults who postpone marriage and family commitments, this period of life represents the opportunity for advanced education and career development, and a time for relatively free spending and enjoyment of leisure. Economist Fabian Linden comments, "This longer period of financially independent young adulthood amounts to an economic, social, and psychological revolution." Many young singles are able to indulge in "the 'me-me-me purchasing cycle' of chic clothes, cars, cruises, and other luxuries. But the free-spending ways halt after they marry, have children, and begin worrying about paying for cribs, condos, and colleges."

For young adults who marry and raise families, leisure begins to center around children, in terms of membership in parent-teacher associations or serving as volunteer leaders or coaches in youth groups and leagues. Often recreation is carried on close to home, in backyard games and picnics; travel, when it occurs, is aimed at national or state parks or family-oriented theme parks, rather than popular singles' destinations or cruises.

Contrary to the assumption that active recreation automatically drops off through the decades of adulthood, Rodney Warnick cites research findings showing that both the 25-to-34-year-old and the 35-to-44-year-old segments of the adult population have higher participation rates in a number of outdoor recreation activities than the younger cohorts of adults aged 18 to 24.

> [P]articipation rates were higher for 25- to 34-year-olds than for 18- to 24-year-olds in such activities as bicycling, swimming, fresh water fishing, salt water fishing, hiking, cross-country skiing, health club membership. . . . This trend carried over to the . . . middle-aged adult segment in activities such as salt water fishing, health club membership, and travel. . . . These changes appear to have occurred in the 1980s. In fact, for probably the first time, evidence now exists that participation rates are higher among older adults, particularly the middle-aged adults, than young adults in a wide variety of activities . . .[31]

Midlife Years

Osgood and Howe describe this period as the "establishment" phase of the life cycle, when men and women settle down, move ahead in a work career, assume increasing responsibility in civic organizations, and become "culture bearers" to the next generation. Now that life is "half over," many men and women reexamine their career goals and family status from a new time perspective, and it is not uncommon to make major life changes at this point.

For Americans, this population consists heavily of the "baby boomers" born in the two decades after World War II. They differ from those who preceded them in that a lower percentage are married and a higher percentage are divorced or have never married. They are better educated and have fewer children, but are unlikely to be able to "catch up" to their parents in terms of real income or net worth. But, as they approach the preretirement years, research indicates that most mid-life Americans are satisfied with their life situation. According to the American Board of Family Practice, an organization of 37,000 family physicians, the majority of Americans view the ages of 46 through 65 very positively, as a time for becoming closer to their spouses, children, and friends: "for most men, middle age is a period of settling and reconciling personal and occupational goals. For most women it is a period of greater independence and freedom."

There was little support for the notion that midlife was a time of crisis or personal anguish, or for the widespread belief that men discard their wives and begin driving fancy sports cars when they enter middle age. For many middle-aged men and women, however, this period does represent a time when they seek to recapture their youth, in terms of nostalgia—attending concerts by 70-year-old singers who were pop idols when they were young, or indulging the fantasy of playing baseball with other men in their forties and fifties, at so-called Dream Weeks at training camps with ex-"pro" athletes.

In general, the baby boomers' role as the psychological center of gravity, to use David Wolfe's term, has not been to influence the nation with a return to the ideals and values of their youth. Instead, boomers have in great numbers become more conservative and even spiritual, in terms of seeking meaning in their lives. Wolfe cites the cover story of a recent issue of *Sales and Marketing Management,* which begins:

> There's strange talk being spoken in the hallways of Corporate America today. It's about inner peace and a desire to gain more from business than a hefty paycheck. . . . Spirituality, folks, is taking hold of the workplace.[32]

Wolfe concludes that the world's preeminent youth culture is steadily becoming middle-aged. And inevitably, it is also becoming an elderly culture.

Leisure and the Elderly

In the late 1980s, the American Association of Retired Persons reported that those aged 65 or older represented 12 percent of the nation's population—a figure that will grow to 20 percent in the century ahead. Jacqueline Morrison points out that medical advances are steadily increasing life expectancy. She writes:

> The number of people over 65 has grown by more than ten times (from 3.1 million to 32.8 million) since 1900. The result is a 75–84 age group that is now fourteen times larger and a 85 and above age group that is seventeen times larger.[33]

Based on this trend, demographers estimate that life expectancy in the United States will continue to climb from the present 75.9 years, with the number of those 85 or older doubling by 2030; by the year 2050, 40 percent of the population will be over age 50. Strikingly, those who reach the age of 100—centenarians—are growing rapidly in number. Proportionately, they are the country's fastest growing age group, numbering over 30,000 today.

Our view about growing old are sharply contradictory. On the one hand, many individuals look forward eagerly to retirement and being able to lead independent, relaxed lives. On the other hand, the elderly are often denigrated in society; to be old has frequently meant to be isolated, no longer a contributing member of the community, ill or disabled, and economically vulnerable.

In the mid-1990s, the *New York Times* noted several current retirement trends:

Las Vegas has now surpassed Florida as the best place to retire, according to a recently published directory, "Retirement Living Communities."

A quarter of newly retired people hold seasonal or part-time jobs.

There are nearly 700 retirement communities in the United States; in the next decades, that number is expected to double.

Americans can now expect to spend a fourth of their lives retired.

Most retirement communities have waiting lists, ranging from six months to ten years.[34]

Aspects of Aging

The reality is that aging is a complex phenomenon that varies greatly from person to person. Gerontologists agree that there are three or more stages of aging, ranging from those who are healthy, mobile, independent, and optimistic, to those who have serious problems of health and/or locomotion and are unable to live independently. Aging is generally regarded as a physiological development, with a gradual slowing of biological functions and breakdown of body systems, along with progressive disabilities of the heart and nervous system and decline of vision and hearing. However, aging clearly has social and psychological components as well, and the degree to which individuals are able to remain active and involved with friends, family, and enjoyable lifestyle pursuits may greatly influence the rate of physical aging. Robert Butler, former head of the National Institute on Aging, points out that apart from such factors as brain disease, cancer, or other kinds of serious illness over which one may have limited control, the difference in one's functional aging often comes down to personal and psychological factors. He writes:

People who are actively involved in life will seem younger than people who are emotionally and physically sedentary. People who are productive stay healthy, and if you remain healthy you're more apt to be productive. . . . Whether it's paid or unpaid work there have to be opportunities to keep people active. . . .[35]

Over the past few decades, many Americans have come to think of aging in an entirely new, upbeat way. In 1997, *Time Magazine* summed it up by saying that older Americans were far from "over the hill. They are taking this hill by storm and they're changing everything from the family to the marketplace." John Greenwald writes that the widening gap between the chronological age of Americans and their psychological, physiological, and cultural age is upending traditional notions of work and family.[36]

The gift of longer life means more time, Greenwald writes, to travel, learn, try out new careers, and give something back to the community. And while it also challenges individuals to prepare themselves physically, emotionally, and financially for an expanded period of years, it has also been accompanied by a sharp reduction in the number of chronically disabled older Americans.

It would be a mistake to assume that all elderly Americans are active, happy, and emotionally secure. Many continue to be isolated, financially dependent, or physically disabled. Studies indicate that three million older Americans today have a serious drinking problem. Robert Stock writes that, as people age, the emotional upheavals that can lead to alcohol dependence often come thick and fast:

> . . . retirement, ill health, loss of loved ones, isolation. The constraints that curb younger drinkers—the fear of losing a job, rejection by a spouse, an arrest for drunk driving—may no longer apply. Many older people are introduced to daily drinking in retirement communities where the social life is built around the happy hour.[37]

Leisure's Value

For many elderly persons, leisure provides the opportunity to enrich their lives and diversify their interests. Their new free-time pursuits may take many forms. Hundreds of colleges and universities offer specially designed summer programs for older persons through the Elderhostel movement, which serves thousands of mature students in short-term courses throughout the United States and abroad. Campus housing and faculty resources provide inexpensive packaged programs covering a wide range of educational and cultural subjects. In some cases, entirely independent programs for elderly persons have been established, and in others they are served side by side with younger students.

Many other older persons have explored the possibilities of computer hobbies and using the Internet to gather information, share interests, and make new friends. Some senior centers have begun computer clubs for their members to learn computer skills and use them both for practical purposes and as a form of recreation. Grodsky and Gilbert describe the role of SeniorNet, a national nonprofit educational organization that has established a national network of 128 learning centers covering thirty-five states to assist the elderly in getting on the Information Superhighway.[38]

Another major form of productive retirement activity for elderly persons consists of volunteering. Hundreds of thousands of individuals in their senior years provide regular assistance in hospitals, community centers, organizations like the Salvation Army, the American Red Cross, Foster Grandparents, and the Service Corps of Retired Executives

In addition to continuing education, travel, and volunteerism, many elderly persons enjoy traditional recreational, social, and sports participation in senior centers, retirement communities, or special leagues. For example, a large retirement community, Sun City, Arizona, operates a network of recreation centers that house sports, arts and crafts, hobbies, and other pursuits, with over 140 chartered clubs in varied leisure activities. In California, Laguna Hills offers its residents over forty-five different pastimes, ranging from aerobics, art, billiards, bocce, bowling, calligraphy, and cards, to stamp collecting, swimming, table tennis, tennis, a therapy pool, weaving, and woodworking.

A major thrust in leisure programming for elderly persons today involves active sports leagues and tournaments. Typically, many cities sponsor softball leagues for those 60 or older. In some cases, they may schedule tennis tournaments in which the combined ages of players on a doubles team must be at least 140 or 150 years. A unique example of such sports programming is the North Carolina Senior Games program (NCSG, Inc.). Formed in 1981, NCSG is a year-round health promotion program for adults 55 and older. In a typical year in the mid-1980s, it sponsored over 200 sanctioned games, with several thousand participants taking part in over forty different events, including basketball shooting, cycling, bowling, croquet, track and field, golf, horseshoes, softball throw, spin casting, swimming, and tennis. The number of competitors in events sponsored by the National Senior Games Association, an affiliate of the U.S. Olympic Committee, rose from 1869 in 1987 to 6828 in 1997 for those ages 60 to 79, and from 102 to 559 for those over 80.

Health Values

Elderly persons benefit from active recreation in several ways. Examining the psychological benefits of participation in leisure pursuits, Tinsley, Teaff, and Colbs identified eight important areas of value for the elderly. These were: (1) *self-expression*, the creative use of one's talents; (2) *companionship* with others; (3) a sense of *power*, involving one's ability to deal effectively with social situations; (4) *security*, based on activities being carried out in safe and familiar settings; (5) *compensation*, satisfying the need for new or unusual experiences that may make up for other losses or gaps in the individual's life; (6) *service* to others; (7) intellectual and cultural *stimulation*; and (8) *solitude*, involving the persons' ability to spend time alone comfortably.[39]

A final important value of active recreation for elderly persons has to do with maintaining health and fitness. Numerous studies have shown that even moderate physical exercise can make a significant contribution to the health of aged persons. One cardiologist suggests that physical activity for older persons should include four basic elements: (1) relaxation; (2) endurance exercises to condition the heart, lungs, and circulation; (3) muscle-strengthening exercises; and (4) stretching exercises to improve joint mobility and reduce the aches and pains that may accompany aging. Physiologist William Evans of the Tufts University Center on Aging states: "There is no group in our population that can benefit more from exercise than senior citizens. For a young person, exercise can increase physical function by perhaps 10 percent. But in an old person you can increase it by 50 percent."

Leisure and the Family

One of the important values of leisure is the opportunity it provides for contributing to family cohesion and for helping parents and children share positive experiences together.

This is particularly important in an era in which the family structure has been weakened, and there is convincing evidence that family life has been threatened by divorce and separation, the high rate of children born out of wedlock, the incidence of sexual abuse of children, and of violence, substance abuse, and other pathologies in the family setting. Such problems are *not* unique to the United States, according to recent reports by sociologists and demographers. In both industrialized and undeveloped nations, the increasing involvement of women in outside employment, accompanied by other changes in family structure and relationships, has been linked to the growth of "troubled" households.[40]

Acock and Demo point out that scholars and the popular media often blame nontraditional families for increasing teenage sexual activity, pregnancy, delinquency, alcohol, and drug use.

> They blame these problems on parents (and typically the mothers) for spending little time with their children and for not instilling the "proper" family values in their children. They point to lax parental control, high levels of family conflict, and "broken homes" [along with] father-absent families.[41]

Typically, critics point back to the television-transmitted image of loving mothers and fathers and their mischievious but obedient children during the 1950s and 1960s. However, such sentimental images of the "traditional" family are simplistic and misleading. Westheimer and Yagoda point out that the "Leave It to Beaver"-type family with two married-for-life parents, the father working and the mother a full-time homemaker, in a comfortable middle-class home was predominant only for a short time, and that even then it represented an unrealistic view of American life.[42] Beyond this, Stephanie Coontz writes that the "golden age" vision of the traditional family is an inaccurate mix of structures, values, and behaviors that never existed in the same time and place:

> The notion that traditional families fostered intense intimacy between husbands and wives while creating mothers who were totally available to their children [combines false images drawn from several different periods]. . . . A related myth is that modern Americans have lost touch with extended-kinship networks or have let parent-child bonds lapse. In fact, more Americans than ever before have grandparents alive, and there is good evidence that ties between grandparents and grandchildren have become stronger over the past fifty years.[43]

Realistically, there *have* been major changes in family structures over the past three decades. Peter Kilborn writes that from 1970 to 1990, the number of married couples with children under 18 shrank from 40 percent of all households to 25 percent. In 1995, he continues:

> Divorce rates have soared, and the number of single-person households climbed from 17 percent of all households to 25 percent, where it, too, has remained. The divorce rate has stabilized since 1990. . . . Another important factor is that couples are also having children later and the number of single-parent families rose by 12 percent from 1990 to 1995.[44]

As indicated, one factor in such changes has been the changing role of women in the economic world, with employed women generally working substantially longer hours than men because of their other important family and household responsibilities.

The pressures of having both parents working, the lack of adequate day-care programs, and increasing numbers of latchkey children—all have contributed to the problems facing families in contemporary American society. Studies have shown that children who are alone at home for eleven or more hours a week after school are twice as likely to abuse alcohol, tobacco, or marijuana as are supervised youngsters. In the late 1980s, two-thirds of all school-age children had working mothers. Many infants now go into group care when they are only a few weeks old. And, although the number of children spending their time in day-care or preschool programs has doubled in recent years, the number of organized day-care facilities is still insufficient to meet the demand.

Within this context, how can leisure and recreation help in the solution of the problems that many American families face today? There has long been a widely shared belief that "the family that prays together stays together," today often expressed as "the family that plays together stays together." Dennis Orthner and Jay Mancini point out that the research literature consistently shows that husbands and wives who share leisure time together in joint activities tend to be much more satisfied with their marriages than those who do not. They write:

> The value that shared leisure experience can have for families has been widely acknowledged. One study found that men and women ranked companionship highest on a list of nine goals of marriage. In another study, a national sample ranked such things as liking the same kinds of activities as more important to marital success than having children or financial security.
>
> By the 1980s, desire for companionship reached almost universal proportions. When asked about their primary leisure objectives, a national sample of adults listed "spending time with your family" and "companionship" as their two most common objectives.[45]

Other surveys during the 1980s shows that 82 percent of parents said that children gave them their greatest satisfaction in life, and that participation in sports and recreation within the family unit ranked second only to television-watching as a common family activity. Laura Szwak cites research findings that show that one of the common characteristics of healthy, functioning families is "doing things together.' According to the survey, joint leisure time was an important element in promoting high quality marital and family life."[46]

In 1991, the Gallup Poll conducted a study that asked a national sample of employed adults whether, if they were offered a job that had significantly higher pay and prestige but that would require considerable time away from their families, they would take it. Only 8 percent said they would take the job without reservations; 59 percent said they would turn it down; 32 percent said that they would accept it with some reservations. Clearly, many Americans recognize that shared leisure time represents an important factor in assuring happy family life.

In 1997, Larson, Gillman, and Richards summarized research showing that different family members—father, mother, adolescents, and younger children—had markedly different expectations and outcomes from shared leisure experiences. They concluded that it was essential that recreation planning be sensitive to the special needs of each group to maximize the benefits of family leisure.[47]

Provision of Family Leisure Programs

Many different types of agencies offer recreation for family groups, including public recreation and park departments, Ys and other nonprofit organizations, employee service and armed forces recreation units, and religious bodies. Various denominations and individual churches in particular emphasize recreational family programming, both as an alternative to less desirable play and to strengthen family ties and encourage involvement in other church functions.

As an example, the Church of Jesus Christ of Latter-Day Saints (the Mormon Church) has been particularly active in supporting family recreation. Clark Thorstenson points out that since its inception, the Church has sponsored wholesome family leisure pursuits to promote family cohesiveness and moral values. He writes:

> As a result, family-centered sports, dance, song, theater, and reunions are regularly conducted in thousands of centers throughout the world as a means of providing spiritual, social and physical outlets for its members. . . . Church organizations sponsor family oriented sports competitions such as basketball, volleyball, soccer, tennis, golf, and softball during weekends and on Saturdays.[48]

In addition, Mormons often purchase mountain land or other suitable property for outdoor recreation for church members. Throughout the year, Monday evenings are set aside for family nights, for families to share varied hobbies and leisure pursuits. The church publishes a 346-page *Family Resource Manual*, including guidelines and examples for taking part in games, sports, and aquatics, cultural and social pursuits, and other forms of family enrichment activities.

Commercial Recreation

In addition to such groups, many commercial recreation businesses have packaged their attractions to appeal more directly to family units. To illustrate, in the mid-1980s, the ski industry throughout the country began to recognize that, with growing numbers of families with young children, the number of single adult skiers was declining and the overall rate of participation was suffering. A number of major ski resorts in New England, the Midwest, and the West have now initiated strategies to appeal to family participation. These include free lift tickets on weekdays for children; on-site nurseries and day-care programs for younger children; other sports and entertainment facilities, including video game rooms; family transportation and lodging packages; and other marketing strategies to appeal to family units.

Tourism organizations have also promoted many types of family-centered trips, including varied adventure programs. According to a 1997 survey of the Travel Industry Association of America, 41 percent of those who went on "soft adventure" trips (biking, horseback riding, canoeing) took along children or grandchildren on their most recent trip, while 18 percent of those who went on riskier outings were accompanied by younger family members.

Varied gambling businesses, including major casinos in Las Vegas and Atlantic City and riverboat casinos on midwestern rivers, have also sought to picture themselves as centers of family entertainment and have advertised a "wholesome" atmosphere and diversified family recreation activities in an effort to draw a wider set of players—with the added purpose of familiarizing children with the casino atmosphere as a place for play and developing a new generation of gambling customers.

What such ventures raise as an issue, of course, is whether the concept of family recreation should legitimately embrace any sort of activity or whether it should be restricted to socially and morally desirable activities that promote healthy family interactions and outcomes. In 1993, two Rockford, Illinois, parents hired a stripper for their son's birthday party. It was an exciting occasion:

> The dancer stripped down to a halter and G-string . . . and the son licked whipped cream off her breasts as the mother looked on. Her 6-year-old daughter and 3-year-old son also were at the party.[49]

Shortly, both parents were brought to court; they received jail time, probation, and a substantial fine. Later, the couple split up and the state took custody of the "birthday boy."

Socioeconomic Trends Affecting Leisure Involvement

As earlier chapters have shown, throughout history social class and wealth have always affected the kinds of pursuits that people engaged in—both in terms of their leisure tastes and preferences and their economic capability for engaging in play. Sociological studies in the United States during the 1920s and 1930s emphasized the impact of social-class identification on youth recreation and membership in organized groups, for example.

Today, the issue of socioeconomic class has become an increasingly important factor affecting leisure choices because of the degree to which most recreational opportunities have had price tags attached to them in recent years.

Social Class Awareness

Despite the historic vision of the United States as a democratic, classless society, there have always been widely understood lines of social class identification, based on wealth, family background, education, racial or ethnic background, and lifestyle factors. That this tradition persists is illustrated in a recent *New York Times* article depicting life in Dixon, Illinois, a city 100 miles west of Chicago. In Dixon, with sprawling new homes with three-car garages springing up in response to the booming economy, families spend lavishly on leisure toys, vacations, and clothes. Dirk Johnson writes:

> Unlike young people a generation ago, those today must typically pay fees to play for the school sports teams or band. It costs $45 to play in the youth summer soccer leagues. It takes money to go skating on weekends at the White Pines roller rink, to play laser tag or rock-climb at the Plum Hollow Recreation Center, to mount a steed at the Horseback Riding Club . . . to go shopping for clothes at Cherryvale Mall.[50]

The *Times* tells how Wendy Williams, a pretty 13-year-old girl in the Dixon Middle School, the child of two working parents—father a welder and mother a part-time cook—has to struggle to maintain her self-esteem. Living in a trailer park, she knows that to be without money is to be left out in so many ways. As she sat in the school bus wearing a cheap belt and rummage-sale slacks, other students paraded past her, wearing designer clothes. One boy stopped and yanked his thumb, demanding her seat. "Move it, trailer girl," he sneered.

Middle-Class Decline

Numerous studies have shown that the majority of Americans tended to define themselves as middle-class, and the attainment of the American dream was largely equated with achieving middle-class status. While this socioeconomic class has been defined both as the statistical middle group in the nation's income scale and as a sociological entity in terms of the way its members are perceived, the reality is that it has been declining over the past two decades as a proportion of the overall population.

Structural unemployment stemming from recessions during the 1980s and in the early 1990s led to many white-collar middle-income workers losing jobs, and downsizing in the mid- and late-1990s displaced many more. During this period, wages tended to rise steadily at the upper and lower ends of the wage scale and more slowly in the middle. Many workers now have lower real earnings—adjusted for inflation—than they did during the 1970s. Tax cuts heavily favored the wealthy, resulting in David Broder's conclusion that the United States has become "the most economically stratified of industrial nations."

Former Labor Secretary Robert Reich describes the long-term trend affecting America's population. Increasingly, he writes, it is being split into three groups:

> An underclass largely trapped in center cities, increasingly isolated from the core economy; an overclass of those who are positioned to profitably ride the waves of change; and in between, the largest group, an anxious class, most of whom hold jobs but who are justifiably uneasy about their own standing and fearful for their children's futures.[51]

Spending by the Rich

The late 1990s showed vivid examples of what Veblen called "conspicuous consumption," lavish spending to affirm one's superior status.

Increasingly, new sports stadiums and arenas are being built with extended sections of new, more expensive seats, while past ticket-holders are pushed back from the action. Elaborate sky-boxes offer privacy, comfort, food and drink, and other amenities for guests of corporations or other clients. Wealthy families seek the best for their children in schools and camps, ballet and figure-skating lessons, clothes, toys, and travel. Parents indulge expensive hobbies, from maintaining costly strings of polo ponies to buying and flying surplus Russian LIGs or Czech L-39s.

Housing for the rich reached a new level of extravagance in the 1990s. Across the country, developers built lavish new homes with luxury features, often on small properties but costing several million dollars or more. An extreme example was found in Southampton, New York, where a wealthy industrialist planned a "mega-mansion," a five-structure dream house on 63 acres:

> . . . 29 bedrooms, 39 bathrooms, a 164-seat theater and a restaurant-size kitchen with five refrigerators, six sinks and a 1500 gallon grease trap [and outbuildings that included] a sports pavilion with two tennis courts, two bowling alleys, and a basketball court; a garage sufficient for 200 cars, and a power plant with four huge water tanks, a 2.5 million-B.T.U. furnace, and a maze of underground tunnels.[52]

Not surprisingly, neighbors—themselves extremely wealthy—opposed the project before the town's Zoning Board and the State Supreme Court, as excessive for single-family use.

Leisure for the Poor

In contrast, recreational opportunities for economically disadvantaged families tend to be severely limited. As Chapter 3 points out, parks, playgrounds, and recreation centers in impacted neighborhoods in many large cities are often poorly maintained and staffed, with limited organized program opportunities.

Buildings are often covered with graffiti, vandalized, and not repaired, and many centers are dominated by teenage gangs and drug-dealers. At the same time, statistics of single-parent families and nonmarital pregnancy are high, with welfare dependency, school dropout, and other problems related to poverty. As Foley and Ward point out, the nonprofit youth-serving organizations that often provide recreation and other social services in American communities typically are absent in such settings—or at best only able to provide a minimum of services.

Through the 1990s, there was little effort to address this disparity—with negative implications for such badly needed services as programming for at-risk youth. Obviously, leisure and recreation are only a part of the total picture of preventing juvenile deviancy. Other services—including improved education, family services, job counseling, substance abuse prevention and treatment, outreach workers, and similar measures—are all essential. However, organized recreation programs designed to meet the needs of at-risk youth must be part of the total prevention effort. Recreation serves a number of important purposes—not simply keeping youth "off the streets" or "filling empty time." Instead, it has the following values:

- Carefully designed, appealing recreation programs serve as "threshold" activities that draw young people into services like those offered by Boys and Girls Clubs, the Police Athletic League, or other organizations that work with problem youth.
- Active sports and games or challenging outdoor trips both fulfill the need for risk and adventure that impels many children and youth and serve to build stronger self-concepts, feelings of sportsmanship and team play, discipline, and accomplishment.
- Citizenship activities, trip programs, and vocationally connected experiences as well as community-service tasks all help to broaden the perspective of young people and

help them build connections with the adult world. Supportive contact with adult leaders can help to change negative or self-destructive values and can impel many at-risk youth into more positive life patterns.

The single example of the need to provide more effective programs designed for at-risk youth is part of the broader picture of using organized leisure services to achieve a wide range of community benefits. It relates to each of the points covered in this chapter: (1) overall population growth, (2) the increase in numbers of specific age groups, (3) problems related to family stability, and (4) social priorities stemming from the decline of the middle class and the growing gap in American society between the rich and poor.

Summary

The issue of overpopulation affects all aspects of national life, including education, housing, the environment, and leisure. While the latest statistics indicate that the rate of population growth will continue to decline during the twenty-first century, the swelling numbers of youth and young adults and the elderly will pose challenges for the recreation, park, and leisure-service movement in the years ahead.

This chapter outlines lifestyle patterns and leisure needs of four age groups: children, adolescents, adults, and older persons. It examines the current trends in family life and describes the value of leisure in building family cohesiveness. It concludes by pointing out the sharp gap that now exists between rich and poor socioeconomic classes, with those in the middle class shrinking in numbers, as well as the implications for leisure policy of these changes.

Key Concepts

1. Overpopulation has generally been regarded as a severe threat to world or national well-being, but the rate of population growth in developed countries has slowed markedly in recent years.
2. Based on shifting birthrates, extended life expectancy, and immigration patterns, the two age cohorts that will require fuller attention from leisure planners in the decades ahead will be youth and young adults and the elderly.
3. The lives of children have become increasingly pressured and uncertain over the past fifteen or twenty years, making constructive play a critical necessity for healthy development. While children in wealthy families often are overscheduled, those in poorer neighborhoods tend to lack adequate leisure opportunities.
4. Teenagers today constitute a uniquely separate social class, often with problems related to sex, drugs, alcohol, and other forms of leisure involvements. Both "relaxed" and "transitional" leisure pursuits make important contributions to teenage life, which, despite public concerns to the contrary, is marked by positive values and social behavior for most adolescents.

5. The adult age group falls into a sequence of development from young adulthood to midlife maturity, with leisure playing an important role at each stage, including enriching family life. Evidence shows that participation in active pursuits actually grows during the middle years of this period.

6. With dramatically growing numbers of elderly persons, it is clear that providing fuller and more varied leisure pursuits for senior citizens will be a major priority for all types of public, nonprofit, and other organizations.

7. While the public and the media tend to overromanticize the image of family life in past generations, the reality is that families have become increasingly fragmented and unstable since the 1960s and 1970s, with resulting needs for expanded and enriched programs to serve new kinds of family structures.

8. Based on recent economic trends, the country has become increasingly split, with richer population groups spending lavishly on personal leisure and poorer groups lacking even the most fundamental recreational facilities and programs in many communities.

Endnotes

1. U.S. Population Growth Stayed Flat in 1997. *New York Times* (January 4, 1998): 13.
2. Acock, A.C., and D.H. Demo. 1994. *Family Diversity and Well-Being*. London: Sage Publications, p. 1.
3. Ditton, R. 1997. Fisheries Professionals: Preparing for Demographic Change. *Fisheries* (20/1): 40.
4. Grant, L., cited in Hines, A. 1998. Population Growth: Two Warring Paradigms. *The Futurist* (January/February): 68.
5. Applebome, P. 1996. Enrollments Soar, Leaving Dilapidated School Buildings Bursting at the Frayed Seams. *New York Times* (August 25): 25.
6. Edginton, C.R., D.J. Jordan, D.G. DeGraaf, and S.R. Edginton. 1995. *Leisure and Life Satisfaction: Foundational Perspectives*. Dubuque, IA: Brown and Benchmark, p. 195.
7. Wattenberg, R. 1997. The Population Explosion Is Over. *New York Times Magazine* (Nov. 23).
8. Sheehy, G. 1996. Am I an Adult Yet? *Utne Reader* (May/June): 62.
9. Osgood, N., and C. Howe. 1984. Psychological Aspects of Aging. *Society and Leisure* (7/1): 176.
10. Bettelheim, B. 1987. The Importance of Play. *Atlantic Monthly* (March): 35.
11. Barnett, L. 1990. Developmental Benefits of Play for Children. *Journal of Leisure Research* (22/2): 138–153.
12. Winn, M. 1983. The Loss of Childhood. *New York Times Magazine* (May 8): 18.
13. Barnett, L., and G. Chick. 1986. Chips off the Ol' Block: Parents' Leisure and Their Children's Play. *Journal of Leisure Research* (18/4): 266–267.
14. Davidson, S. 1988. Kids in the Fast Lane. *New York Times* (October 16): 52.
15. McNeal, J. 1998. Tapping the Three Kids' Markets. *American Demographics* (April): 37–41.
16. Kivel, B. 1998. Adolescent Identity Formation and Leisure Contexts. *Journal of Physical Education, Recreation and Dance* (January): 36.
17. Wartella, E., and S. Mazzarella. 1990. A Historical Comparison of Children's Use of Leisure Time. In *For Fun and Profit: The Transformation of Leisure Into Consumption*, ed. R. Butsch. Philadelphia: Temple University Press, p. 174.
18. *Ibid.*, p. 187.
19. Weinberg, S., 1998, review of Hersch, P. *A Tribe Apart: A Journey Into the Heart of American Adolescence*, in *Philadelphia Inquirer* (Apr. 12): Q–1.
20. Kleiber, D., R. Larson, and M. Csikszentmihalyi. 1986. The Experience of Leisure in Childhood. *Journal of Leisure Research* (18/3): 175.

21. Shaw, S., L. Caldwell, and D. Kleiber, 1996. Boredom, Stress, and Social Control in the Daily Activities of Adolescents. *Journal of Leisure Research* (28/4): 274–292.

22. Dornbusch, S. 1989. The Sociology of Adolescence. *Annual Review of Sociology* (15): 249.

23. Calloway, J. 1991. Leisure and Youth: Make the Connection. *Parks and Recreation* (November): 57.

24. Whitman, D. 1997. The Youth "Crisis." *U.S. News and World Report* (May 5): 24.

25. Goodstein, L., and M. Connelly, 1998. Teen-Age Poll Finds a Turn to the Traditional. *New York Times* (April 30): A–20.

26. Finnegan, W. 1998. Prosperous Times Except for the Young. *New York Times* (June 12): A–21.

27. Osgood and Howe, *op. cit.,* p. 184.

28. Bronner, Ed. 1999. In a Revolution of Rules, Campuses Go Full Circle. *New York Times* (March 3): A–1.

29. McGuire, F., F.D. Dottavio, and J. O'Leary. 1987. The Relationship of Early Life Experience to Late Life Leisure Involvement. *Leisure Science* (9): 255.

30. Scott, D., and F. Willits, 1989. Adolescent and Adult Leisure Patterns: A 37-Year Follow-up Study. *Leisure Sciences* (11): 323–335.

31. Warnick, R. 1987. Recreation and Leisure Participation Patterns Among the Adult Middle-Aged Market from 1975 to 1984. *Journal of Physical Education, Recreation and Dance* (October): 49.

32. Wolfe, D. 1998. The Psychological Center of Gravity. *American Demographics* (April): 17.

33. Morrison, J. 1996. Crisis or Comfort? *Parks and Recreation* (March): 89.

34. Retirement. (1995). *New York Times Magazine* (September 17): 24.

35. Butler, R. 1984. Cited in Today's Senior Citizens, Pioneers of New Golden Era. *U.S. News and World Report* (January 2): 52.

36. Greenwald, J. (1997). Age Is No Barrier. *Time Magazine* (September 22): M–9.

37. Stock, R. 1996. Alcohol Urges the Old. *New York Times* (April 18): C–1.

38. Grodsky, T., and Gilbert G. 1998. Seniors Travel the Information Superhighway. *Parks and Recreation* (June): 70.

39. Tinsley, H.E., J.D. Teaff, and S. Colbs, n.d. *The Need Satisfying Properties of Leisure Activities for the Elderly.* Carbondale, IL: Southern Illinois University, pp. 2–3.

40. Lewin, T. 1995. Family Decay Global, Study Says. *New York Times* (May 30): A–5.

41. Acock and Demo, *op. cit.,* p. 3.

42. Westheimer, R., and L. Yagoda, 1998. *The Value of Family: A Blueprint for the 21st Century* (New York: Warner).

43. Coontz, S. 1992. *The Way We Never Were* (New York: Basic Books): 9.

44. Kilborn, P. 1996. Shifts in Families Reach a Plateau, Study Says. *New York Times* (November 27): A–16.

45. Orthner, D., and J. Mancini, 1990. Leisure Impacts on Family Interaction and Cohesion. *Journal of Leisure Research* (22/2): 126.

46. Szwak, L. 1988. Leisure and the Changing American Family. *Journal of Physical Education, Recreation and Dance* (April): 27.

47. Larson, R., S. Gillman, and M. Richards. 1997. Divergent Experiences of Family Leisure: Fathers, Mothers, and Young Adolescents. *Journal of Leisure Research* (29/1): 78–97.

48. Thorstenson, C. 1984. The Mormon Commitment to Family Recreation. *Journal of Physical Education, Recreation and Dance* (October): 50.

49. Party Theme Results in Jail for Parents. *Inquirer Wire Service,* Rockford, IL, August 27, 1993.

50. Johnson, Dirk. 1998. When Money Is Everything, Except Hers. *New York Times* (April 14): A–1.

51. News in Brief: A New Profile of Middle Class. *Employee Services Management* (May/June 1995): 4.

52. Gross, J. 1998. Millionaire's Mega-Mansion Shocks Even the Hamptons. *New York Times* (August 23): 34.

7 People II: Racial and Ethnic Influences on Leisure

As a result of the political and social changes of recent decades, cultural pluralism is now generally recognized as an organizing principle of this society. In contrast to the idea of the melting pot, which promised to erase ethnic and group differences, children now learn that variety is the spice of life. . . .

They learn that . . . the unique feature of the United States is that its common culture has been formed by the interaction of its subsidiary cultures. It is a culture that has been influenced over time by immigrants, American Indians, Africans (slave and free), and by their descendants. American music, art, literature, language, food, clothing, sports, holidays, and customs all show the effects of the commingling of diverse cultures in one nation.[1]

We now turn to an examination of several other demographic elements in American life that have had a powerful influence on leisure values and behavior. The first of these has to do with race and ethnicity, factors that have played a key role in determining the social status and lifestyles of many Americans. This chapter explores earlier American attitudes with respect to race, ethnicity, and national origin, such as the harsh biases against people of color and those from southern and eastern Europe. It reviews the influence of the melting pot approach, which has largely been replaced by a multicultural view of American life and education. Four minority populations—African Americans, Hispanic Americans, Native Americans, and Asian Americans—are examined in terms of the role leisure has played in their lives and the impact they have had on other Americans' use of free time.

As this chapter will show, there has been significant progress in the way racial and ethnic minorities have gained a measure of equality in the United States over the past half-century, in economic, social, educational, and recreational terms. At the same time, there continue to be major tensions and areas of conflict in race relations as we enter the twenty-first century.

Definitions of Race and Ethnicity

The term *race* is frequently misused; we tend to think of people who share common languages or religious beliefs or who have similar national origins as belonging to the same racial group. However, such factors have little to do with race. Instead, a race is a statistical aggregate of people who share a composite of genetically transmissible *physical* traits, such as:

> skin pigmentation, head form, facial features, stature, and the color, distribution, and texture of body hair. Since gross similarities are to be noted among human populations, many attempts have been made to classify the people of the world racially. Estimates of racial types range from three—Caucasoid, Mongoloid, and Negroid—to thirty or more.[2]

In contrast, *ethnicity* involves having a unique social and cultural heritage that is passed on from one generation to another. Ethnic groups are often identified by distinctive patterns of language, family life, religion, recreation, and other customs that differentiate them from other groups. To illustrate the point, Americans of different European origins would normally be regarded as of the same racial stock—Caucasoid. However, they would have different ethnic backgrounds because of their distinctive customs, values, or cultural traits.

In the recent years, the concept of race has become increasingly challenged. Historians have pointed out that until comparatively recently, while people have always commented on physical differences among strangers, they did not categorize them systematically as members of different races. Following European conquests of other continents, the prevailing notion that people were divided into separate groups that had distinctive inborn characteristics as well as exterior differences was widely accepted. The Darwinian view of such groups falling into different places along a scale of social evolution, with more advanced societies showing a higher level of intelligence, morality, and other desirable traits was used to justify slavery, colonialism, and even the massacre of "inferior" or more "primitive" groups.

Today, social scientists, particularly biological anthropologists, tend to believe that race is no longer a valid way of distinguishing among different groups of people. Indeed, the notion of there being three primary races—Caucasoid, Mongoloid, and Negroid—obviously is useless, given the immense number of subgroups under each heading and the degree of admixture within each group.

A recent statement by the American Association of Physical Anthropologists, designed to provide guidelines for UNESCO and other international organizations, states that:

> Pure races in the sense of genetically homogeneous populations do not exist in the human species, nor is there evidence that they have ever existed in the past history of the human family. Hereditary potentials for overall intelligence and cultural development do not appear to differ among modern human populations, and there is no hereditary justification for considering one population superior to another.[3]

Despite such views and the effort to develop new categories for census or related purposes, such as biracial or multiracial, the notion of race is still widely accepted, and many social or economic problems are generally referred to in racial terms today.

Prejudice, Discrimination, and Racism

Hess, Markson, and Stein identify three factors that serve to keep people apart, based on racial or ethnic differences; *prejudice, discrimination,* and *institutional racism.* The first two are primarily individual reactions, while the third involves a widespread structural arrangement or behavioral system:

> *Prejudice* literally means "prejudging" without knowledge. Thus, ethnic, racial, religious, or other social categories are *stereotyped.* A stereotype is an image in which a single set of characteristics, favorable or unfavorable, is attributed to an entire group. Stereotypes are overgeneralized; that is, behavior that may be true of some members is taken as typical of the whole group.[4]

One major purpose of prejudice is to improve one's own position in competition for such benefits as jobs, wealth, or housing, at the expense of another group. This is done through practices of discrimination.

> Whereas prejudice is a set of attitudes, discrimination is the practice of treating people unequally. The two are closely related. That is, prejudice often leads to discrimination. Discrimination, in turn, reinforces prejudice in a vicious circle that limits opportunity and produces a self-fulfilling prophecy.[5]

Finally, institutional racism involves actual practices of discrimination that are based on a larger structure of societal norms and behavior and that are reinforced by both formal and informal agents of social control in areas such as housing, education, job opportunity, and leisure.

It should be stressed that throughout America's history prejudice and discrimination have affected not only people of color, but also those of European origin or of certain religious affiliations. Terms like *dago, kike, honky,* or *wop* illustrate such attitudes; during their early periods of migration, the Irish were often greeted by signs like "No Irish need apply." Reactionary politicians frequently leveled charges of "Papist" against their opponents, meaning that they were tools of the Roman Catholic church. Although Jews were generally well accepted in the American colonies, by the latter part of the nineteenth century, anti-Semitism was widespread in social circles and the business world.

Within a mindset of total Anglo-Saxon superiority, ethnocentrism flourished, and immigrants from central and southern Europe were regarded as second-class citizens. Racial and ethnic prejudices found a home in the Know-Nothing political parties that opposed the immigration arriving on America's shores throughout the nineteenth century and virulently expressed their hatred for Catholics and Jews. It continued for a major part of the twentieth century, as Congress extended a ban on Asian immigrants that had been enacted in the 1880s and established new formulas that sharply favored the admission of northern Europeans from such countries as Sweden, Germany, and the British Isles.

While discrimination affected all minority groups, it was most severe against people of color. Those coming from European countries could normally become Americanized and gain a degree of economic security within a generation or two, but African Americans whose families had been in the country for hundreds of years and who had helped build the nation and fight in its wars continued to be excluded from full citizenship.

Through the early years of the new republic, despite our fighting against the British in the Revolution and the War of 1812, admiration for them tended to be widespread, particularly among the upper classes, who held the conviction that it was important to be white, Protestant, and of Anglo-Saxon heritage. Sociologist Digby Baltzell points out that during the nineteenth century a closed WASP elite came to dominate the United States in terms of banking, major corporations, education and religion, literature, politics, and other elements of culture.

Linked to American admiration for Great Britain was a tacit acceptance of that nation's role as a colonial power, which embodied an ideology of racial superiority—later to be described by Rudyard Kipling as "the white man's burden." This ideology held that whites were racially superior, and that it was their mission to rule the colored peoples of the world.

The "Melting Pot" Ideal

In contrast to this ethnocentric view, a different thrust in American life, literature, and politics was the concept of the "melting pot"—the idea that America's greatness stemmed from the contribution of newcomers of many nationalities who would all become blended into a new and unique citizen, the American. The melting pot idea stemmed from the very first days of the republic, when a naturalized New Yorker of French origin, Jean de Crève-coeur, wrote in 1782 of individuals of many nations being "melted" into a new race of men. Much later, in 1908, a play titled *The Melting Pot* was a smash success on Broadway. Its hero, a Russian-Jewish immigrant who had fled from persecution, exulted in his new country, praising America as "God's crucible," where all the nations of Europe were melting and reforming, despite past "blood hatreds and rivalries."

The melting pot vision opposed the idea of having "hyphenated" Americans who maintained even a vestige of their old loyalties and customs. Only English was to be taught in schools, and settlement houses and other agencies sought to help new immigrants become assimilated as quickly as possible. Under its pressures, the children of immigrants learned to be ashamed of their parents and grandparents, who spoke with accents and were perceived as "foreign."

By the mid-twentieth century, however, it was apparent that many Americans continued to retain ancestral ties and loyalties, often through national folklore societies or religious affiliations. Beyond this, the melting pot idea had never really applied to Americans of other than European origin. Indeed, miscegenation—the intermarriage or interbreeding of whites with those of color, including African Americans, Native Americans, and Orientals—was illegal by statute in a number of states. The great Supreme Court justice, Thurgood Marshall, commented, "The dream of America as the great melting pot has not been realized for the Negro; because of his skin color he never even made it into the pot."

Cultural Pluralism

A new concept came into being: *cultural pluralism*. It held that the United States was really a checkerboard or mosaic of different minority groups, and that it was strengthened, rather than weakened, by its continuing diversity. It sought to promote favorable attitudes toward those of different European origins and to create a hospitable climate toward improving race relations generally throughout the United States. For the first time, serious questions were raised about the place of African Americans and other nonwhites within the American mosaic.

Until the 1940s only a few scholars or political leaders like W.E.B. DuBois and Marcus Garvey had fought to promote black pride and a sense of unity among Americans of African ancestry. However, as the civil rights movement gained momentum in the 1950s and 1960s, a new doctrine of "black is beautiful" began to be preached. There was increased interest in African art, history, religion, and folklore, and when the television series "Roots" captured a huge, multiracial audience in its portrayal of a single African American family's history from slavery days to the present, interest was redoubled.

The Drive Toward Multiculturalism

It was clear that the nation's educational system had presented a rigidly one-sided picture of American life. One writer, Ji-Yeon Mary Yuhill, expressed an Asian American child's view:

> I grew up hearing, seeing, and almost believing that America was white. . . . The white people were everywhere in my 1970s Chicago childhood: founding fathers, presidents, explorers, and industrialists galore. The only black people were slaves. The only Indians were scalpers. . . .
>
> I never heard one word about how Asian immigrants were among the first to turn California's desert into fields of plenty. Or about Chinese immigrant Ah Bing, who bred the cherry now on sale in groceries across the nation. Or . . . that Asian immigrants were the only immigrants denied U.S. citizenship, even though they served honorably in World War I. All the immigrants in my textbook were white. . . .
>
> So when other children called me a slant-eyed Chink and told me to go back where I came from, I was ready to believe that I wasn't really an American because I wasn't white.[6]

Writing in 1990 in *The American Scholar*, Diane Ravitch, Chancellor of the University of Texas, summed up the background of the controversy: that for years, schools and colleges had attempted to neutralize issues related to race, religion, or sexuality largely by ignoring them:

. . . textbooks minimized problems among groups and taught a sanitized version of history. Race, religion, and ethnicity were presented as minor elements in the American saga; slavery was treated as an episode, immigration as a sidebar, and women were largely absent. The textbooks concentrated on presidents, wars, national politics, and issues of state. An occasional "great black" or "great woman" received mention, but the main narrative paid little attention to minority groups and women.[7]

Another writer described the spirit in which "Americanization" was conducted in the schools, as part of the "melting pot" approach:

Far from benignly insisting on immigrants learning English, living by American laws and earning citizenship, the Americanization movement was nativist and coercive. Central to the movement were an insistence that immigrants speak no language other than English, a wholesale assault on immigrants' culture and customs, and the deportation of alien "radicals" who expressed unpopular views.[8]

Beyond such educational approaches, the reality was that many elements in the culture tended to promote racial stereotyping and prejudice. Feagin and Vera point out that racialized ways of feeling and acting—particularly with respect to antiblack prejudice—are widely disseminated by parents, peers, the media, and the educational system:

They are passed along from generation to generation. . . . The broad availability of racial categories, prejudices, and myths helps to explain, to an important extent, how many new immigrants to the United States quickly adopt negative images of African Americans [or hold] antiblack prejudices and stereotypes even before they set foot in this country . . . imbibed from U.S. movies, television programs, and publications, which are now viewed in every country around the globe.[9]

Proponents of new multicultural approaches began to condemn as "Eurocentric" the entire system of education, with its emphasis on the writings of great white, male classicists like Plato, Aristotle, Milton, and Shakespeare, and to urge that major portions of it be replaced by materials drawn from other cultures, races, and religious traditions.

Resistance to Multicultural Pressures

A number of scholars came out in defense of classical education and against the new trend toward "political correctness"—the compulsive avoidance of any statement or even phrase that might offend the new multicultural orthodoxy. Apart from their resistance to what they viewed as the unconscionable rewriting of history, such traditionalists sought to defend what they considered to be the great treasures of world literature and art. They feared that the emphasis on the contributions of each separate racial or ethnic group in American society would mean that the nation would be fragmented and would lose its core of common values.

On the other hand, those who argued for overthrowing the traditional content of American education saw the need to resist the "patriarchy" of the white, male Eurocentric elite that had dominated women and minorities in the past. By the early 1990s, it appeared that a consensus was developing; while the great literature and art that had characterized Western cultural education would *not* be abandoned, there would be a greater effort to present fully and fairly the contributions of all the cultural groups that made up the American mosaic. Beyond this, it would be imperative to give a more honest picture of the nation's history, including the aggressions and cruelties that had been part of American "manifest destiny" and economic expansionism.

Additionally, more and more schools and colleges recognized the need to provide positive learning experiences that promoted fuller intergroup understanding and appreciation. This involved not only the teaching of ancient history or literature, but a realistic emphasis on recent history and current events—recognizing that such instruction ran the risk of being attacked as propaganda or "brainwashing" efforts.

Beyond the issue of black/white relationships, other population trends made this trend inevitable. In April 1990, a *Time* cover story, "Beyond the Melting Pot," made it clear that in the rapidly approaching twenty-first century, racial and ethnic groups in the United States would outnumber whites for the first time. It predicted that the "browning of America" would alter everything in society, from politics and education to industry, values, and culture. Demographers reported that within twenty years, Hispanics would be the nation's largest minority group, and that the substantial influx of Asians meant that there were more Muslims in the United States than Episcopalians. Indeed, religion linked to ethnicity was altering the face of popular culture throughout America, with Hindu temples, Muslim mosques, Buddhist shrines, and other Eastern religious centers springing up around the nation.

With most immigrants coming from Asian and Hispanic countries, with higher birthrates:

> . . . demographers are predicting that the U.S. before long will have to redefine just who its minorities are. In 1950, for example, 75 percent of all the minorities in the U.S. were African Americans. Hispanics now number about 24 million, and by 2010 they will have surpassed blacks in number.[10]

Leisure and Ethnicity: A Challenge

Why is the nation's growing diversity and the drive toward multiculturalism particularly relevant to the study of leisure and the promotion of recreational services in American life?

One answer is that leisure and recreation can represent a positive force toward achieving fuller intergroup understanding and more constructive relationships among Americans of different racial and ethnic origins.

In the past, this view of the role of community recreation was presented uncritically by authors in the field of recreation and leisure. For example, educators like Harold Meyer and Charles Brightbill argued that recreation provided a powerful influence in the "assimilation" of immigrant groups and achieving "social well-being" among those of different races. Programs of Americanization and the constant process of "infiltration and blending" (a clear reference to the melting pot idea) were said to find in recreation a strong ally.

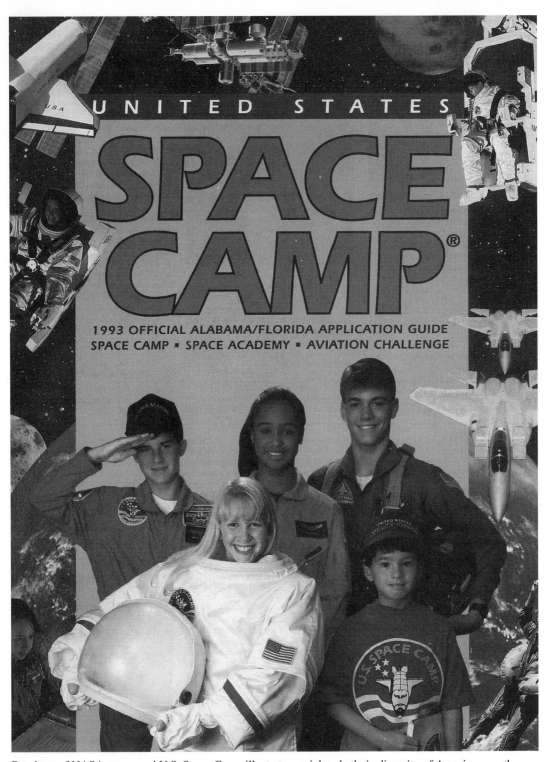

UNITED STATES

SPACE CAMP®

1993 OFFICIAL ALABAMA/FLORIDA APPLICATION GUIDE
SPACE CAMP ■ SPACE ACADEMY ■ AVIATION CHALLENGE

Brochure of NASA-sponsored U.S. Space Camp illustrates racial and ethnic diversity of American youth.

Similarly, a respected researcher in the recreation and park field, George Butler, claimed in a widely used textbook that community recreation was an important tool in promoting democracy and overcoming the gulf between different races and social classes:

> The young man who excels in swimming or basketball is recognized, regardless of his creed or color, by followers of these sports, and the woman who can act or paint scenery is welcomed by the drama group, without reference to her social position. The banker and the man on relief are found singing in the community chorus. . . .[11]

But were Americans ever as colorblind or unconcerned about race or socioeconomic status as Butler's statement suggests? The reality is that race has historically been a powerful force in dictating one's lifestyle patterns and social roles. African Americans were deprived of leisure and forced to work under harsh and cruel circumstances as slaves, and later were barred from many forms of recreational opportunity—by law, community custom, and the inadequate provision of facilities and programs in black neighborhoods.

We must now ask—does institutional racism still exist in recreation and leisure and, if so, in what form? Do members of ethnic and racial minorities differ from the larger white population in their leisure interests and behaviors? How have members of different minority groups contributed to the national culture in such leisure-related fields as sports, the arts, and popular entertainment? To what degree does leisure serve as a catalyst for improving intergroup understanding or for providing channels for social mobility or career development for African Americans and other minority groups?

Leisure Involvements of African Americans

Some critics may object to singling out any racial or ethnic groups for special study or concern. Opponents of affirmative action, for example, sometimes argue that while the United States was guilty of widespread racial discrimination against African Americans in the past, this is no longer the case. Today, they say, the "playing field" is level for all.

Certainly, considerable progress has been made in recent years. In the last decade or two we have seen the first black presidential candidate, first black astronaut, first black mayors of many major cities, and numerous other evidences of positive change in the nation's racial philosophy and practice.

Many athletic clubs or other sports organizations that formerly discriminated blatantly against blacks and other minorities—such as the New York Athletic Club, the Augusta National Golf Course, or the West Side Tennis Club, formerly home of the United States Open Tennis Championship—have either changed their policies or lost influence on the national scene.

However, in many respects, African Americans continue to be second-class citizens. Racial discrimination in housing is endemic, despite efforts to eliminate red-lining and other real estate practices that bar blacks from traditionally white neighborhoods. A 1991 Federal Reserve Board report shows that racial and ethnic minorities, particularly blacks, are rejected for mortgages at a far higher rate than whites, even when they are in the same income categories. While it is true that many African Americans have moved up the economic ladder, roughly a third of blacks are still mired in poverty. Even among those who have reached management positions in American businesses, few have achieved the highest ranks of responsibility. That this situation has continued to the present is documented by two research studies in the late 1990s that show that, having made significant progress until about 1975, African American workers have suffered from substantial wage inequality with comparison with whites during the 1980s and 1990s.[12] According to a 1998 Urban League report, a striking "wealth gap" continues between blacks and whites.

In terms of health, while the longevity of African American men and women has improved in recent years, on average they die about six years younger than whites. Far fewer blacks, Mexican Americans, and Puerto Ricans than whites have private health insurance, and elderly African Americans have greater difficulty in being admitted to nursing homes—despite the fact that they have the same Medicaid reimbursement eligibility as whites.

Brigid Schulte confirms that the health gap is widest for African Americans in practically every type of illness and cause of preventable death but suicide. African Americans suffer and die younger, faster, and at a higher rate than whites:

> . . . the biggest killer [for blacks] is high blood pressure, which leads to greater rates of stroke, heart attack, and kidney failure. . . .
> . . . Although a mother's death during childbirth is rare in this country, black women die in childbirth at four times the rate of white women, according to the federal Centers for Disease Control and Prevention. . . . whites are two-thirds likelier than nonwhites to receive kidney transplants and when hospitalized for pneumonia, whites are likelier than blacks to receive intensive care.[13]

Another major area of institutionalized racism is found in the American criminal justice system. The National Commission on Crime and Justice reported in June 1991 that persons of color and the poor are subject to disadvantages at every stage of the justice system. A study of the National Prison Project of the American Civil Liberties Union reported that minority-group individuals typically lacked adequate legal assistance and were penalized by much harsher sentences than whites, for similar infractions. Linked to such disparities were widespread practices of police brutality toward persons of color.

Striking evidence of such discriminatory policies was shown in the mid-1990s, when federal statistics showed that prosecution for drug offenses was markedly influenced by race:

> Blacks account for more than 90 percent of federal prosecution for crack [cocaine] offenses and whites for less than 4 percent, the U. S. Sentencing Commission found. So that must be because more blacks than whites use and sell crack, right?
> Wrong, says the U.S. Department of Human Services, which found in 1993 that 46 percent of all crack users were white, while 38 percent were black. White dealers are either being ignored or, by prosecutors' decision, being tried in state courts, where penalties are sharply lower.[14]

Even middle- and upper-class African Americans are subject to discriminatory police policies in many communities, where black drivers of luxury vehicles are often picked up "on suspicion," and well-to-do residents are often stopped while walking on streets near their homes, simply because of their color. When the widespread racist practices of the New Jersey state police system were exposed in 1999, many African Americans commented that white troopers had created a new traffic offense—DWB ("Driving While Black").

Racial Barriers to Leisure Participation

Turning more directly to leisure-related issues, much of the racist segregation of the past in community recreation has been eliminated through legislation and court decisions. Through the 1970s and 1980s, however, resistance to the integration of varied types of recreation facilities continued.

In 1972, for example, the Supreme Court upheld the right of private clubs, such as the Loyal Order of Moose, to exclude blacks from membership, despite lawsuits that sought to deny such clubs from having state-issued liquor licenses. On the other hand, in 1973 the Supreme Court ruled that privately owned community pools that customarily served those living close by might not exclude black neighborhood families. In another decision, the court ruled that an Arkansas amusement park had illegally excluded blacks from entering, because it was a "public accommodation" involved in interstate commerce and therefore forbidden by the Civil Rights Act of 1964 to discriminate on racial grounds.

Practices in Nonprofit and Private Settings.   Most voluntary, nonprofit organizations that had tended to be racially segregated before World War II accepted the principle of desegregation, and some, like the Young Women's Christian Association, have dedicated themselves vigorously to the elimination of racism in all their programs and facilities.

In contrast, there continued to be numerous examples of discriminatory policies in commercially operated recreation businesses. For example, in the 1970s and 1980s, it was revealed that in suburban Washington, DC, home of the nation's capital, the exclusive Chevy Chase Country Club permitted black-skinned members of the foreign diplomatic corps to join, but refused to allow black Americans—even the city's mayor—to be admitted. Numerous other prestigious clubs have continued to practice racial exclusion—a policy highlighted in the press in 1990, when the Shoal Creek Country Club in Birmingham, Alabama, scheduled to host the Professional Golf Association championship, was revealed as having a whites-only membership.

There have been other examples of private businesses such as dance studios or swim clubs continuing to exclude blacks until compelled to do so by court decisions. A leading example came in the late 1980s, when a U.S. District Court found that U.S. Health, Inc., in Towson, Maryland, operator of a successful chain of fitness spas, had engaged in widespread practices of discriminating against black applicants who sought to join its clubs. Following court action, U.S. Health accepted a consent order documenting that it had committed the following types of violations of civil rights law: (1) employees at the Holiday clubs had been instructed to discourage black persons from joining and to make it difficult for them to schedule appointments; (2) black persons were often told about the most expensive membership options and were not informed of favorable financing methods; (3) salespersons were reprimanded for selling memberships to black persons and often were denied commissions for such sales; and (4) black members who did join were treated rudely to discourage them from attending the clubs or recommending them to other black persons.

Mardi Gras: A "White" Celebration.   As another example of how long-standing traditions of racial exclusion continued to be challenged within the sphere of leisure activity, the discriminatory practices of the famous New Orleans Mardi Gras celebration came under concerted attack in the late 1980s. Historically, Mardi Gras had been carried on by "krewes" (clubs formed by the city's white male aristocracy) that paraded in the streets every year before Lent, wearing the elaborate costumes of kings, lords, and jesters. Membership in the krewes was controlled by unwritten laws—there might be no blacks, no Jews, no women, no Italians.

Through the years, the white krewes had constituted an inner circle of prestige and power, where many of New Orleans' most influential business leaders met and exchanged contacts, constituting a *de facto* chamber of commerce. However, by the late 1980s the city had become 61 percent black, with an African American–dominated City Council and a black mayor. Unwilling to accept the existence of a publicly assisted institution like Mardi Gras in which all but white Christian males were barred from the elite clubs, the City Council passed an ordinance that banned krewes from discrimination on the basis of race, sex, religion, disability, or sexual orientation.

Comparative Studies of Leisure Involvement

Over the past three decades, a number of studies have examined racial or ethnic influences on leisure behavior. Some have focused primarily on the involvement of a minority group within a particular sphere of activity or on comparing one racial or ethnic population with another. Others have dealt with several different groups, or have combined the issue of race with gender or social-class factors.

As examples of such studies, Steven Philipp has examined race and gender differences in adolescent peer group attitudes;[15] Bialeschki and Walbert did a historical analysis of women of different racial and class backgrounds in the "new" South;[16] and Shinew and Arnold measured the influence of race, gender, and income level on the use of public parks in the Chicago, Illinois, metropolitan area.[17]

Research Focusing on African Americans.   Many other research studies have focused more sharply on the leisure patterns of African Americans, either separately or in contrast to white Americans.

For example, a study of consumer expenditures conducted by the Wharton School of Finance in the 1950s showed significant differences in black and white spending on such items as admissions, radio and television purchases, and other leisure pursuits. The 1962 Outdoor Recreation Resources Review Commission found that African Americans engaged in outdoor recreation activities like camping or hunting far less often than whites.

A study by Short and Strodtbeck in 1965 examined the leisure behavior of several hundred black and white youthful gang members in Chicago. This report showed distinctly different patterns of involvement based on race. Black gang members tended to be more frequently involved in antisocial activities related to physical violence and heterosexual activity. On the other hand, white gang members were more frequently involved in homosexual activity, the use of hard narcotics and alcohol, gambling, auto theft, and other kinds of delinquent acts. A 1967 study by Kraus examined participation in public recreation and park programs in the tristate metropolitan area of New York, New Jersey, and Connecticut. It found marked differences between black and white urban and suburban residents in such activities as sports, cultural programs, and activities for specific age groups.

A number of other comparative studies were carried out in the decades that followed. In 1985, Stamps and Stamps reviewed seventeen different studies that examined African Americans' leisure in terms of urban-suburban, regional, or social-class factors or compared them to white populations.[18] In summarizing their findings, they reported: (1) southern blacks usually participating in inexpensive, close-to-home forms of leisure; (2) the leisure patterns of blacks persisting over time, even after migration from rural to urban areas; (3) a heavy involvement in church activities for all African Americans, regardless of class; and (4) middle-class blacks typically participating in such activities as bridge, travel, and both participation and spectator involvement in sports, comparable to whites. In other studies, Stamps and Stamps found a higher participation rate by blacks than whites in group-oriented pursuits, and a higher rate for whites in outdoor activities such as winter sports, camping, waterskiing, and golf.

Ethnicity/Marginality Perspectives. In such comparative studies, the question arises— are differences between ethnic and racial groups due to innate or inherited cultural traits or to other environmental factors?

Hutchison suggests two possible theoretical explanations for them: *ethnicity* and *marginality*. He writes:

> The ethnicity perspective argues that an identifiable set of black activities results from a distinctive black subculture—a set of cultural patterns which are somehow different from that of the majority of white Americans. This is a cultural explanation for intergroup differences, and involves a complex interplay of social values, social organization, and normative elements passed from one generation to the next through the socialization processes of the family, local schools, and community.[19]

In contrast, the marginality perspective suggests that the different values and leisure behavior of American blacks stem from their generally disadvantaged position in American society—more limited income, inadequate provision of recreational opportunity, and other social factors. Illustrating the marginality perspective, West found that black residents tended to use Detroit city parks more than whites, and that whites from Detroit used parks in the wide tricounty regional area more than blacks. Poorer access to transportation as well as feelings of being unwelcome or unsafe in the regional parks because of interracial prejudice were apparent reasons for African American residents failing to make use of the broader park system.

In some cases, traditional cultural behaviors or practices may be deliberately revived or even created to promote a distinctive culture. For example, in the 1960s and 1970s, many communities established courses, workshops, exhibitions, and events dealing with African art, music, history, religion, and other aspects of black culture. An example of such efforts is the festival of *Kwanzaa*, a seven-day-long non-religious celebration of black culture that has been accepted as a form of holiday celebration by more than five million African Americans. Originated in Los Angeles in 1966, *Kwanzaa* (a Swahili term meaning "first fruits of the harvest") stresses the importance of the black community and family and is based on the *Nguzo Saba*, a framework of seven principles designed for black people to live by through the year. Examples of these principles are: *umoja* (collective work and responsibility), *kujich-agulia* (self-determination), and *imani* (faith). Patterned after various African agricultural festivals, Kwanzaa is intended to help black people rescue and reconstruct their own history and culture.

In the late 1990s, Myron Floyd urged that the ethnicity/marginality approach be expanded to reflect a variety of other influences—social, economic, and regional—on leisure behaviors, as well as the growing differences *within* racial or ethnic populations.[20]

A number of research studies have begun to examine such issues. For example, Michael Woodard focused on the influence of regionality on the leisure behavior of American blacks, summarizing earlier reports showing that social life in the South relied heavily on the home, church, and fraternal halls, while in the North, there was more emphasis on leisure activities in the streets, in schools, and commercial settings like pool or dance halls. Woodard also reported that the most popular leisure activities among urban black Americans were domestic pursuits, such as socializing with friends or family, radio and television, having barbecues, and other low-cost and communal activities.[21] In 1997, Outley, Floyd, and Shinew studied the effects of regionality, socioeconomic status, and race on issues related to park use—including activity preferences and constraints.[22]

Other Social Trends Affecting African Americans.   Over the past two decades, a number of other social trends among African Americans have been reported that have direct impact on their involvement in leisure pursuits.

For example, there is growing evidence that as a greater number of African Americans have entered the managerial or professional ranks in American society, a sharp cleavage has grown between them and the much larger group of working class or economically disadvantaged blacks. Shinew, Floyd, McGuire, and Noe examined this trend in a study of class polarization of African Americans and its impact on leisure.[23]

In some suburban communities, where large numbers of African Americans have purchased homes, relationships between blacks and whites are often positive with a high level of integration in recreation activities. In others, where African Americans are in a distinct minority, they often tend to be socially isolated. In such settings, organizations like Jack and Jill, a long-established social club for children of the black middle and upper class, provide a positive outlet for youth. Marianne Rohrlich writes:

> From its beginnings as a purely social organization [with a reputation for elitist, color-conscious, and bourgeois attitudes] Jack and Jill has become one of the largest African American philanthropic groups. Its foundation has more than $3 million in

assets. Foundation grants are distributed in the black community for children's welfare, women's health care, and school enrichment programs.[24]

A number of other trends affecting African Americans have included the following: (1) clear evidence that far fewer blacks than whites own computers or are involved in their use, with studies showing that many tend to view cyberspace as a predominantly white, male domain; (2) a strong trend toward mutually accepted racial segregation on American college campuses, with growing incidences of tension and occasional conflict; and (3) that many young urban blacks in particular have become a "study in alienation," with cynicism and a prevailing disbelief in the future that leads to drug use and careless exposure to AIDS.

Other Leisure Aspects: Sports, the Arts, and Television.   Three other elements of popular culture have become increasingly important in the lives of black Americans. The first of these, the success of black athletes, has proven to be a major channel for skilled young African Americans, many of whom have achieved wealth and fame in the professional leagues.

History of Blacks in Sport.   African Americans suffered harsh discrimination in many areas of opportunity during the past two centuries—including sport. While many blacks were successful athletes during the early and middle nineteenth century, they were frozen out of professional horse racing, which they had dominated, by the early 1900s, by edict of the Jockey Club.

When the National Association of Base Ball Players was formed in 1858, there were many black ball players in organized baseball. In 1867, the same year the Ku Klux Klan was established, the members of the National Association—all northerners at this point—met in Philadelphia and decreed that blacks should be totally banned from the sport.

In the 1880s, blacks organized several professional baseball teams, a number of which regularly barnstormed the country year after year, often playing against white teams in exhibition games. In addition, separate Negro leagues were established. Despite the fact that many black players were recognized by sports fans as outstanding performers, segregation enforced by both association edicts and state Jim Crow laws prevented black athletes from playing on white professional baseball teams. In football, an occasional black athlete was permitted to play on college teams during the early 1990s, including Paul Robeson, a top-ranked student who went on to become a world-famous singer, actor, and social activist.

A highlight of African American progress toward equal opportunity in sports came with the striking victories of the great track star, Jesse Owens, at the 1936 Olympics in Berlin—an event that infuriated Adolf Hitler and confounded his theories of Aryan racial superiority. The reign of Joe Louis as a superb heavyweight champion led to fuller acceptance of blacks in boxing. After Branch Rickey brought Jackie Robinson, who had starred in basketball, baseball, football, and track at the University of California at Los Angeles, to the Brooklyn Dodgers, racial barriers began to break down in both college and professional sports.

In the period from the 1960s through the 1990s, the greatest American sports idols included such names as Muhammed Ali, Henry Aaron, Jim Brown, Wilt Chamberlain, Michael Jordan, Willie Mays, Bill Russell, and hundreds of other outstanding black stars.

In such sports as tennis and golf, which tended to be nurtured in private clubs and were regarded as middle- or upper-class pastimes, there began to be outstanding professionals like Althea Gibson and Arthur Ashe in tennis, and Charlie Sifford and Lee Elder in golf, but even here, black tournament players frequently met humiliation or discrimination in terms of housing arrangements, as well as the lack of sponsors or lucrative advertising contracts. Not until the emergence of such brilliant young stars as Venus and Serena Williams in tennis, and Tiger Woods (actually a mix of several "racial" strains) in golf, were African American athletes fully accepted in these sports.

Negative Elements of Sports Success.   Despite their dramatic success in college and professional sports, an argument can be made that many young African Americans are severely exploited through sports, and that covert discriminatory practices continue to operate throughout the sports establishment.

David Wiggins points out that the first black athletes on white college campuses were an elite group of individuals who came for the most part from middle- or upper-class families that placed a heavy emphasis on education as preparation for professional success. In the 1960s and 1970s, however, many poorly prepared young black athletes were admitted to colleges throughout the country. Often they came from inferior ghetto schools and had limited academic skills or motivation. Entering colleges that had formerly admitted few African Americans, they were often academically neglected, socially isolated, and permitted to play out their eligibility and leave school without having made real progress toward a degree.[25]

Ignoring their examples and the widely publicized odds against young athletes getting scholarships to college or beyond that, making it into the professional ranks, great numbers of young blacks let sports dominate their lives—at the cost of paying little attention to school work and foreclosing the possibility of other kinds of promising employment.

In addition to such practices, a number of studies have also shown that positions of leadership and authority in sports have been held chiefly by white males, as evidenced by the decades-long unwillingness to hire black quarterbacks in professional football.

Much attention has been drawn recently to the reluctance of college and professional sports teams owners or administrators to hire African Americans in head coaching roles. In the late 1980s, the percentage of black head coaches at predominantly white institutions was as follows: baseball, 0; football, 1.5; women's basketball, 3.4; men's basketball, 10.9. Between 1989 and 1992, nineteen head coaching jobs opened up in the National Football League. All but one went to white men, despite the fact that over 60 percent of the players in the league were African Americans. In the National Basketball Association, in 1992, 80 percent of the players were black—but there were only two African American coaches.

In the spring of 1993, as professional athletes representing the baseball, football, and basketball players' unions formed a coalition with the heads of the NAACP, the national Urban League, and the Southern Christian Leadership Conference, national attention focused more sharply on the need to eliminate racist practices in professional sports. Yet, in 1997, when eleven new head coaches were hired by National Football Leagues teams, not a single African American was selected, and few of the key coordinator positions were filled by blacks. Similarly, on the college ranks, in Division I of the National Collegiate Athletic Association, in other than historically black colleges the proportion of African American athletic directors in 1998 was 2.8 percent—eight of 288.[26]

African Americans in the Arts and Popular Entertainment. While sports are the most obvious area in which blacks have made a strong impact on American life, they have also been preeminent in the fields of the arts and music, dance, and stage entertainment.

Musical Influences. Historically, when black slaves were brought to America, they brought with them distinctive African cultural practices that they linked with American customs to create unique kinds of folk expression. In music, both spirituals and secular songs were part of an oral tradition that expressed the religious beliefs of slaves during the pre-Civil War period. They evolved a type of music called the blues, based on both traditions, that dealt with the personal and social concerns of African Americans. Later, a new, lighter and more improvisatory form of black music emerged, influenced by nineteenth-century dance, military band, and ragtime music. Called jazz, it flourished in New Orleans, later moving to the northern cities, where it was played by white musicians and was called Dixieland music.

Among black audiences, gospel music, an emotional form of religious song, and so-called rhythm and blues music continued to appeal. Black artists like James Brown and Aretha Franklin offered gospel and soul music that was derived from African American musical traditions. In addition, a number of black musicians were able to overcome white prejudice and gain recognition in the field of classical music, including Marian Anderson, Leontyne Price, Paul Robeson, and Andre Watts, a leading concert pianist. In so-called "popular" music, African Americans have had an immense influence on jazz, swing, rock and roll, rap, and currently popular "hip-hop" music.

Dance. In colonial days, African-born slaves danced to entertain their masters, and often would play the fiddle or banjo as well. A number of dances created by black slaves were alter transformed into popular social dances of the late nineteenth and early twentieth centuries, such as the Cakewalk, Turkey Trot, Black Bottom, and Ballin' the Jack. African American dance forms also became the basis for many minstrel show routines, although, ironically, blacks were usually barred from performing in such shows. Instead, white performers in these popular stage presentations usually were made up in exaggerated blackface, and performed in comic routines that ridiculed blacks as lazy, superstitious, and cowardly.

Black dancers were able to perform in segregated theaters or on African American vaudeville circuits during the early twentieth century and in time a number of black dancers, singers, and musicians were accepted more widely in all-black musical revues.

In the post-World War II period, many black choreographers and dancers emerged in the modern dance movement, a twentieth-century form of concert dance. Despite these successes, few blacks have entered the more exclusive field of traditional ballet, an aristocratic art form that has been identified with upper-class audiences and board members in the United States. A key exception was Arthur Mitchell, who became a leading black dancer with the New York City Ballet and went on to found the Dance Theater of Harlem.

Literature and Fine Arts.   Black writers who have achieved fame included Richard Wright, author of *Black Boy*; James Baldwin, author of *Giovanni's Room* and *The Fire Next Time*; and Ralph Ellison, author of *The Invisible Man*. Alex Haley's *Roots*, which led to a tremendously popular television miniseries, along with works by black militants Eldridge Cleaver and Malcolm X, helped to focus the eyes of white America on issues surrounding race in modern society. More recently, a number of African American women have become popular authors, including Alice Walker, Toni Morrison, and Paula Marshall.

Through the nineteenth and early twentieth centuries, there were relatively few African American artists; some of the more successful ones traveled to Europe to study and pursue careers. Beginning in the 1930s, a number of black painters, including Jacob Lawrence and Romare Bearden, began to capture critical acclaim. During the Depression, numerous other black artists were employed in the Federal Art Project; they painted murals and taught art in community centers around the country.

Radio, Film, and Television.   In early radio and film programming, African Americans were presented in extremely limited and demeaning roles that reflected their subordinate role in American society at large. While there were a number of comedy shows that involved blacks, the most popular one was "Amos and Andy," a daily program written and acted by two white men, which ridiculed blacks as impractical, lazy, and pompous. The first silent films tended to portray blacks in negative ways, a prime example being "Birth of a Nation," which showed them as ignorant and brutal creatures after the Civil War and fanned antiblack hostility across the nation. Too often, African Americans were depicted as shuffling, stupid, and cowardly menials. In the 1940s and 1950s, films began to deal more realistically with blacks and the issue of race relations in American life.

The period of the 1960s and 1970s took a different turn. Under the impact of the civil rights movement and the urban race riots, black males began to be perceived as threatening and dangerous, and a series of films portrayed them as gangsters and "macho" men—in so-called blaxploitation films. Others showed them in more sympathetic roles in films about prizefighters, adventure, and war exploits. These themes continued in the treatment of blacks in films of the 1980s and 1990s with a new factor entering in—the emergence of a new group of young African American directors.

In the 1980s a young black filmmaker, Spike Lee, produced a number of entertaining films that reached a broad audience and began to open the door for other African American directors like John Singleton and Mario Van Peebles, who in turn created films that showed the harsher and more realistic side of urban ghetto life.

Television followed much the same course as motion pictures, with the early roles given to blacks perpetuating racial myths and stereotypes, or presenting an unrealistic picture of their lives. Gradually, a conscious effort was made to cast African Americans in more positive and diversified roles. Popular shows in the 1960s and 1970s showed blacks and whites together as buddies in adventure series, interracial friendships, or adoptive families—all at a time marked by tremendous racial tension in the society at large.

The long-running, highly rated Bill Cosby sitcom depicting the Huxtable family was clearly intended to counter the prevalent negative images of African Americans by showing stable, loving, and affluent black parents and their endearing brood. However, some critics commented that the show totally disregarded the social problems that affected the rest of black America. A research study by two University of Massachusetts professors found that the Huxtables had apparently led many white Americans to believe that African Americans had made it—and that racial injustice no longer needed to be addressed in the United States.

Relatively few television problems, apart from occasional documentaries and such series as "All in the Family" and "I'll Fly Away" dealt honestly with problems of racial discrimination and hostility. Although talk-show hosts like Oprah Winfrey have proved popular with white and black audiences alike, the overall treatment of African Americans on television has tended to be superficial and misleading. Some critics comment that many black young people are presented as dim-witted and ridiculous, and that the realities of life for the struggling black poor are simply ignored on television, or stereotyped on police "reality" shows as criminals.

Blacks as Consumers. In terms of cultural tastes, blacks are less interested or involved than whites in the more "highbrow" forms of culture, such as opera, serious drama, or orchestral music—which may reflect both inherited ethnic taste and socioeconomic status.

A unique factor that influences African American behaviors negatively is the intensive target marketing of consumer products like alcohol and tobacco at minority-group youth. As one drives along any major avenue into inner-city neighborhoods today, one sees an unrelenting lineup of billboards advertising beer, cigarettes, and varied forms of hard liquor. Featuring popular entertainers, sports stars, or models in alluring poses, many of the ads are deliberately manipulative. For example, malt liquor makers have used rap artists like the popular Ice Cube with pitches aimed at under-21 audiences, with sexually slanted messages. A given malt liquor "will put you in the mood and make you wanna go oooh!" or "get your girl in the mood quicker."

In the late 1980s, the Center for Science in the Public Interest issued a report sharply critical of the liquor industry for targeting blacks, whose death rates for illnesses relating to smoking and alcoholism are significantly higher than those of whites. In cities like Chicago and Philadelphia, neighborhood task forces and clergymen have joined forces to protest targeting of black and Hispanic American Youth in low-income neighborhoods. Such practices represent an extension of a long-standing tradition—that poor neighborhoods, particularly those where minority-group populations live, were often places where city fathers permitted vice to exist. In such settings, houses of prostitution, speakeasies, and illegal gambling activities could all flourish, protected by bribes to the police. It was assumed that, if such enterprises could be confined geographically, other parts of the city would be protected. What it usually meant was that the Harlems of the nation were places where whites could go for illicit forms of pleasure. Today, this is still a common practice with respect to the drug trade. In some cities, white suburbanites drive regularly into black and Hispanic neighborhoods to satisfy their need for crack cocaine or heroin.

Historically, racial stereotyping has been evident in many other areas of popular culture, including such diverse consumer products as children's dolls or newspaper comic strips. In the past, dolls often reflected "slave" images, such as Aunt Jemima or Black Sambo types. More recently, major toy companies have brought out attractive and realistic African American dolls. Similarly, major crayon companies now produce "multicultural" colored crayons that reflect the skin tones of various racial or ethnic groups. Finally, a number of popular comic strips in daily newspapers are now drawn by African American artists and feature sympathetic black characters.

Leisure and Hispanic Americans

Although African Americans represent the most visible and numerous racial or ethnic minority in the United States, there are obviously other important minority populations that have unique leisure values and interests.

One of these groups is the Hispanic American population—often referred to as Latinos. Although they come from many different ethnic and racial strains and usually prefer to be identified in terms of their specific national origins (as Cubans, Mexicans, Colombians, Puerto Ricans, or Dominicans), most Latinos tend to be proud of their Spanish ancestry. For example, the October 12 holiday, Columbus Day, is known throughout the Spanish-speaking world as *Día de la Hispanidad* (Hispanic Day) or *Día de la Raza* (Day of the Race). Although the majority of Hispanics in American speak English as their main language and consider themselves loyal citizens of the United States, Nielsen surveys indicate that three out of four American Hispanics between ages 18 and 49 watch Spanish-language television.

In terms of social, economic, and political advancement, the picture is a mixed one for Hispanic Americans. Many, particularly those of Puerto Rican, Mexican, or other Central or Latin American backgrounds, are below the poverty line, labor as migrant workers, and are poorly educated. On the other hand, for those who have been in the United States for a generation or more, growing numbers have been successful in the business and professional worlds. Mireya Navarro writes about Miami and Dade County, Florida:

> The mayors of the city and county of Miami, the county police chief, and the county state attorney are all Cuban-born or of Cuban descent. So are the president of the largest bank, the owner of the largest real estate developer, the managing partner of the largest law firm [and many state and Congressional legislators].[27]

Despite such successes, many Hispanic Americans continue to be stereotyped in the entertainment media as illiterate wetbacks or Cuban American drug lords. To understand the leisure roles of Latinos, one should examine separate ethnic blocs, which vary greatly from each other. James Abreu, for example, describes the lives of Mexican Americans in southwestern rural villages and small towns as heavily influenced by traditional customs and by affiliation with the Catholic Church. Their culture tends to be a unique blending of Indian, Spanish, Mexican, and Anglo elements. Religious holidays and church fiestas, including nativity plays (simple folk dramas that were used by early Spanish missionaries to instruct newly converted Indians), are frequently held. Rodeos and horse-racing events are popular forms of entertainment. Family activities, including traditional foods and music, are common. Many youths enjoy sports like boxing and basketball, while middle- and upper-class Latinos are gradually adapting to the dominant Anglo pursuits, such as tennis and golf.[28]

In contrast, leisure activities of the young in the inner-city areas of such cities as Los Angeles, San Antonio, and El Paso tend to be less constructive. In crowded *barrios* (the term *mi barrio* refers equally to "my gang" and "my neighborhood"), poverty and unemployment are common. Mexican American youth are slow to assimilate and tend to join fighting and drug-using gangs at an early age, affiliating with *klikas* or age-cohort groups. Research suggests that efforts made to transform these groups into social and sports groups emphasizing baseball, boxing, or other club activities have often proved unsuccessful.

A number of other studies have examined the lives of Mexican Americans in other regions and cities of the United States. Some yielded research findings showing that Mexican Americans typically valued vacations and free time more than whites or African Americans, and that their leisure usually involved extended-family and large group pursuits. Beyond this, Hispanic activities made heavy use of neighborhood leisure facilities and programs, and followed cultural traditions by having sharply segregated gender- and age-groupings. Among all Hispanic American populations, the most popular sports activities tend to be baseball and boxing, with less interest in football and basketball, which place a premium on the player's size. These interests reflect a carryover from Caribbean and Latin American origins, where baseball is a major interest and boxing has proven to be a career choice of many Hispanic youths. While Mexican American groups differ from region to region, they generally acknowledge common background ties with respect to cultural history, music, folk heroes, and food. These are illustrated in the *Cinco de Mayo* patriotic holiday that is celebrated in many Spanish-speaking communities.

The enthusiasm of many Hispanic Americans for sport—particularly baseball—was linked with ethnic pride in 1998 and again in 1999, when Cuban Americans hailed the role of Orlando (El Duque) Hernández, an outstanding pitcher who had fled from Castro's Cuba, in helping the New York Yankees win the World Series. Also in 1998, the feat of Sammy Sosa, a dark-skinned, Spanish-speaking Dominican in breaking the home run record that had existed for many years in a head-to-head race with Mark McGwire, claimed the allegiance of many on ethnic grounds:

> For those who are picking a champion, race often seems to play a role. Latinos, whites, and blacks speak of choosing "one of our own" or "someone like us. . . ."
>
> In Latino neighborhoods across the country, Dominican flags are flying and Latinos of every origin are soaping Sosa's name and uniform No. 21 onto windows. In South Florida, Cuban radio stations have been preaching that all Hispanics should support Sosa.[29]

In terms of outdoor recreation, a number of studies have examined the differences between participation patterns and interests of different groups of Hispanic Americans, such as those who were born in the United States, in Mexico, or in other Central American countries. Other studies have compared the interests, group makeup, and campsite preferences of Hispanic Americans, Anglos, and Asian park visitors to the Angeles National Forest in Southern California. In a study of three different groups of Los Angeles residents' outdoor recreation interests, designed to develop effective visitor management strategies for urban user groups, Debbie Chavez contrasted the interests of Anglos, Hispanics, and African Americans.[30] In a 1997 study, Pawelko, Drogin-Rodgers, and Graefe examined the dynamics, relationships, and constraints of Hispanic Americans visiting scenic and recreation rivers in the Northeast.[31]

Increasingly, as Hispanic Americans grow in numbers and political influence, Hispanics are making their voices heard on issues of public policy. In numerous West Coast cities, such as Santa Monica, California, public recreation departments have developed extensive programs to serve Latino populations, including senior citizens and parent-education bilingual programs, sports, excursions, and other cultural pursuits.

On a broader scale, Hispanic Americans have made a strong impact on American culture through their popular music and dance. Latin American dance music—particularly drawn from Cuba and Puerto Rico, such as the rumba, merengue, mambo, pachada, and lambada—has for long been featured at resorts and on cruise ships, in nightclubs and movies, and on television. Latino musicians and singers like Ritchie Valens, Jose Feliciano, Linda Ronstadt, and Gloria Estefan have had a huge influence on American popular music, and Latino-themed restaurants, radio stations, and publications are growing in numbers.

Other impacts on American culture include Latino contributions to literature and motion pictures. Today, there are a number of recognized Latin American and Central American authors, like Gabriel García Marquez and Pulitzer Prize-winning Oscar Hijuelos, who are contributing to contemporary literature. Although they have been generally neglected or treated in a distorted fashion in the popular media, Latinos are today being more thoughtfully portrayed in such films as "La Bamba," "Stand and Deliver," "American Me," and "Born in East L.A."

Native Americans and Leisure

A third major minority population in the United States consists of American Indians—frequently referred to as Native Americans or first Americans. Straussfeld writes that for centuries, white people have perpetuated two contrasting myths about Native Americans: "In one myth the Indian is idle, heathen, and deficient in every respect. In the other he is a 'noble Savage' whose natural way of life reveals the deficiencies of Anglo-American society."[32]

To illustrate, much of America's folklore and published literature contains references to the "noble red man"—as in the novels of James Fenimore Cooper, or the radio and television character of Tonto, the Lone Ranger's faithful companion. A famous author and naturalist, Ernest Thompson Seton, founded a popular organization called Woodcraft Indians and a Woodcraft League near Santa Fe, New Mexico, in the early 1900s. In contrast to the materialism and treachery he found in white civilization, Seton wrote glowingly of the Native American's character:

> Whereas the redman believed in many gods, he accepted "one Supreme Spirit." The redman revered his body and his parents, and he respected "the sacredness of property" such that theft was unknown. . . . For the redman, the "noblest of virtues was courage," and he never feared death. . . .[33]

Despite this widely shared view, American Indians have also been depicted in popular American culture as bloodthirsty, cruel, and treacherous. In pulp magazines, cheap novels, television, and movies, the ongoing war between settlers or U.S. soldiers and savage Apaches has been a staple of childhood play and adult entertainment. For many years the genocidal slogan, "the only good Indian is a dead Indian," justified efforts to exterminate the various Indian tribes in the United States, if not by actual massacres, deliberate starvation, or economic policy, then by crushing their culture and forcing them to assimilate. Deloria and Cadwalader write:

> In language that today makes one cringe, the Indian Rights Association in 1885 said that "the Indian as a savage member of a tribal organization cannot survive, ought not to survive the aggressions of civilization." These friends of the Indian believed that only assimilation could save the Indian from extermination. Many of them also believed in the superiority of the white man's way of life.[34]

There were consistent efforts to wipe out Native American culture by banning religious dances and other ceremonials as primitive and degrading. Various tribes were doomed to live on barren reservations; widespread illiteracy, disease, and alcohol became commonplaces of Native American life. In recent years, with a growing sense of militant pride, many tribes have strongly reaffirmed their heritage, disclaimed early treaties that exploited or manipulated them, and revived their ancient languages and traditions. A number of Indian tribes have successfully sued local and other governmental units to recover their rights to large land areas in eastern states, salmon and steelhead fishing rights in the Pacific Northwest, and water rights elsewhere.

Native Americans in Sports and Outdoor Recreation

When the first English settlers came to North American shores, they found tribes of the Algonquin nation playing games similar to modern soccer and field hockey. The most distinctive of all the North American Indian games was *lacrosse*, a ball game played with sticks netted on one end with strips of deer or squirrel skin. Baker describes lacrosse, which became a popular school and college sport for many white Americans, as: "a 'little war,' a mock military struggle in which warrior athletes tested their courage, endurance, and skill.

The game was surrounded with religious ceremonies designed to obtain the favor of the gods who supposedly bestowed health and fertility on victorious tribes."[35]

In modern times, a number of Native Americans became outstanding athletes. Of these the most famous was Jim Thorpe, a brilliant track star and football player. When Thorpe won the decathlon in the 1912 Olympics at Stockholm, King Gustav called him the "world's greatest athlete." Thorpe is credit with the success of the early National Football League; he was the first big-name athlete to play professional football, and the first president of the American Professional Football Association, later to become the NFL. It is generally recognized that the new league started from ground zero with Thorpe and grew into a billion-dollar industry.

Another influence of American Indians on the nation's leisure has been in the realm of outdoor creation—hunting and fishing, woodcraft, and forest survival skills. These became an important part of the organized play of many American boys and girls and also proved to be a source of revenue for Indian tribes that were able to use their lands and streams to serve hunting and fishing parties of white visitors. A number of tribes operate tourist shops and concessions in national parks and forests.

Revival of Native American Cultural Forms

With the recent growth of interest in native cultures and traditions, varied Native American art forms have gained popularity among whites. The American Indian Dance Theater, founded in Colorado in 1987, has toured in the United States and abroad with great success. The company presents versions of dances performed by eighteen of the nation's 430 recognized Indian tribes, chiefly from the Southwest and the northern plains—the Zuni Rainbow dance, the Buffalo dance, the Hoop dance, the Eagle dance, and Shawl dances for women.

The dance company's success reflects the overall resurgence of interest in Indian culture in recent decades. Today, large powwows (three- or four-day gatherings) are held regularly around the country, particularly in the western states, with less stress on single tribes and more on the Indian people as a group. Such festivals or jamborees include both traditional dance, music, folk arts, and ceremonials, and other works that are developed today based on past themes and styles (see Figure 7.1). Linked to this revival has been a growing trade in Native American arts and crafts—Kachina dolls, Navajo rugs, Zuni pottery, and other artifacts—with large-scale Native American trade shows that are held in major exhibition halls around the country.

Greater efforts are being made to preserve Native American languages that, given the impact of television, radio, and increased mobility for young people, are under threat of dying out in many tribes. Similarly, tribal organizations are being formed to protect archaeological sites and promote land use and resource management approaches that are keyed to Native American religious beliefs concerning nature, wildlife, and wildlands. McDonald and McAvoy write that one of the strongest values held by Native Americans is the

> . . . sense that humans are either inseparable from a revered nature, or at least that there is a clear and reciprocal inter-dependent relationship with all of creation. Since

9TH ANNUAL
AMERICAN INDIAN
ARTS FESTIVAL
OCTOBER 10, 11 & 12 11AM TO 6PM

JURIED SHOW & SALE
* Spectacular Aerial Dance Atop A 100 Foot Pole!
* "Dance of the Mother Earth"! * World Famous Hoop Dancer!
* Alligator Wrestling! * Live Wolves Show!
* 40 Tribal Nations * 100 Native Artists & Performers!
* Continuous Performances! * American Indian Foods!

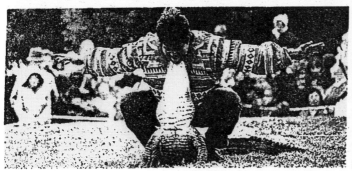
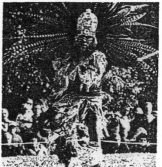

Coupon
Admit one child 12 or under Free
with a paid adult at full admission price!
*** OR ***
Receive $1 OFF adult admission!
With this AD!

This offer good for Oct. 1992. May not be combined with
any other offer or promotional discount.

**RANKOKUS INDIAN
RESERVATION**
Westampton Twp.
Burlington County, NJ
(609) 261-4747

Adults: $6.00
Seniors &
Children: $3.00
Group Rates!
No Pets or Videos Please!
(cameras are allowed)

DIRECTIONS
From Philadelphia & South Jersey: take Route 295 North to Exit 45 A. Follow signs to Reservation.(3/4 of a mile on right)
From Trenton & North Jersey: take Route 295 South to Exit 45 A. Follow signs to Reservation. (3/4 of a mile on right)

FIGURE 7.1 Example of Native American art show and festival.

all is sacred, and infused with spirit, there is a much more egalitarian view of human relationship with nature, rather than the dominant or stewardship view taken by most Euro-Americans.[36]

Tribal Gambling Enterprises

A unique development over the past two decades has been the development of lucrative gambling casinos for outsiders on many Indian reservations.

Based on their right of self-government on reservations, a number of tribes initiated high-stakes Bingo games early in the 1980s. In 1982, although some states attempted to control or limit Indian bingo, the federal appellate courts ruled that if a state allowed any Bingo gambling—and forty-two states did—it had no authority to control it on Indian reservations. By 1985, the practice had spread to at least eighty-five reservations in eighteen states, ranging from Maine's Penobscots to North Carolina's Cherokees and California's Morongos.

Encouraged by their success with Bingo, numerous tribes have gone ahead to develop huge gambling casinos—often with outside funding and technical expertise. By 1998, Indian gambling had become a $7 billion-a-year industry, federal officials say, with 185 tribes running 285 gambling operations in twenty-eight states. Two of the leading casinos are in Connecticut: the Foxwoods Resort, owned by the Mashantucket Pequots, a tribe of 380 members, and the Mohegan Sun, owned by the Mohegan tribe of 1100—ancient rivals of the Pequots. These ventures are huge in scope and income:

> About 250,000 square feet [the Foxwoods Resort is] the nation's largest, with 4428 slot machines, 308 table games, a 3000-seat Bingo hall, Keno, and an off-track betting center [and the Mohegan Sun] is about 170,000 square feet, third largest in the nation.[37]

The Foxwoods Casino, situated as it is in a heavily populated area, is the world's most profitable casino, with more visitors annually, at least 20 million, than the combined populations of New York City, Los Angeles, and Chicago and an estimated income of over $1 billion in a recent year. Decades ago, the Pequots were on the brink of extinction, with only nine members listed in the 1910 U.S. Census; in the 1970s, only one Pequot lived on a reservation that had shrunk to 200 acres. Today, the tribe—whose members may be as little as one-sixteenth Pequot—is immensely wealthy. In addition to lavish housing, security gates, and community facilities, members qualify for employment and training opportunities, free medical care, free child care and graduate school, and substantial annual dividends from casino profits.

In addition to providing jobs in the casino itself for both tribal members and outsiders, many Indian gambling ventures around the United States have yielded funds used to develop a range of other business ventures. These include boatyards and ship construction companies, theme parks and hotels, museums and cultural centers, and a host of other enterprises designed to promote tribal economies and employment.

In many cases, Indian tribes went to great lengths to gain the right to establish casinos. In Duluth, Minnesota, a former Sears store was certified as an Indian reservation belonging to the Fond du Lac Chippewa tribe, solely to allow the operation of a casino downtown. And in 1998, the City Commissioners of Wildwood, New Jersey, a beach resort town, voted to transfer a 2.5-acre municipal parking lot to the Delaware tribe of western Oklahoma to operate a gambling casino. The rationale was that the Oklahoma tribe was descended from Indians who had been pushed out of New Jersey in the 1830s. While the proposal remained in litigation, the Oklahoma Delawares responded promptly with a law-suit claiming all of Wildwood and thousands of acres around it that they claimed had been taken in violation of a 1790 federal law.

Social Conditions and Leisure Pursuits

Meanwhile, what of the social conditions and leisure pursuits of the mass of Indian tribes that do not have profitable gambling casinos? In an article on the Arapaho tribe on the Wind River Reservation in Wyoming, Swick describes such social problems as widespread unemployment and a heavy reliance on drinking and gambling as leisure activities. Approx-imately 30 to 40 percent of the children on the reservation are born with fetal alcohol syn-drome Despite these social pathologies, traditional ceremonies continue to be held by the Arapaho tribespeople, and basketball thrives in the local high school gymnasium and com-munity center.

In the late 1990s, the Arapaho sought to develop a variety of new enterprises to im-prove conditions on the reservation. In addition to such present ventures as a truck stop, a laundromat, a printing company, and a construction concern, they seek to take fuller advan-tage of the $1.6 billion a year that tourists spend in Wyoming:

> Under consideration are a dozen more enterprises, including a trading post, a recre-ational vehicle park, a hunting outfitter's service, a fast-food outlet, and expanded gambling operations [to help the tribe] cash in on its lands, its culture and its scenic location.[38]

Research on Native American Leisure. In a study of off-reservation leisure, Carol Panc-ner and Maureen McDonough, with a grant from the U.S. Forest Service, examined a group of Native Americans living in the Chicago Metropolitan area. They found that many of their leisure pursuits were similar to those of the population at large—including picnicking and driving for pleasure—but with a much higher emphasis on team sports, including base-ball, volleyball, and basketball. About three-fourths of those studied reported taking part in Indian powwows during the year and engaging in such traditional pursuits as tribal danc-ing, beadwork and other crafts, and storytelling.[39]

In a report on the Navajo Nation in New Mexico, home to one-fifth of America's one million Native Americans living on reservations, James Brooke points out that, in addition to problems of alcohol and drug abuse, unemployment, crime, and a teenage suicide rate that is three times the national average, health statistics for Navajos have plummeted. About one-quarter of the tribe's young people are obese, thanks to a sedentary lifestyle, and a high percentage have diabetes.[40] In response, a new wave of interest in running—a traditional Indian pursuit with close ties to religious beliefs—has been developed by Wings of Amer-ica, a youth program based in Santa Fe, New Mexico. Although Native American running clinics have been held across the country, Navajo teenaged runners have been especially successful in national cross-country championships and see the sports as vital to their de-veloping health, pride, and positive cultural identity.

A final aspect of the role of Native Americans in contemporary culture has to do with the way their image is presented in current films and television programs. Strenuous efforts have been made to eliminate the distorted and bloodthirsty portraits of the past and to have more honest and realistic treatment of Indians—played, whenever possible, by actual Native Americans. Similarly, in the fall of 1991, a number of Native American activists demanded that baseball fans stop their parodying of Indian customs (wearing headdresses, waving tomahawks, and mimicking Indian warwhoops and chants) during the World Series battle between the Atlanta Braves and the Minnesota Twins—and, beyond that, that college and professional teams stop calling their sports teams by such names as Braves, Indians, Chiefs, and Redskins. During the 1990s, many sports teams acceded to such requests.

Asian Americans and Leisure

A fourth important racial or ethnic subgroup to be considered involves Asian Americans. Elements of this overall population have lived in the United States since the last century, when Chinese were imported to work on railroad gangs and Japanese were brought to Hawaii and the West Coast as cheap farm labor.

Following a period in which they were not permitted to enter the United States, in recent years there has been an immense influx of new residents from varied Eastern countries—Thais, Vietnamese, Filipinos, Koreans, Indians, Cambodians, Japanese, and Chinese. Steven Holmes writes that though people of Asian descent comprised only 3.7 percent of the American population, Asians made up 36.6 percent of immigrants to the United States in the mid-1990s. He continues:

> . . . they also have special memories and fears: The United States Government interned many people of Japanese descent in camps during World War II, and Asians are the only ethnic group this century to have been specifically barred by law from entry or naturalization.[41]

Unlike the earlier waves of immigration, these newcomers differ widely in terms of their education and professional status. Many are investors and businesspeople who quickly purchase properties or businesses, or work hard and are able to build new enterprises through mutual cooperation.

Varying Backgrounds of Asian Immigrants

The stories of Asian success in America are impressive; the East has replaced Europe as the leading foreign source of U.S. engineers, doctors, and technical workers. From 1975 to 1985, the number of full-time Asian faculty members in U.S. colleges nearly doubled and the number of capable Asian students in universities skyrocketed, so that a number of top schools felt compelled to establish quotas limiting the number admitted each year in order to maintain racial balance among students.

However, this picture is deceptive. Not all Asian American students are super-achievers; many of them are only average, and they suffer from excessive pressure to excel. A study of Asian American youth by the U.S. Department of Health and Human Services showed that the suicide rate among Chinese Americans aged 15 to 24 was nearly 37 percent higher than the national average; among Japanese American youth, it was 54 percent higher. Beyond that, many new immigrants meet ethnic hostility. Korean merchants are threatened by black militants, Vietnamese shrimp fishermen are fired at off the Louisiana coast, and newcomers from Southeast Asia, such as Cambodians and the Hmong, with rural backgrounds and limited education and technological skills, find great difficulty in learning English, getting jobs, and surviving in urban ghettos.

Gang Youth

There is evidence that the tide of immigration from Asia has resulted in a wave of crimes by youth gangs who practice extortion on Asian merchants, operate gambling rings, manage imported prostitutes, and engage in almost random violence. To a degree, this is understandable in the light of the history of Asian immigrants in America. Distrustful of the police and the courts, many early Chinese settlers joined *triads* (Chinese secret societies) and *tongs* (self-help associations) in major cities, which governed the operation and protection of gambling, drug trafficking, and other crimes, but which also had a degree of standing and legitimacy in the Asian community. However, many of the new immigrants are not willing to be controlled by the tongs. They often have difficulty speaking English, are failing in school, and are recruited to join gangs when they are as young as 14. They see the

> easy money and exciting life of the gangs as a sharp, pleasant contrast to that of their parents, both frequently working two or three low-paying jobs in restaurants, laundries, or garment sweatshops. . . . There are flashy cars, [and] available women and guns [are] stashed in communal gang apartments.[42]

Stimulated by the lurid and exciting portrayal of gangsters in popular Chinese movies and videotapes, for many young Asians crime represents an attractive way of life—in a sense, an exciting game or sport. School for them represents a dead end, and they feel that no matter how they attempt to assimilate they will always be perceived as racially different and will not be accepted by the larger society. However, gang youth represent only one segment of the Asian American community. By far the greater number are moving steadily toward integration in American life, and leisure represents one of the channels for this development.

Asians in American Culture

The role of Asian Americans in American culture has often been marked by distortion in the popular media of entertainment. Often the images of Orientals in magazines and movies are deliberately manipulated to conform to national policy and public concerns.

For example, Dr. Fu Manchu, a brilliant but diabolical villain, appeared in the period around World War I, when Asian workers were seen as a threat to native labor, and the term *Yellow Peril* became popular. When more severe immigration restriction laws were passed and the threat of the Yellow Peril passed, detective Charlie Chan (actually played by a white actor in yellowface), became a hero in movie thrillers.

In terms of popular literature, a number of best-selling novels, including works by Pearl Buck and James Michener, have improved public understanding of Asian Americans. Recently, several writers of Chinese and Japanese descent, including Gus Lee, Maxine Hong Kingston, Amy Tan, and Gish Jen have written successful novels and collections of short stories that tell the stories of Asian Americans' transition from being first-generation foreigners in a strange and different culture to becoming "ordinary" Americans in their second and third generations here.

In a comprehensive article on Asian Americans in the United States, *Time* describes the pursuits that different groups are enjoying in California: Filipino cheerleaders in Daly City; Japanese tennis players in San Francisco; Cambodian soccer players in Long Beach; and Korean girls in a beauty contest in Los Angeles. Asian American athletes like tennis champion Michael Chang and Olympic Gold-medal winner, figure skater Kristi Yamaguchi, have become increasingly visible. From a reverse perspective, millions of Americans have become enthusiasts of varied forms of Eastern exercise and martial arts disciplines, ranging from *yoga* and *tai chi chuan* to *karate* and *kung fu*. Similarly, in 1991, Atlantic City casinos introduced such traditional Chinese gambling games as *pai gow* and *sic bo*, hoping to appeal to regular gamblers and to attract more Asian bettors.

There is evidence that gambling represents a particularly serious problem for many Asian Americans. Suzanne Sataline refers to it as their "age-old problem" and their newest. From *mah-jongg* in China to *hwatoo* in Korea, or the *pai gow* tables of Atlantic City, she writes:

> . . . the game of chance has seduced Asians for generations, a pastime as rooted in the cultures as their fabled work ethic.
>
> [In New Jersey and Pennsylvania] lawyers, prosecutors, and community leaders say that in the last two years they have seen more and more East Asian immigrants forced into bankruptcy, turning to loan sharks, even embezzling from business associates, because of gambling.[43]

Research on Asian American Leisure Patterns

A number of research studies have examined the values and behaviors of different groups of Asian Americans. For example, Berryman and Yu analyzed the relationships among self-esteem, acculturation, and recreation involvement of recently arrived teenaged Chinese immigrants and found that self-esteem and acculturation were positive factors in promoting active leisure involvement and associating with non-Chinese friends.[44] Similarly, Tirone and Pedlar studied the lives of teenagers and young adults living in Canada, with family backgrounds in India, Pakistan, and Bangladesh. As members of the younger generation moved in leisure activities from the "small community" of their families to the "greater society," leisure involvements sometimes led to conflict between older and newer values and customs.[45]

Leisure in the Lives of White Ethnics

Finally, although this chapter has focused on four major groups of racial or ethnic populations that are primarily nonwhite (recognizing that many Hispanic Americans have strains of African or Indian ancestry), it should also consider the leisure lives of "ethnic" Americans of varied national backgrounds.

Particularly in political reporting, the term "white ethnic" is often used to describe individuals of Southern or Central European background—often "blue collar" or working class. Each such group, when it came to the United States, brought with it unique folk characteristics. For example, Malpezzi and Clements describe nine aspects of the lives of Italian Americans who migrated to the United States in the late nineteenth and early twentieth centuries—their conversation; life-cycle customs; calendars of holidays and celebrations; supernaturalism; folk medicine; recreation and games; stories and storytelling practices; drama, music, and dance; and "foodways."[46]

They go on to describe such traditional games as *bocce* and *mora*, wedding customs, and the informal but effective systems of health and life insurance that Italian Americans established through community clubs. Obviously, to the degree that such ethnic groups have assimilated into the larger American culture by intermarriage and by living in communities that have no particular ethnic character, their lives have generally become indistinguishable from the typical ones of the overall society. However, when clusters of families from a given nationality continue to live together, generation after generation, they tend to retain customs and traditions of the past.

Although much of the old snobbery is gone, ethnic identity continues to be linked to social class exclusiveness in American life and to serve as a bar to acceptance in clubs, resorts, or other aspects of leisure involvement. This was illustrated in the experience of an outstanding figure-skating couple, Rocky Marval and Calla Urbanski—he a truck driver, she a cocktail waitress—who represented America at the 1992 Winter Olympics in France. There was a time, Marval remembers, when he could not be admitted to the best skating clubs in Philadelphia and Wilmington. His real name is Rocco Marvaldi, and his family has been in the meatpacking business for years. When he was ten, the Marvaldis applied for membership in skating clubs in Philadelphia and Wilmington, but were promptly rejected.

> "They were social clubs," Marval said. "If you weren't in their social circles, if you weren't white Anglo-Saxon Protestant, you weren't accepted in."
>
> That is partly the reason he now skates under the name Marval. "A little less ethnic," he said.[47]

In some cases, actual discrimination or the anticipation of it may cause white ethnics to avoid rejection by maintaining "ethnic enclosure," in Stodolska and Jackson's terms, by avoiding interactions with the mainstream—as shown by an analysis of the leisure behaviors of members of the Polish community in Edmonton, Alberta, Canada.[48]

Hispanic Heritage Celebration 1983

Sunday, July 10th, 4 to 8 PM
Tibbetts Brook Park, Yonkers, N.Y.

Featuring:
- **Johnny Colon Orchestra and East Harlem Workshop Band**
- **Hispanic Delicacies**
- **Spanish American Folk Lore Dance Group**
- **The Menudo Babes**

Admission is free
Parking charge $1.00 before 5 PM

Please bring blankets or chairs

Rain site: Westchester County Cente
White Plains, N.Y.

Co-Sponsored by:

Andrew P. O'Rourke
County Executive
Joseph Caverly
Commissioner
Department of Parks
Recreation and Conservation

Westchester County

Westch
Co

Slavic Heritage Celebration

Sunday, July 31, 1983   1 PM — 7 PM
Tibbetts Brook Park, Yonkers

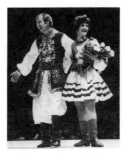

Featuring:
- **Pilsner Brass Band**
- **Limbora Slovak Dancers**
- **Ukrainian Band—Evatra (Bonfire)**
- **Harvest Moon Ball — Polish Polka Champions**
- **Troika Russian Balalaika**
- **Cultural Exhibits and Slavic Food**

Rain site: Lemko Hall, 556 Yonkers Ave, Yonkers

Free admission
Parking charge $1.00 before 5 P.M.

Co-sponsored by:

Joseph M. Caverly
Commissioner
Department of Parks,
Recreation & Conservation

Westchester County

United Slavonian American League
President: Nicholas Benyo
Chairman: Paul Kubawsky
Co-Chairmen: Stephen Trusa
Dorothy Turchinsky
Hon. Chairman: Andrew P. O'Rourke

FIGURE 7.2   During the 1980s and 1990s, many public leisure-service agencies, as in Westchester County, NY, sponsored programs celebrating varied national and ethnic cultures (above and facing page).

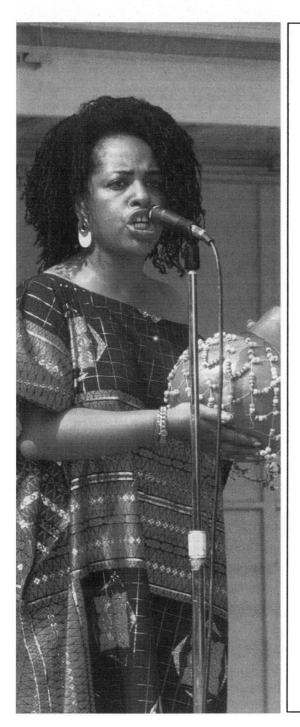

Cultural Events

"Celebrate the Earth" Day
Sunday, April 20 — 11 a.m. to 4 p.m.
Lasdon Park and Arboretum, Somers

African-American Heritage Celebration
Sunday, June 29 — 1 p.m. to 7 p.m.
Kensico Dam Plaza, Valhalla

Slavic Heritage Celebration
Sunday, July 13 — 1 p.m. to 6 p.m.
Tibbetts Brook Park, Yonkers

Irish Heritage Celebration
Sunday, July 13 — 1 p.m. to 8 p.m.
Ridge Road Park, Hartsdale

Italian Heritage Celebration
Sunday, July 20 — 2 p.m. to 8 p.m.
Kensico Dam Plaza, Valhalla

New York Philharmonic Outdoor Concert
Saturday, July 26 - 8 p.m.
Westchester Community College, Valhalla

Polish Heritage Celebration
Sunday, July 27 — 1 p.m. to 6 p.m.
Kensico Dam Plaza, Valhalla

Hispanic Heritage Celebration
Sunday, August 10 — 1 p.m. to 7 p.m.
Kensico Dam Plaza, Valhalla

Yiddish Heritage Celebration
Sunday, August 17 — 5 p.m. to 8 p.m.
Kensico Dam Plaza, Valhalla

Arab Heritage Celebration
Sunday, August 17 — 1 p.m. to 7 p.m.
Tibbetts Brook Park, Yonkers

Ukrainian Heritage Celebration
Sunday, August 25 — 2 p.m. to 7 p.m.
Tibbetts Brook Park, Yonkers

Muscoot Bluegrass Minifest
Sunday, August 31 — 12 noon to 4 p.m.
Muscoot Farm, Somers

Croton Point RiverFair
Croton Point Park, Croton-on-Hudson
Saturday and Sunday, September 13 & 14

The Great Car, Truck and Motorcycle Show
Sunday, October 5 — 11 a.m. to 4 p.m.
Playland Park, Rye

Westchester Ballet Company's Production of "The Nutcracker"
Friday and Saturday, December 19 & 20
Westchester County Center, White Plains

"Say Happy New Year!" Alcohol-free Party
Wednesday, December 31 — 9 p.m. to 1:30 a.m.
Westchester County Center, White Plains

Call for admission and/or parking fees. For a complete "Park-it" calendar of events, call 242-PARK.

Gradually, such patterns of social class and ethnic snobbery have declined in America. At the same time, many young white Americans—particularly those of lower-class background who live in disadvantaged urban neighborhoods—continue to display resentment of other racial minorities. Often this stems from fear of economic displacement in the tightening job world or from ethnocentric resistance to "outsiders." Particularly among members of white gangs in fringe neighborhoods where other forms of constructive play are lacking, racial disputes offer a break from boredom and represent an ugly kind of play. The commander of a Philadelphia community intervention task force comments: "They pick fights, they drink, they fight, they destroy property. They go out looking to start racial incidents." Black or Hispanic families that move into neighborhoods where such gangs exist are likely to be harassed—to have their windows smashed, their tires flattened, threats whispered in their ears.

White Ethnics as a Growing "Underclass"

Typically, when the term *underclass* is used, it refers to socially and economically disadvantaged members of racial or ethnic minorities. However, there is strong evidence that substantial sectors of white ethnic groups are now joining the underclass.

In the mid-1990s, studies showed that growing numbers of urban slum residents, plagued by delinquency and crime, drugs, adults out of work, teenagers having babies out of wedlock—living in ghettolike tracts where 40 percent or more of the residents are below the official poverty line—are white. The Urban Institute reported that during the 1980s, this population grew by 85 percent, particularly in older industrial cities marked by the loss of manufacturing and the migration of jobs out of central city areas.[49]

What this suggests is that poverty must not be thought of, either in urban or rural settings, as a racial or ethnic minority problem. It affects the entire society—with race relations being one of its important components—as disadvantaged, hopeless people fall victim to their own frustration and strike out against each other.

The evidences of racial tensions are many. In some high schools throughout the United States, white students have responded to the establishment of ethnic minority student clubs by forming their own "European American" clubs—designed to promote the "educational and social advancement of European American students."

A variety of racially linked problems may face public recreation and park agencies in large cities today. In one typical community, African American youth protested vehemently against the assignment of a white leader to their neighborhood community center, and other groups challenged public funding assistance given to rowing clubs that were primarily white in membership. In other situations, conflicts may arise when minority-group members seek to use the tennis courts, pools, or other facilities in neighboring communities or township areas.

Demographers report that "white flight," which originally meant middle-class white families leaving cities for the suburbs, increasingly involves whites leaving metropolitan areas entirely and moving to more rural regions in states like Colorado, Idaho, Montana, and Nevada.

The implication for recreation, park, and leisure-service agencies is that they must accept the challenge of working in communities marked by tensions between and among different racial and ethnic populations. For all groups, recreation programs can offer a means of overcoming racial antagonism and promoting positive relationships among ethnic factions in American society. Many public recreation and park agencies have been active in this respect, sponsoring intercultural festivals, workshops, and celebrations, or offering programs that encourage goodwill and develop pride and self-understanding among minority group members.

However, such programs must be carefully designed, with the input of diverse ethnic representatives, social agencies, churches, and political and special-interest groups. Sharon Washington writes:

> It is essential to have a balanced representation of people of color and whites to provide an equitable starting place for planning and negotiation. Programs that reflect local values and interests may elicit greater involvement [and] networking within the community can provide a wealth of information, resources, and creativity that can benefit the parks and recreation program and the community.[50]

Summary

Race and ethnicity are defined in this chapter, along with such terms as prejudice, discrimination, and institutional racism. Their impact on American life through the centuries is discussed, with emphasis on the high status assigned to those of European background, particularly from the British Isles. The melting pot ideal and the later multicultural or cultural pluralism approaches are examined, with implications for the leisure involvement of African, Hispanic, and Asian Americans, as well as Native Americans.

Each such group is described in terms of its involvement in sport, outdoor creation, and popular culture. With respect to Native Americans, the contrast between the wealthy tribes that have established lucrative gambling casinos and those living on poverty-stricken reservations is shown. The chapter concludes with a discussion of white ethnics living in "underclass" neighborhoods in central cities and an overview of the problems of racial or ethnic conflict that face recreation and park agencies in these cities. Throughout, the point is made that the United States is steadily becoming a society in which people of color will constitute a majority, rather than a minority population.

Key Concepts

1. Although the concept of race has been challenged by anthropologists in recent years, in the popular mind it continues to play an important role and to be linked to patterns of prejudice and discrimination in various areas of life—including leisure.

2. Following a period in which racial and ethnic prejudice was widespread, the goal of achieving a "melting pot" in American society, in which all races and social groups might be blended, was widely voiced. However, this goal has been largely abandoned; instead, the thrust is toward achieving cultural pluralism, in which the traditions and contributions of all racial and ethnic groups would be taught and valued.

3. African Americans, as the nation's most prominent racial or ethnic minority, have made remarkable advances, but still are considered to be discriminated against in terms of health care, economic opportunity, the justice system, and other social systems.

4. Sports, along with the entertainment world and various aspects of the arts, have provided an important channel for African Americans to progress in national life.

5. In the ethnicity/marginality explanations for different leisure values and behaviors of racial or ethnic minorities, it is now apparent that other factors, such as regional differences or economic status, also play an important part.

6. Hispanic Americans, although they identify themselves primarily in terms of their country of origin, also feel themselves part of a larger Latino society. As with African Americans, sports and involvement in the arts and entertainment provide Hispanic Americans with a vehicle for achieving pride and economic success.

7. Asian Americans are also extremely diverse in terms of their national backgrounds. Today, unlike the earlier generations of Chinese and Japanese immigrants who were largely of the laboring class, many Asians come as successful business and professional persons, and students from such backgrounds tend to achieve well in American schools. In general, they are adapting rapidly to American popular culture and leisure pursuits.

8. Native Americans, or "first Americans," have had a sharply split identity—both positive and negative—in American folklore and literature. Similarly, the success of tribes owning gambling casinos contrasts sharply with the poverty and social pathologies affecting many other Indians on isolated, rural reservations.

9. Finally, the term "ethnic" also applies to many whites who have tended to keep their distinct cultural traditions alive, rather than blend totally into American culture. In a growing number of cases, urban whites living in high-unemployment areas constitute an "underclass" today—making it clear that poverty is not a uniquely racial minority problem.

Endnotes

1. Ravitch, D. 1990. Multiculturalism: E Pluribus Plures. *The American Scholar* (January): 339.

2. Rose, P. 1964. *They and We: Racial and Ethnic Relations in the United States.* New York: Random House, pp. 7–8.

3. Engler, R.E., Jr. 1995. *The Challenge of Diversity.* New York: Harper and Row, p. 269.

4. Hess, B., E. Markson, and P. Stein. 1988. *Sociology.* New York: Macmillan, p. 249.

5. *Ibid.,* p. 250.

6. Yuhill, J.M. 1991. Let's Tell the Story of all America's Cultures. *Philadelphia Inquirer* (June 30): 7–E.

7. Ravitch, *op. cit.*, p. 338.

8. Law, A. 1998. Letter to Editor, *New York Times* (May 31): 10.

9. Feagin, J.R., and H. Vera. 1995. *White Racism: The Basics.* New York: Routledge, p. xi.

10. America's Immigrant Challenge. Special Issue, *Time Magazine,* Fall 1993, p. 3.

11. Butler, G. 1959. *Introduction to Community Recreation.* New York: McGraw-Hill, p. 59.

12. Mason, P. 1998. Race, Cognitive Ability, and Wage Inequality. *Challenge* (May/June): 63–84.

13. Schulte, B. 1998. Solving Puzzles of Why Minorities Fare Poorly. *Philadelphia Inquirer, The Health Gap* (August 9): A–1, A–18.

14. Editorial: Crack and Consequences. 1995. *Philadelphia Inquirer* (September 2): A–6.

15. Philipp, S. 1998. Race and Gender Differences in Adolescent Peer Group Approval of Leisure Activities. *Journal of Leisure Research* (30/2): 214–232.

16. Bialeschki, M.D., and K. Walbert. 1998. You Have to Have Some Fun to Go Along with Your Work: The Interplay of Race, Class, Gender and Leisure in the Industrial New South. *Journal of Leisure Research* (30/1): 79–100.

17. Shinew, K., and M. Arnold. 1997. The Relationship of Gender, Race and Income to Leisure Constraints. *NRPA Leisure Research Symposium*, p. 69.

18. Stamps, S.M., and M.B. Stamps. 1985. Race, Class and Leisure Activities of Urban Residents. *Journal of Leisure Research* (17/10: 40–55.

19. Hutchison, R. 1988. A Critique of Race, Ethnicity and Social Class in Recent Leisure-Recreation Research. *Journal of Leisure Research* (20/1): 15.

20. Floyd, M. 1998. Getting Beyond Marginality and Ethnicity: The Challenge for Race and Ethnic Studies in Leisure Research. *Journal of Leisure Research* (30/1): 3–22.

21. Woodard, M. 1988. Class, Regionality and Leisure Among Urban Black Americans. *Journal of Leisure Research* (20/2): 87–105.

22. Outley, C., M. Floyd, and K. Shinew. 1997. Effect of Regionality, Socioeconomic Status, and Race on Selected Leisure Activity Preferences Among African Americans: Preliminary Findings. *NRPA Leisure Research Symposium*, p. 5.

23. Shinew, K., M. Floyd, F. McGuire, and F. Noe. 1996. Class Polarization and Leisure Activity Preferences of African Americans: Intragroup Comparisons. *Journal of Leisure Research* (28/4): 219–232.

24. Rohrlich, M. 1998. Feeling Isolated at the Top, Seeking Roots. *New York Times* (July 19): 9–1.

25. Wiggins, D. 1994. *Glory Bound: Black Athletes in a White America*. Syracuse, NY: Syracuse University Press.

26. Naughton, J. 1998. Black Athletic Directors Remain a Rarity in NCAA's Division I. *Chronicle of Higher Education* (July 3): A–29.

27. Navarro, M. 1999. Miami's Generations of Exiles Side by Side, Yet Worlds Apart. *New York Times* (February 11): A–1.

28. Abreu, J. 1987. Leisure Programming for Hispanics. *Parks and Recreation* (December): 52–54.

29. Dedman, B. 1998. It's a Race, But Is It Also About Race? *New York Times* (September 20): SP–3.

30. Chavez, D. 1992. *Ethnic Group Activities: A Survey of Los Angeles Residents*. Riverside, CA: U.S. Forest Service, Recreation Research Update (October).

31. Pawelko, K., E. Drogin-Rodgers, and A. Graefe. 1997. Ethnic/Cultural Origins and Its Impact on River Recreationists' Experiences: The Case of Hispanic-Americans. *NRPA Leisure Research Symposium*, p. 6.

32. Straussfeld, D. 1984. In *The Aggressions of Civilization: Federal Indian Policy Since the 1980s*, ed. S. Cadwalader and V. Deloria. Philadelphia: Temple University Press, p. 20.

33. Mechling, J. 1985. In *Meaningful Play, Playful Meaning*, ed. G.A. Fine. Chicago: Human Kinetics, p. 50.

34. Cadwalader and Deloria, *op. cit.*, p. xii and jacket.

35. Baker, W.J. 1988. *Sports in the Western World*. Urbana and Chicago: University of Illinois Press, p. 71.

36. McDonald, D., and L. McAvoy, 1997. In Countless Ways for Thousands of Years: Native American Relationships to Wildlands and Other Protected Places. *Trends* (33/4): 35.

37. Rabinovitz, J. 1996. Place Your Bets: A New Casino. *New York Times* (October 11): B–1.

38. Swick, T. 1991. In the Land of Cowboys and Indians. *New York Times* (June 16): 6–H.

39. Pancner, C., and M. McDonough. n.d. *Use of Urban Recreation Resources by Native Americans*. East Lansing: Michigan State University and U.S. Forest Service.

40. Brooke, J. 1998. Indians Revive a Running Tradition. *New York Times* (August 2): 20.

41. Holmes, S. 1996. Anti-Immigrant Mood Moves Asians to Organize. *New York Times* (January 3): A–1.

42. A Tide of Asian Immigration Brings Wave of Gang Crime. 1991. *New York Times* (January 5), p. 20.

43. Sataline, S. 1996. With Asian Casino Games, Much at Stake. *Philadelphia Inquirer* (April 29): B–1.

44. Berryman, D., and P. Yu. 1996. The Relationship Among Self-Esteem, Acculturation, and Recreation Participation of Recently Arrived Chinese Immigrant Adolescents. *Journal of Leisure Research* (28/4): 251–273.

45. Tirone, S., and A. Pedlar. 1997. Assimilation and Conflict: Leisure Experiences in the Lives of South Asian Adolescents in Canada. *NRPA Leisure Research Symposium*, p. 2.

46. Malpezzi, F., and W.M. Clements. 1992. *Italian-American Folklore*. New York: August House.

47. Longman, J. 1992. Skating Pair Defies Skeptics. *Philadelphia Inquirer* (February 9): C–9.

48. Stodolska, M., and E. Jackson. 1997. Incidents and Implications of Ethnic Discrimination in Leisure. *NRPA Leisure Research Symposium*, p. 4.

49. Whitman, D., and D. Friedman. 1994. The White Underclass. *U.S. News and World Report* (October 17): p. 44

50. Washington, S. 1990. Provision of Leisure Services: To People of Color. *Journal of Physical Education, Recreation and Dance* (October): 38.

8 People III: Gender, Sex, and Leisure Lifestyles

What are little boys made of?
What are little boys made of?
Frogs and snails, and puppy dogs' tails,
That's what little boys are made of.

What are little girls made of?
What are little girls made of?
Sugar and spice, and everything nice,
That's what little girls are made of.

Anonymous

Half a century after [publication of the best-selling Kinsey Report on sexual behavior in the human male] courses examining the origin and meaning of sexual identity have appeared in nearly every catalogue of American liberal arts colleges, and the area is still growing. Unlike the short health classes taught at colleges in the past, what is now available permits students to specialize in sexuality, especially as a cultural phenomenon.[1]

Beyond such demographic variables as age or ethnicity, another element that influences leisure in American society is gender, seen both as biological identity and as a set of values and behaviors. This chapter reviews the degree to which the constraints that were placed on women and girls in various areas of daily life—education, careers, family roles, social and political affairs—also limited their participation in leisure in the past. It examines the impact of the feminist movement and the progress made by females in sports, outdoor recreation, and other recreational pursuits. It goes on to discuss the special place of leisure in the lives of men and boys, of lesbians and gay men, and finally, the role of sex as a form of popular recreation.

Meanings of Sex and Gender

The terms *sex* and *gender* are often used in ambiguous and contradictory ways. Schur suggests that true sex roles—such as wet nurse or sperm donor—are biological and can only be played by members of one biological group, male or female. On the other hand, the word *gender* should be used to refer to masculine or feminine characteristics or roles, based on the sociocultural and physiological shaping, patterns, and evaluating of female and male behavior. According to this usage, most "sex roles" are, strictly speaking, "gender roles."[2]

Extending this discussion, one's biological membership in one sex or another—male or female—customarily results in gender identification within a system of normative behavior that society has developed through the years. One's gender role is not established at birth

> but is built up cumulatively through experiences encountered and transacted—through casual and unplanned learning, through explicit instruction and inculcation. In brief, a gender role is established in much the same way as is a native language.[3]

Historical Subordination of Women

Throughout history, the gender roles of women have been subordinated to those of men in varied spheres of life activity—education, careers, political, and family circumstances. The French novelist and philosopher, Simone de Beauvoir, points out that legislators, priests, philosophers, and scientists have all argued that the subordinate position of women is willed in heaven and advantageous on earth:

> Since ancient times, satirists and moralists have delighted in showing up the weaknesses of women. . . . For instance, the Roman law limiting the rights of women cited "the imbecility, the instability of the sex," just when the weakening of family ties seemed to threaten the interest of male heirs.[4]

She goes on to point out that in the sixteenth century, St. Augustine stated that "woman is a creature neither decisive nor constant," and Clement of Alexandria wrote, "Every woman ought to be filled with shame at the thought of being a woman." Nor were such attitudes confined to Western cultures. The Confucian Marriage Manual held that typical female behaviors were "indocility, discontent, slander, jealousy, and silliness," and Napoleon Bonaparte summed up the feelings of his age:

> Nature intended women to be our slaves. They are our property, we are not theirs. They belong to us, just as a tree that bears fruit belongs to a gardener: What an insane idea to demand equality for women . . . they are nothing but machines for producing children.[5]

Despite such views, in some societies women did hold positions of prestige and honor, and their status has fluctuated through the ages. The ancient Egyptians had women as deities and rulers, as did the Greeks and Romans. Elizabeth I of England, Catherine the

Great of Russia, and, most recently, Indira Ghandi of India, Golda Meier of Israel, and Margaret Thatcher of Great Britain were all powerful national leaders. Anthropologists suggest that in the early periods of humankind's existence, women had relatively equal work and influence. During later agricultural eras, when families were tied to farms, males came to have a higher degree of dominance; in the modern industrial period, with women becoming more economically independent, they have gained a fuller degree of social equality.

Jean Schroedel points out that women during the colonial period in America had the same rights as men to own land, enter occupations, marry whomever they wished, and vote if they met the property qualifications. However, after the Revolutionary War, the British legal theory—that husband and wife were one person and that women therefore had no legal standing—gained credence. Schroedel writes:

> Within twenty years only white men could vote in any part of the United States. Women were also beginning to be excluded from professions such as law and medicine, which they had previously practiced. This trend culminated in an 1873 Supreme Court decision upholding the right of a state to exclude women from the legal profession because "the natural and proper timidity and delicacy which belongs to the female sex evidently unfits it for many of the occupations of civil life."[6]

Sexual Vulnerability and the "Double Standard"

Application of English common law in the United States meant that husbands had control of wives' persons, beatings included, control also of their children and all of a wife's property at marriage unless protected by a previously created trust, as well as numerous other restrictions. The assumption that women were "timid" and "delicate" did not apply to working-class women, who labored up to sixteen hours a day, while their wealthier sisters led lives of enforced idleness in the home or were restricted to the function of supervising servants. Indeed, despite the great concern about "protecting" women during the nineteenth century, slave and lower-class women led sexually vulnerable lives at all times.

During the Industrial Revolution, prostitution became inevitable for many poor women who were drawn into sexual commerce because of their vulnerability or domestic disaster. Thrown on their own resources, young widows and country girls in the city faced desperate economic choices because most women's work paid too poorly to provide decent food, clothing, and shelter. Without any form of social support, they were often forced into prostitution and condemned by polite society—although men who patronized them were not treated with equal scorn.

Impact of the Feminist Movement

In the United States, there were two important waves of the women's liberation, or feminist, movement: (1) The first, with roots in the abolition and temperance movements, claimed the Married Women's Property Acts of the 1860s as its first success, and then went on to achieve passage of the Nineteenth Amendment, which granted women suffrage, in 1920; and (2) the modern era of the movement, which began in the early 1960s, when many women who had gained a degree of independence by working during World War II and volunteering in the civil rights and anti-Vietnam War movements became activists in women's causes. Authors like Betty Friedan, Kate Millett, and Germaine Greer sought to establish the intellectual respectability of feminism by presenting a new theory of unisexism. Talk of inborn differences in the behavior of men and women became unfashionable, even taboo. Many of the differences—such as male domination of fields like architecture and engineering—were the direct result of social conditioning or environmental pressures, rather than inherent differences between the sexes, it was argued. Gorman writes:

> Women did the vast majority of society's childrearing because few other options were available to them. Once sexism was abolished, so the argument ran, the world would become a perfectly equitable, androgynous place, aside from a few anatomical details.[7]

It was recognized that, in terms of personality, women were usually more intuitive, sensitive, and nurturing, while men were less emotional but better able to perform tasks like reading maps or thinking in three dimensions. However, feminist writers argued that differences in mental abilities, emotional makeup, or even physical skills were the product of past centuries of conditioning. Anthropologist Helen Fisher wrote:

> for two millions years, women carried around children and have been the nurturers. That's probably why tests show they are both more verbal and more attuned to nonverbal cues. Men, on the other hand, tend to have superior mathematical and visual-spatial skills because they roamed long distances from the campsite, had to scheme ways to trap prey, and then had to find their way back.[8]

Other scientists supported the view that gender traits have been conditioned over time by cultural practices. If men are less adept at recognizing emotions, it is a "trained incompetence," according to Harvard psychologist Ronald Levant. Young boys were told to ignore pain and not to cry, a carryover from the need for them to separate from their mothers, learn to fight, and ultimately engage in hand-to-hand warfare.

Changing Views of Gender-Related Traits

More recently, biologists, psychologists, and other social and behavioral scientists began to document significant differences between males and females that appeared to be innate, rather than culturally induced. At birth, the skeletons of girl babies are slightly more mature than those of boys, while boys pass girls in this respect by the end of the first year. At the age of 2, boys begin to show signs of greater aggressiveness. At 3, a female edge in verbal ability disappears, but returns by 10 or 11. Boys show superiority in spatial skills at the age of 8 or so, and at 10 or 11 start outperforming girls in mathematics.

During adolescence, girls fall behind in body strength, spatial skills, and mathematics, while gaining superiority in verbal skills. Conceding these differences between the sexes, some investigators continue to develop evidence that many behavioral differences are the result of conditioning of boys and girls. Harvard psychologist Carol Gilligan has noted the phenomenon of young girls in the preadolescent years who are confident and outspoken, but who, on entering the teen years, become less certain, bury their knowledge, experience self-doubt, and even panic in affirming their views. They are "confident" at eleven, "confused" at 16.

Role of Play in Gender Acculturation

Childhood play has a significant impact on the shaping of gender-related values and behavior. In the past, it was assumed that parents or nursery school teachers would help children learn their "proper" gender roles. Little boys would be given guns and bows and arrows and encouraged to play at vigorous and combative games. Little girls were given dolls, sewing kits, and cooking equipment. Such childhood play emphases seem, however, to reflect children's choices as well as adult encouragement. In play laboratories, young boys appear to spontaneously favor sports cars and Lincoln logs, while girls are drawn more to domestic toys like dolls and kitchen equipment. Gorman writes:

> . . . another generation of parents discovered that, despite their best efforts to give baseballs to their daughters and sewing kits to their sons, girls still flocked to dollhouses while boys clambered into tree forts. Perhaps nature is more important than nurture after all.[9]

Leisure in the Lives of Women

As shown in earlier chapters, women were historically limited by the stereotyped view of them as fragile and sensitive, and by the prudery of the times that placed respectable women on a pedestal.

Sociological studies found that during the early decades of the twentieth century, most middle- or upper-class women tended to do volunteer community work, patronize the arts and cultural activities, or engage in other leisure pursuits. Lower-class women, whether or not they had paid employment, usually had heavy homemaking responsibilities with only occasional breaks for sociability with other women. Kathy Peiss writes:

> Women had to fit their entertainment into their work rather than around it. Washing the laundry, supervising children at play, or shopping at the local market, women might find a few moments to socialize with neighbors. . . . Given the task-oriented nature of their [daily lives,] married women's leisure was intermittent, snatched between household chores. . . .[10]

In a study of the lives of farm women, Henderson and Rannells found that their dominant memories were of hard work with relatively little free time, but that they had experienced feelings of pleasure, satisfaction, and self-fulfillment from having contributed to their families' survival:

> The work of the women on the farm provided social interaction whether it was with the family, spouse, neighborhood or community church members. . . . To adhere to

the strong work ethic, women often used household obligations as a way to fulfill leisure needs. For example, corn-husking, maple sugar gathering, harvesting, quilting parties and other sewing tasks provided women with [the] opportunity to socialize with other women and get out of the isolation of their homes.[11]

Growing Leisure Opportunities

During the nineteenth century, Peiss points out, there was a prevailing "public order" that kept women out of most commercially provided social activities and settings. Saloons, for example, primarily served men, who used them not only for drinking and socializing, but also as informal employment agencies and for union and political meetings. Women were not welcome in such settings.

In time, other forms of commercially sponsored amusement became open to women. The legitimate theater began to provide a more wholesome setting that women might attend, along with other more respectable types of music halls—in contrast with vaudeville and burlesque theaters, which were considered disreputable kinds of entertainment. A new "Sunday-school" circuit of entertainment developed, which guaranteed circumspect language and subject matter, to encourage respectable family attendance.

Role in Organized Programs.   During much of this period, girls and women were given far less support in terms of organized recreation programs and were regarded as inferior to boys and men with respect to their leisure interests and group capabilities. A 1953 publication of the National Recreation Association described the "problems" faced by leaders of female recreation groups:

> It is usually more difficult to lead girls' groups than boys' groups. They need more personal attention, more help in getting started and more encouragement to keep going. Girls do not respond to highly organized competitive activities as well as boys do. They respond better to small group organization where individual interest is developed into individual achievement. Strange as it may seem, many girls need help in accepting with pride their role as women and an appreciation of the special responsibilities which will be theirs because they are women.[12]

In many public recreation departments, programming for boys and girls was sharply divided, with boys having more athletic and active pursuits and girls being encouraged to participate in the arts or homemaking activities. In Philadelphia during the 1930s, and other cities as well, swimming in city pools was strictly segregated, with alternate days of the week assigned to each sex.

An early study of leisure in community life was conducted in Westchester County, New York, in the mid-1930s. It examined the work and free-time patterns of eight different population groups—laborers, white-collar workers, high school and college students, professional and executive personnel, housewives, and the unemployed. Housewives were found to have the most leisure (9.2 hours per day) and laborers the least (5.7 hours), based on the principle that women's unpaid tasks in the home, such as cooking, cleaning, or child care, should not be regarded as work.

A half-century later, Susan Shaw examined sixty married couples in Canada, and found that men had significantly more leisure time than their wives on weekends, with only minor differences during the week. Reluctance to regard unpaid housework as "real" work also affected the analysis in Shaw's study. She writes:

> since paid employment is recognized as "work" and is restricted to particular working hours for most people, men have considerable access to leisure during their "non-work" hours, and especially during weekends. Unpaid work, on the other hand, is often "hidden," is not restricted to particular days or times . . . and is thus more likely to impede access to leisure independent of the day of the week.[13]

John Shank explored the lives of professional women, both married and single, in their twenties and thirties, who lived under severe time pressures and had little discretionary time. For them, leisure satisfaction—when they were able to achieve it—was most directly associated with the sense of relaxation and recuperation that it was able to provide from the stress and strain of their daily lives. For these women with heavy work schedules and children and homes to care for:

> leisure was conceptualized as a time for self-directed activity that would result in feelings of renewal, revitalization and stability. It was a time for self-nurturance. Regardless of the form, whether jogging or sewing, [it] became the "glue" or "mortar" that held their lives in a balanced state. Having an aspect of her life, a "space" devoted to herself alone . . . contributed to [a respondent's] feeling "whole," "centered," and "individuated."[14]

Similarly, in a study of the meaning of leisure for women in the United Kingdom, Eileen Green found that—particularly when shared with other women—leisure provided the opportunity for women to review their lives, develop a fuller sense of their own identities, gain stronger feelings of empowerment, and resist sexist pressures or stereotyping.[15]

The issue of job status was explored by Allison and Duncan, who studied two kinds of women: professional and blue-collar. They found that professional or high-status career women tended to get a feeling of satisfaction, immersion in the activity, and personal reward from their work, while women in lower-level jobs did not achieve the same kinds of emotional values and sought them in leisure.[16]

In other recent studies, Frisby, Crawford, and Dorer examined the issue of helping low-income women gain fuller access to sport and fitness recreation programs,[17] and Keane, Whyte and Shaw explored the factor of crime and violence in inhibiting women from taking part in community leisure pursuits.[18]

Masculine/Feminine Orientations and Leisure.   Other research studies have examined the degree to which leisure activities were commonly regarded as masculine or feminine. Kenneth Gruber had male and female college students rate a list of leisure pursuits according to their perceived masculinity or femininity. Activities identified as masculine generally involved a degree of competition and physical contact or risk, including such pursuits as auto racing, wrestling, pole vaulting, handball, and skydiving. Feminine activities included cooking, interior decorating, ballet, sewing, knitting, and embroidery. So-called neutral activities, suitable for both sexes, included archery, golf, bowling, tennis, swimming, and bridge.[19]

In a related study, Gentry and Doering examined the sex-role orientations of 200 male and female college students to determine how their choice of leisure pursuits related to their degree of masculinity, femininity, or androgyny (having a high degree of both masculine and feminine traits; see page 195). They found distinct differences between male and female students in their leisure choices, with the androgynous respondents tending to be more active overall in their leisure than the other two groups.[20]

Women in Leisure-Service Field

Another subject that has recently been explored with respect to gender involves career opportunities for women in the recreation, park, and leisure-service field.

Leandra Bedini points out that thousands of women—often hailing from backgrounds in education, group work, and nursing—worked in settlement houses and other big-city settings during the late 1800s and early 1990s.[21] Known as "play ladies," they were the first therapeutic recreation specialists, with a special emphasis on serving indigent and disabled populations. Many other women found positions in the same period, as volunteers and then as paid leaders in public playgrounds, day camps, and recreation centers.

Through the years, women tended to hold chiefly program leadership positions, while men held upper-level management posts, particularly in recreation and park executive positions. Henderson and Bialeschki reported a steady growth through the 1980s and early 1990s in women entering the broader field.[22] Although some women have moved into higher-level managerial or executive positions, particularly on municipal, county, or state levels, they tend to be underpaid in comparison with men on the same job levels. In other research studies, Arnold and Shinew document that, in the late 1990s, women remained significantly underrepresented in upper-management positions in public recreation, park, and leisure-service agencies.[23]

Women in Sports

Clearly, one of the key areas of leisure involvement in which girls and women have been deprived of equal opportunity for participation in the past was sports. Why was this the case?

Simply stated, the sports field, with its emphasis on power, strength, and courage, has historically been viewed as a masculine domain. Sabo and Pantopinto describe football as a critical channel for boys' gender-identity development. Many of the meanings that coaches attached to football revolved around such themes as:

> . . . distinctions between boys and men, physical size and strength, avoidance of feminine activities and values, toughness, aggressiveness, violence and emotional self-control. Sometimes the coach's masculine counsels were overt: "Football is the

closest thing to war you boys will ever experience. It's your chance to find out what manhood is all about."[24]

In reviewing their past experiences in sports, adult men agreed that football helped them achieve success in later life. Football had been a realistic training for the business world. A law student remembered his coach's emphasis on hard work and competition: ". . . he taught us benefits we'll carry for the rest of our lives. We have to learn to be competitive, because it is a competitive world. You have to be a real tough bastard to get to your goal."

Recognizing such meanings in sport, many women felt it offered an ideal medium through which girls and women might gain in self-confidence and feelings of empowerment. Through sports they might show that they were strong, courageous, and in control of their own lives and bodies. One writer summed it up: "I have long believed that physical fitness is the key to woman's emancipation . . . in marathon races, martial arts, or basketball, women are showing that they are not quitters, nor creatures of inferior potential."[25]

Some feminists stressed the potential values of sports in helping women learn principles of strength, cooperation, and solidarity in other areas of life, and thus to transform politics, business, or family life into less oppressive social constructs. Feminist values applied to sports might, in Bialeschki's words, reveal to each woman her real potential and help her overcome the limitations imposed on her by an arbitrary social code. As late as the 1970s, however, the prejudice against women taking part in active sports in the United States was widespread. Gilbert and Williamson wrote in 1973:

> There is no sharper example of discrimination today than that which operates against girls and women who take part in competitive sports, wish to take part, or might wish to if society did not scorn such endeavors. No matter what her age, education, race, talent, residence or riches, the female's right to play is severely restricted. The funds, facilities, coaching, rewards and honors allotted to women are greatly inferior to those granted men. In many places absolutely no support is given to women's athletics, and females are barred by law, regulation, tradition or the hostility of males from sharing athletic resources and pleasures.[26]

Historical Background

However, women have not always been totally excluded from sports. Allen Guttmann points out that throughout history, women have rowed, wrestled, swum, boxed, fenced, shot arrows, raced horses, and played various team games. He writes: "There has never been a time when girls and women were wholly excluded from sports and there have certainly been times and places where their involvement was almost as extensive . . . as the men's." In some cases, women have defeated men at their own games, or have broken cycling or long-distance swimming records. However, Guttmann continues, sports were often used as a form of sexually oriented entertainment by upper-class male spectators:

> Italian prostitutes in the fifteenth and sixteenth centuries raced on foot for minor prizes. Male spectators would frequently "trip them and send them sprawling to the ground . . ." an activity considered good sport . . . Throughout nineteenth-century

France, working-class women boxed and wrestled, sometimes stripping to the waist and fighting in front of a drunken mob.[27]

Such practices were cited as the reason for excluding women from the first modern Olympics in Athens in 1896; Pierre de Coubertin felt that providing sexual entertainment for men was not the true purpose of sports. Despite such concerns, during the Victorian era many women did take part in varied forms of athletics and outdoor recreation. In mid-nineteenth-century America, women began attending sports events like horse racing, base-ball, and other athletic contests, in specially built ladies' stands. Women's schools and colleges introduced gymnastics, dancing, and varied games and exercises; gradually such activities as conquet, tennis, horseback riding, swimming, ice and roller skating, and bicy-cling became popular pastimes.

Elsewhere, men were not permitted to watch women competing because to be seen "sweating" or engaging in vigorous activity would not be "ladylike." And, invariably, fears were expressed that women might become too "masculine" if they played sports too seri-ously. Protesting against women's playing cricket, for example, a British newspaper pleaded, "Let our women remain women instead of entering their insane physical rivalry with men."

Through the early years of the twentieth century, organized sports for girls and women grew at a limited pace. In 1936, only 17 percent of seventy-seven schools surveyed reported female varsity athletics, although about three-quarters of respondents sponsored playdays or "telegraphic meets" (schools competing at a distance, with "wired" results).

In many ways, discrimination against girls and women in sports was part of a larger pattern in schools and colleges. Sue Durrant points out that before the 1970s, certain classes or courses of study were limited to males and others to females. Males could often live off campus and did not have closing hours in residential halls, while females were required to live in dormitories with stricter rules. Different dress codes were enforced according to gen-der, and women's dormitories were supplied with ironing boards and sewing machines, while men's dormitories were given recreational facilities and equipment. Durrant continues:

> In physical education and athletic programs, it was not unusual to find males using new equipment and facilities while females used the "hand-me-downs"; for the boys' teams to have specific team uniforms while the girls used their physical education uniforms; for girls to have their team practices early in the morning or at night while the boys had the use of all facilities immediately after school; or for the college men's teams to travel by bus or airplane while the women's teams went in cars dri-ven by the coaches and players.[28]

Growth of Women's Athletics

In the post–World War II years, girls and women pressed for fuller sports opportunities. In 1966, the Commission on Intercollegiate Athletics for Women (CIAW) was created by the Division for Girls' and Women's Sport (DGWS) of the American Association for Health, Physical Education and Recreation, to sponsor national championships and sanction women's intercollegiate athletic events. This led to a revolution in women's athletic competition; over the next six years, national championships were established in seven sports: golf, gymnastics, track and field, badminton, swimming, diving, volleyball, and basketball. However, hampered by lack of financial resources, this organization was replaced in 1971 by the Association for Intercollegiate Athletics for Women (AIAW), an organization requiring institutional membership with annual dues.

The women's sports movement was immeasurably aided by the enactment of Title IX federal legislation in 1972, which prohibited discriminatory practices on gender grounds in schools and colleges that received federal assistance. Over the next decade, the AIAW grew to be the largest intercollegiate athletic governance organization in the nation, with a membership of 973 institutions. Christine Grant writes:

> Colleges and universities increased their offerings of women's sports from 2.5 sports per school for women in 1973 to 6.48 in 1979. . . . In approximately the same time frame, budgets for women's athletic programs grew from 1 percent to about 16 percent of the total athletic budget.[29]

The growth of interest in women's sports was accompanied by increased television coverage of girls' and women's athletics. In the late 1970s and early 1980s, the NBC and ESPN networks acquired television rights to women's gymnastics and basketball championships, and there was increased coverage of professional tennis and golf tournaments for women, along with their expanded role of Olympic and other international competitions. However, the 1980s also saw a number of setbacks in organized sports for women. In the summer of 1982, the National Collegiate Athletic Association (NCAA), a powerful, predominantly male organization with major influence over all collegiate sports activities, established a number of Division championships in women's sports. Unable to compete with the NCAA in offering expense-paid competitions, the AIAW terminated its operations.

During the 1980s, women's sports in schools and colleges suffered a number of other setbacks. The percentage of women coaching women's sports teams declined markedly in sports such as basketball, tennis, and volleyball, and in thirty-five mergers of formerly separate male and female athletic departments, only one woman was named to head the combined departments following a merger.

Through the 1990s, a number of court cases forced major colleges and universities to restore or provide additional athletic opportunities for women, as in a major lawsuit that compelled Brown University to continue to offer women's gymnastics and volleyball, based on a ruling by the U.S. Supreme Court. At the same time, a 1997 report on gender equity by the NCAA showed that there had been modest gains in scholarship, coaching, and recruiting spending for women's sports, but that fuller equity was at least ten years away.

Health Issues

During the 1970s and 1980s, many of the older myths regarding the dangers of active sports competition were dispelled. One excuse for discouraging women from taking part in vigorous athletics had been that their "fragile" bodily makeup—particularly their reproductive systems—would be affected. By the late 1970s, however, there was considerable evidence that these beliefs were poorly founded.

Specifically, research demonstrated that fears of damage to women's ovaries or breasts through active play were not justified. While girls are more loose-jointed than boys, making them more susceptible to injuries affecting muscles, tendons, and ligaments, such risks can be minimized with proper training. Although cessation of the menstrual cycle may occur among women runners, gymnasts, dancers, or ice skaters with rigorous training schedules, the cycle normally returns with the cessation of heavy work; even pregnant women safely engage in many activities during the first two trimesters, and with careful supervision, in the third.[30]

Strikingly, there has been a strong surge of interest in competitive athletics by older women, with thousands in their fifties, sixties, and beyond discovering their athletic selves in sports such as rowing, soccer, swimming, and softball.

Confronting Gender Barriers

Increasingly, girls and women have challenged gender-segregation practices in sports, and in a number of cases have successfully played on formerly all-male teams. Jan Felshin and Carole Oglesby point out that in the post–World War II era, high school girls played in boys' baseball leagues, on high school football teams (chiefly as field-goal kickers), and on mixed teams in field and ice hockey. Writing in 1986, they summed up coeducational sports examples in the New York–New Jersey–Connecticut tristate area:

> In Connecticut high schools last year, 11 girls played on boys' soccer teams, 159 swam on boys' swim teams, and 98 ran on boys' cross-country squads. In New Jersey, boys' ski teams had 125 girls on them. Between 100 and 150 high schools fielded coed teams in cross-country, indoor track, and tennis. An additional 98 high schools had mixed bowling teams, and in golf, 81 did.[31]

In addition to such examples, over the past two decades there was been considerable progress in having girls admitted to community sports teams and leagues that were traditionally all male. In Canada, for example, a 12-year-old girl fought to be able to play in an all-boy ice hockey league sponsored by the Ontario Hockey Association, taking the case to the Ontario Supreme Court. In the United States, a number of lawsuits sought to compel the Little League youth baseball organization to admit girls to competition. In June 1974, Little League gave in and changed its charter to incorporate girls. However, it also organized a softball league, which, while not officially restricted to girls, serves them primarily. Relatively few girls have joined boys' baseball teams, and in some cases they have been denied access by local independent athletic associations. Where discrimination has been persistent and overt, cases have been taken before commissions on human relations, city councils, and law courts.

As an example of such lawsuits, the Southern California chapter of the American Civil Liberties Union has sued the City of Los Angeles for discrimination in the facilities and services offered to girls' softball leagues, compared to boys' baseball leagues.

> City-owned fields used by boys' leagues have three to five diamonds, electronic scoreboards, backstops, outfield fencing, batting cages, dugouts, bullpens, bleachers, and concession stands. By contrast, the softball players say, the fields they use lack

not only these perks [which are essential for gaining advertising or sponsorship and food-sales revenue] but also smooth and safe playing surfaces.[32]

Apart from school, college and community programs, growing numbers of girls and women are now competing professionally. In the mid- and late-1990s, two professional women's basketball leagues were formed, although only one, the Women's National Basketball Association, has continued to operate—with many of its coaches and directors men with past National Basketball Association backgrounds.[33] In 1998, the National Soccer Alliance was set in motion with eight women's teams across the country. And uniquely, women prize fighters—while viewed as a marketing "gimmick" by some—have been featured on a number of major boxing cards and have aroused considerable fan interest.

Resistance to Girls and Women in Sports

Not surprisingly, the rapid growth of female participation in sports has met opposition from some male-dominated groups. Women, too, express concern about their daughters, fearing that they will lose their femininity. One mother described her feelings as she watched her daughter, who had been only marginally interested in athletics, who fumbled the ball and tittered in embarrassment, gradually become a "jock"—earning varsity letters in cross-country, soccer, basketball, and softball. Gradually, the mother realized that sports had transformed her daughter—that she had become an intense competitor, and an assertive, confident person.

The mother confessed that what amazed her and made her hold her breath in wonder and hope was both the ideal of sports and the reality of a young girl not afraid to do her best:

> I watch her bringing the ball up the court. We yell encouragement from the stands, though I know she doesn't hear us. Her face is red with exertion, and her body is concentrated on the task. She dribbles, draws the defense to her, passes, runs. A teammate passes the ball back to her. They've beaten the press. She heads toward the hoop. Her father watches her, her sisters watch her, I watch her. And I think, drive, Ann, drive.[34]

The unspoken threat for many parents is the identification of women athletes with lesbianism. Often the charge has economic as well as personal implications for women athletes. On the professional golf or tennis circuits, for example, the stakes are high. Traditionally, the unwritten contract between professional athletes and sponsors demanded in effect that they promised to be or act heterosexual in exchange for corporate sponsorship. In recent years, as a number of leading women athletes have been identified through palimony lawsuits and extensive press coverage as lesbian, the public has faced this issue, and these athletes have maintained their popularity.

Research into Gender Roles of Athletes

Some scholars have investigated this issue by studying the personality traits of female athletes and nonathletes. Kathleen O'Connor and James Webb, for example, examined four groups of female athletic competitors in different sports and one group of nonathletic female students. They found that the personalities of the athletes differed significantly from nonathletes on four of twelve personality traits—intelligence, radicalism, self-sufficiency, and control. Beyond this finding, the research also showed that there were distinctly different personality traits among the women in the four different sports—basketball, swimming, tennis, and gymnastics.[35]

Another study, by Joan Duda, sought to measure the relationship between goals and actual behavior of male and female undergraduate team athletes.[36] Goal choices, between mastery or social comparison emphases, were influenced by gender; females were less oriented to social comparison-based sports than men were. In a related study, Craig Wrisberg examined the gender-role orientations of male and female coaches in basketball—a masculine-type activity. While male coaches endorsed masculine traits to a greater extent than female coaches did, Wrisberg concluded that the gender endorsements of the two groups were not "appreciably different."[37]

Women in Sports Careers

In the past, those who worked in such sports-related jobs as professional athletes, coaches, officials, journalists or commentators were largely male, just as college and professional sports were largely male. In the late 1980s, Joy Defensi and Linda Koehler pointed out that women have increasingly been finding jobs in sports, athletics, and fitness agencies as public relations, marketing, and program managers. At the same time, they stress that 97 percent of combined (male and female) college athletic programs are governed and managed by men, and that women are consistently underrepresented in high-profile management positions.[38]

However, growing numbers of women have entered the sports field as journalists and commentators. Lisa Rubarth points out that the surge of women's athletics following the passage of Title IX led to greater acceptance of women in a formerly male domain, including

> opportunities for women to gain experience covering women's sports and hopefully to move into covering men's sports. It has been easier for women to gain employment as sportswriters and sports information directors covering women's sports, but the entrance into covering men's sports has been hard-fought. And the battle is still not over.[39]

One point of conflict has involved the right of women to obtain access to locker rooms of professional teams to conduct post-game interviews as male reporters routinely do. In a widely publicized case, Lisa Olson, a sports reporter for the *Boston Herald*,

> charged five football players of the just-defeated New England Patriots with sexual harassment for making sexually suggestive and offensive remarks to her when she entered their locker room to conduct a post-game interview. The incident amounted to nothing short of "mind rape," according to Olson.[40]

Following this episode, the team and the five players were fined $25,000 each, and the National Organization of Women called for a boycott of Remington electric shavers because its president, who also owned the Patriots, had ridiculed Olson's complaint.

Male resistance to women having a bigger role in sports is illustrated also in the case of Pam Postema, who had worked for thirteen years as a minor-league baseball umpire before she was released after the 1989 season. Postema had graduated from umpire school in 1977, rated seventeenth in a class of 130, and had progressed steadily through the minors to triple-A ball in the Pacific Coast League. In her last active years, she was chief of her umpiring crew and was selected to work in All-Star Games. However, with her unwillingness to accept a job as supervisor of minor-league umpires in lieu of a promotion to the majors, she was released. In a lawsuit against the organized baseball system, Postema claimed that she had consistently been the victim of sexual harassment and discrimination. Among her charges were that:

> Players and managers "on numerous occasions" called Postema a four-letter slang word for female genitalia. Players and managers repeatedly told her that she should be cooking or cleaning instead of umpiring. One major-league pitcher . . . said that if Postema became a big-league umpire, it would be an affront to God and contrary to the Bible.[41]

Beyond such attacks, Postema was frequently spit on during arguments and had to endure more verbal abuse than male umpires had to face. Occasionally she was kissed on the lips by managers when they brought their starting line-ups to the plate. In her lawsuit, she charged that the baseball establishment knew of such sexual harassment and had encouraged it to keep her from becoming a big-league umpire.

In contrast, in 1997, when the National Basketball Association signed two women, Violet Palmer and Dee Kantner, who had officiated college and professional women's basketball and who had gone through NBA training programs and preseason play successfully, to full refereeing contracts, there was little outcry from men. While some players questioned their competence or ability to handle confrontation and foul language, there was little difficulty during the season.

> "Adjudicating is not a gender thing, it's an expertise thing," said Marcy Weston, the NCAA national coordinator of women's basketball. "And they have it."[42]

Participation in Other Physical Recreation Pursuits

Apart from their growing involvement in all types of sports, many girls and women have entered physical recreation activities that were regarded as masculine domains. For example, thousands of women today compete in triathlon competitions that combine swimming, biking, and running—including the famed Ironman Triathlon held in Hawaii, which features a 2.4-mile ocean swim, a 112-mile bicycle ride, and a 25-mile, 385-yard marathon. Of 500,000 participants in various triathlons each year, by the mid-1980s, approximately 16 percent of competitors were women. At the 1992 winter Olympics, far more American women competitors than men won gold medals.

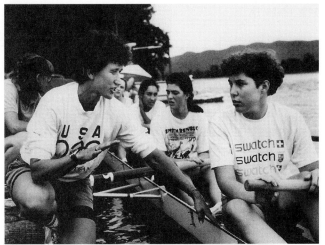

Girls and women engage in sport and varied outdoor recreation pursuits, as shown in teen basketball tournament in Westchester County, New York, crew competition at Smith College, and bicycling event in Portsmouth, Virginia. Woodswomen, Inc. sponsors numerous outdoor adventure clinics and trips for participants of every age.

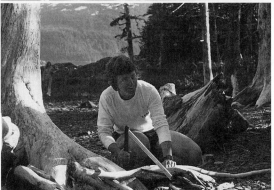

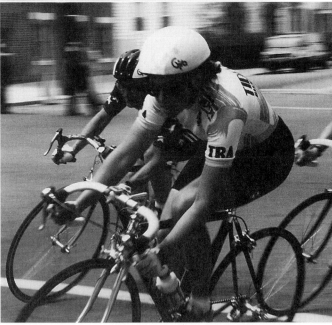

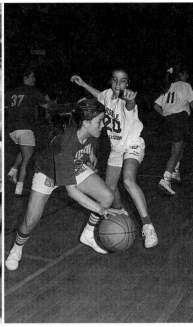

Individual women competitors have won such grueling competitions as the annual Iditarod dog-sled race, and an all-women group of British adventurers recently formed an expedition to make a hazardous journey of 600 miles, pulling their own 140-pound sledges across icy terrain, to reach the North Pole. Other women have formed all-female crews for transatlantic yachting races and similar challenging competitions. In 1991, a woman jockey, Gwen Jocson, achieved fame by completing her apprenticeship as the leading young rider—male or female—in the country. The famed woman jockey, Julie Krone, who retired in 1999, won over 3,500 races during a long, brilliant riding career.

Club Memberships.   As in their exclusion from many sports activities, through the years many women have been barred from membership in varied male-only clubs and service organizations. Because such membership societies often are places where influential people in the community establish friendships and make key business decisions, the inability to be part of them represents an important area of exclusion for business and professional women. A number of cities, including New York, San Francisco, and Washington, have passed antidiscrimination laws that forbid barring individuals from membership on sexual, racial, or religious grounds, unless such clubs are clearly private.

On American university campuses, such prestigious societies as Skull and Bones, the secret enclave at Yale University, and the all-male eating clubs at Princeton have yielded under pressure and opened their doors to women. In the late 1980s, many other service groups, such as Rotary International, Moose, Elks, Lions, and Kiwanis, were compelled by Supreme Court decisions to modify their exclusionary policies. Even today, many leading golf clubs continue to bar women as members; in some cases they force them to apply for membership under their husband's name, or restrict their hours of play during the week.

Needs-Oriented Programming.   As a final example of contemporary leisure program trends for women, many nonprofit organizations that had formerly conformed to the traditional stereotypes of feminine behavior and personality now have adopted a broader and more needs-oriented programming approach. Typically, Girl Scout and Girls Club programs now deal with such elements as consumer education, career development, health problems like bulimia and anorexia, sex and teenage pregnancy, drug abuse, and other problems of youth. Similarly, the Young Women's Christian Association now offers many classes and workshops that relate to the changing role of women in the job world and family life. More and more adult education classes and support groups focus on problems of divorce and single parenting, home maintenance, investment and financial planning, assertiveness training, stress management, sexual harassment, and other needs of women in contemporary society.

Men and Leisure

Although this chapter has focused primarily on women's role in sports and other forms of leisure activity, any gender-related discussion must also consider the role of men in contemporary culture. Paradoxically, the effort made by women over the last thirty years to press for fuller opportunities and status has also caused men as a group to examine their own situation.

While the assumption has traditionally been that men are the stronger sex, in many respects they are more fragile. About 106 male babies are born for every 100 female; yet throughout life they have a higher mortality rate, so that after 50, women increasingly out-number men. Even within the womb, embryonic males suffer from a higher rate of mortality than females. Boys are more susceptible to stress than girls at every age and suffer more from childhood infections and a number of other serious diseases throughout their adult years.

But what of their lives in society? In recent years, a number of observers have concluded that many men are being devastated psychologically and physically by the American socioeconomic system. More and more men over the last several decades have been caught up in a disturbing spiral of self-destruction, addiction, and homelessness. Andrew Kimbrell writes:

> While suicide rates for women have been stable over the last twenty years, among men—especially white male teenagers—they have increased rapidly. Currently, male teenagers are five times more likely to take their own lives than females. . . . America's young men are also being ravaged by alcohol and drug abuse . . . at three times the rate of women of the same age group. More than two-thirds of all alcoholics are men and 50 percent more men are regular users of illicit drugs than women.[43]

Kimbrell suggests that a sense of hopelessness among America's young men is not surprising; real wages for men under 25 have declined over the last twenty years, 60 percent of all high school dropouts are male; and the growth of unemployment and homelessness all contribute to a sense of desperation among many men.

Some writers suggest that the mass media present men with a confusing image of superathletes, superstuds, and superwinners in business—when their real lives are not anything like this. Kimbrell agrees that modern men are entranced by this "simulated masculinity," whereas in real life, most men lead relatively insecure and powerless lives in the factory or office. He concludes that the disparity between their real lives and the macho images of masculinity presented by the popular media of entertainment confuses and confounds many men.

In a recently published text, *American Manhood: Transformations in Masculinity From the Revolution to the Modern Era* (Basic Books, 1993), historian Anthony Rotundo traces the prevailing views of manhood over the past three centuries. He describes three key stages: (1) the emphasis on "communal manhood" in colonial New England, in which a man's worth was measured in terms of his usefulness to his community; (2) "self-made manhood," in which social status was determined by a man's achievements in economic or political terms; and (3) "combative manhood," with emphasis on the individual's competitive toughness—qualities valued during two World Wars and the Cold War of the late twentieth century.[44]

Male Responses to Need for Identity

In recent years, men have explored a variety of ways of affirming their own identity, given the pressures and uncertainty of contemporary life. Lacking real physical challenges and dangers, many men engage in high-risk sports; play mock war games or survival contests like Paintball or Laser Tag, wearing camouflage, bug spray, and war paint; or identify with the professional sports teams they admire, wearing their uniforms and supporting them, sometimes violently.

Still others ridicule their own masculinity. In the town of Roslyn, Washington, a group of men have organized an annual "Manly Man Festival." They parade in pickup trucks, covered wagons pulled by women, dump trucks, motorcycles, go-carts and "Spam-mobiles." To show their masculinity, in a June 1998 festival, they

> . . . flexed, grunted, swaggered, and strutted. They showed off their biceps and tool belts [the more elaborate and laden with tools the better]. They drank Bud, ate Spam, smoked cigars, and generally behaved in a manner befitting their gender [in a deliberately buffoonish way].[45]

The Husbandry Concept. Some men have been attracted to the philosophy expressed by poet Robert Bly in his book, *Iron John*. His view is that true male authenticity began to decline in the Industrial Revolution when fathers left their sons and went to work in factories. At this time:

> The communion between father and son vanished, the traditional connection, lore passing from father to son. And with it went the masculine identity, the meaning and energy of man's life, which should be an adventure, an allegory, a question.[46]

When boys were raised by women, according to this view, they were co-opted by a female view of masculinity and could only respond softly to the challenges of modern life. As a means of regaining their lost "maleness," at Bly's "Wild Man" encampments men are encouraged to cry, to shriek, to drum and stamp on the earth, returning symbolically to their earlier selves as cavemen and primitive warriors. Just as the women's movement encouraged women to explore their relationships with their mothers in therapy groups and other support relationships, so men are encouraged to overcome their inarticulateness about their fathers with each other. One critic argues that men must regain a sense of *husbandry*, defined as "a sense of masculine obligation—generating and maintaining stable relationship to one's immediate family and to the earth itself . . . as provider, caretaker, and steward."[47]

Mannis concludes that a rebirth of husbandry can help reawaken the male spirit from alienation and isolation, and heal the spiritual wound that many men now suffer. While not all men are familiar with these ideas, certainly a much greater number of them are looking at the business of being male in a new light. Whereas men's magazines used to present an image of maleness in macho terms of naked women, sports cars, pop culture, and conspicuous consumption, newer publications aimed at male audiences are emphasizing articles on health, psychology, relationships, and children. Increasingly, men are feeling freer to define themselves in their own terms and to admit, for example, that they are not interested in sports. Whitson comments that sports were historically considered invaluable in helping men identify with each other and develop the qualities of judgment, courage, endurance of pain, team play, and leadership that were considered critical in the achievement of manhood. Today, however, these values are less important than they were, and other values—

such as sensitivity, tolerance, the ability to express emotion, and even gentleness—are regarded as appropriate for men as they are for women.[48]

Sharing Family Tasks.   This shift in gender-based roles is illustrated in recent research showing that men are assuming a growing share of family-based responsibilities, including child care, based on late-1990s studies by the Families and Work Institute, a nonprofit research group. Blue-collar workers, particularly men in municipal and service jobs, are especially involved in child care, according to other Labor Department studies reported in 1997.

Group Associations and Fraternity Life

Another aspect of the leisure interests of men has to do with their traditional involvement in closed groups—particularly secret societies, lodges, fraternities, and other exclusive orders and clubs. Fraternities on college campuses have long been regarded as an integral part of campus life, featuring sports, dances, drinking, and nostalgic memories of brotherhood that, once established, last through a lifetime.

Today, the fraternity system accomplishes much good. Its members often raise money for charities, work as tutors, and assist in neighborhood social programs. But, in recent years, there has been increasing evidence of the negative role played by many fraternities. Mann writes:

> What, in an earlier age, passed for selective admission standards and spirited frat-house behavior today go by different, more accurate names. At colleges large and small, fraternities are accused of violent and vulgar racism, sexism and anti-Semitism. The "innocent hazing" of decades ago has degenerated into poisonings, beatings, burnings and burials. Drunkenness and hedonistic excess are rampant. Gang rape is not uncommon.[49]

The incidents were reported in the nation's press by the hundreds. At Middlebury College in Vermont, the brothers of Delta Upsilon hang a mutilated female mannequin from the balcony during a two-day party; the armless, faceless mannequin drips red paint from its breasts, and a sexual slur is written across its back. Antiblack racism is blatant; on Martin Luther King's birthday, a University of Colorado fraternity distributes a poster of a black women with the caption "Come Play with Me." At George Washington University, Delta Tau Delta circulates fliers advertising a "White History Week" party as a protest to the observance of an official "Black History Month." Says the flier: "Come Help the Delts Celebrate White History Week! Did you know George Washington was a White Man?"[50]

What does all this have to do with leisure? However such attitudes or practices may be viewed by psychologists or sociologists, the reality is that they are a form of fun for the fraternity brothers who share them. Dangerous forms of hazing, such as forcing pledges to drink endlessly as part of initiation (occasionally a pledge dies from choking on his own vomit), or branding pledges with the fraternity's insignia on the bare chest with a red-hot iron (as some black fraternities have done) are all part of the game.

Nowhere has this been more evident than in the way many fraternities regard sex as a form of play activity. With increased national concern about sexual harassment and abuse, one of the most disturbing revelations of the late 1980s was the publicity given to the practice of group sex in fraternity parties, where the "brothers" single out a young girl—often naive or emotionally unstable—ply her with drinks or drugs, and then isolate her in a room where they take turns having sex with her. The practice, which has been widely found in collegiate circles, and which many fraternity members have accepted as a social norm, is called "pulling train," because the men involved line up like freight boxcars, waiting to take their turn. The woman may have passed out, be incoherent, or be caked in her own vomit. She may also be resisting the assault—but it does not matter to the men.[51]

Within a new climate of increased sensitivity and respect for women, such practices are now challenged and, along with hazing abuses, often penalized by university disciplinary action or suspension of the fraternity's charter by national offices. On many college campuses efforts are made to help both male and female students understand their implications and develop more honest and respectful codes of sexual conduct.

Apart from such efforts to counter sexist practices, there has been a gradual shift in public thinking about such issues as sexual preferences and lifestyle. In part, this shift has been based on a recognition that the principle holding that there are two distinct gender orientations—masculine and feminine—is no longer an unquestioned verity.

Androgyny in Popular Culture

The concept of *androgyny* (drawn from the Greek *andro* [male] and *gyne* [female] represents both a universal image that has existed for centuries in folklore, myths, and fairy tales and a contemporary rethinking of social beliefs that arbitrarily separate and define people by their biological identity. Jay Mechling suggests that

> the tendency is to move away from the bipolar approach—that is, one that poses masculinity and femininity as extreme ends of a single dimension—toward a dualistic approach that sees masculinity and femininity as quite separate qualities of self-concept, qualities that can vary independently and appear in every individual. The dualistic approach entertains the possibility of psychological androgyny in persons whose self-concept includes both masculine and feminine desirable traits.[52]

To illustrate, a widely used test of personality, the Bem Sex-Role Inventory (BSRI) identifies a number of traits that have traditionally been regarded as masculine (e.g., "Acts as a leader," "Assertive," and "Self-reliant") and others that are thought of as feminine (e.g., "Compassionate," "Gentle," or "Sensitive to the needs of others") along with other traits that are regarded as neutral—belonging no more to one sex than to the other. Based on the BSRI system, four types of individuals may be identified: (1) *androgynous* persons, whose self-concept is above the median on both masculine and feminine traits; (2) *masculine* persons, whose self-concept is above the median or masculine but below on feminine traits; (3) *feminine* persons, who are above the median on feminine and below on masculine traits; and (4) *undifferentiated* persons, whose self-concept falls below the median on both sets of traits.

Thus, androgyny may be understood as a concept that treats people simply as human beings without arbitrary expectations based on biological gender. There are numerous examples of androgynous behavior or personalities within the world of popular culture. For example, a considerable number of both male and female rock stars who appear in television music video are almost indistinguishable with respect to sexual identification, in terms of their appearance, makeup, hairstyles, or costumes. The concept of androgyny may also be illustrated through examples of role reversal—what happens when members of one group move ahead aggressively to play the role that had traditionally been held by members of the other group.

An example may be found in the relatively new custom of women attending shows in which men strip. As *Time* points out, "peeling" in public for pay has long been a familiar form of entertainment, but beginning in the 1970s, in nightclubs large and small across the country and in places that certainly were not feminist strongholds, the men were doing the grinding and bumping, and the women were watching. Some see the phenomenon as a "mockery" or a "liberation" thing; one viewer explains "why he believed women enjoy watching men strip in public, [citing] the 'get back' factor—the thrill that women get from turning the tables on men by treating them as sex objects."[53]

In another example of role reversal, anthropologist William Arens described how football, as a "bastion of male supremacy," with its emphasis on muscle, power, and speed, was symbolically invaded by women—and how men responded:

> In an informal game between females in a Long Island community, the husbands responded by appearing on the sidelines in women's clothes and wigs. The message was clear. If the women were going to act like men, then the men were going to transform themselves into women. These "rituals of rebellion" involving an inversion of sex roles have often been recorded by anthropologists.[54]

The intricate nature of gender identification in leisure pursuits is illustrated in football, marked by a militant, intensely *macho* atmosphere (evidenced in part by the exaggeratedly male uniform: enlarged head and shoulders, a narrow waist, and skintight pants accented by a metal codpiece). Despite, or perhaps made possible by, this overt masculinity, men are permitted by custom to engage in frequent gestures of physical affection, handholding, hugging, and bottom-patting.

Leisure and Alternative Sexual Lifestyles

Any discussion of sex, gender, and leisure would be incomplete without a consideration of homosexuality. While there remains a powerful degree of disapproval of this form of sexual identification and behavior—particularly within conservative religious denominations—many people now accept the view that homosexuality is not an illness or a crime, but is the lifestyle of millions of men and women who lead responsible and creative lives within the overall society.

The term *homosexuality* is usually used to describe a close identification or attachment to members of one's own sex, which usually includes both emotional and erotic elements. It may involve a total and exclusive involvement in homosexuality as a lifestyle, or it may exist side by side with heterosexual marriage or relationships. It may also include sexual encounters in which participants do not regard themselves *as* homosexuals, as in prisons where individuals seek the only available sexual outlets as an expedient.

Once fiercely condemned by religious and civil authorities and even punishable by execution, homosexuality has also been an accepted part of human behavior in societies throughout history—present in all cultures and condoned in many of them. Historian David Reynolds points out that the free, easy spirit of pre–Civil War America made passionate intimacy between people of the same sex:

> . . . quite common. Surviving letters and diaries show that men often confessed love to each other, embraced, slept together, kissed. Women did the same. But the very historians who have unearthed these private documents are loath to call such activity homosexual in our sense of the word.[55]

For several decades in the twentieth century, homosexuality was defined as a form of mental illness in Western society, due in part to the writings of the famous psychoanalyst, Sigmund Freud. Yet, in the mid-1930s, when it became evident that the Nazis sought to exterminate homosexuals, Freud wrote to the mother of a gay man, "Homosexuality is assuredly no advantage, but it is nothing to be ashamed of, no vice, no degradation, it cannot be classified as an illness." Despite this conclusion, many of Freud's followers condemned and ridiculed homosexuality in the decades following World War II, and sought to "cure" it, as aberrant behavior.

Mid-century research suggested that some men in every society—usually between 5 and 10 percent—were drawn to homoerotic pursuits. More recent research suggests that the number is lower, although a 1989 study by researchers affiliated with the National Academy of Sciences found that 20 percent of American men had had sex with another man at least once. The percentage of homoerotic women is assumed to be smaller, although more women are believed to be bisexual than men. The causes of homosexuality are not known, although many psychologists believe that a distant or punitive father is often linked to male homosexuality. There is increasing evidence that homosexuality may be a matter of genetic heritage, rather than parenting, based on an extensive study of identical twins conducted at Northwestern University and the Boston University School of Medicine. There has also been evidence that "gayness begins in the chromosomes," with research showing that a cluster of brain cells that may guide sexual drives is twice as large in heterosexual males as in homosexual males.[56]

On the other hand, some lesbian activists argue that lesbianism is as much as feminist statement as it is a sexual one. Whatever the origin, in 1976 the American Psychiatric Association agreed that homosexuality was not necessarily related to pathology, other than in one diagnostic category: "persistent and marked distress about one's sexual orientation." Beyond that, psychiatrists tend to agree that sexual orientation is difficult to change, and that change is not intrinsically desirable.

For many years gays were forced to live "in the closet," hiding their orientation for fear of legal or economic reprisal. A major change occurred in American society at the end of the 1960s, when crowds of homosexuals rioted violently following a police raid on the

Stonewall Inn, a popular gay bar in New York City. The Gay Liberation Front was formed in New York a few days later, and similar groups throughout the country began preaching "gay pride," lobbying for pro-homosexual candidates and legislation, and establishing a gay press that sprang up almost immediately.

Since that time, homosexuals have made remarkable progress in terms of their legal standing and recognition as a political and social force. Many colleges and universities have authorized gay student organizations that publish materials and hold events freely. Homosexual faculty members are widely employed, and courses in gay studies are part of the movement toward intercultural education.

Continued Resistance to Homosexuality

On several powerful levels, however, resistance to homosexuality continues. Among the major religions, including the Presbyterian Church, the Episcopal Church, the United Methodist Church, and the Southern Baptist Convention, during the 1990s national bodies issued reports or policy statements condemning such practices as permitting gay priests or ministers to hold posts, performing same-sex marriages, or other policies supportive of homosexual lifestyles.

When, in 1997, the Southern Baptist Convention called for a boycott by members of its 41,000 churches nationwide of all Disney attractions and products because of Disney's allegedly "Christian-bashing, family-bashing, pro-homosexual agenda," the boycott had little effect.

The Catholic church, which has had numerous homosexual priests and nuns within the church through history, has struggled with this problem, not only because such individuals have violated their vows of celibacy but also because there have been a substantial number of cases of catastrophic lawsuits based on the sexual abuse of children by members of the clergy. The church has continued to strongly affirm its opposition to homosexuality. In a statement sent in June 1992 to U.S. Catholic bishops, the Vatican described homosexuality as an "objective mental disorder," comparing it to mental illness, and affirmed its support for discrimination against gay people in public housing, family health benefits, and the hiring of teachers, coaches, and military personnel. In the same year, considerable opposition was expressed to the use of textbooks and course materials depicting homosexual family relationships favorably, which had been introduced for use in the elementary grades in some states.

In the summer of 1998, a coalition of conservative Christian groups placed full-page ads in several major newspapers promoting a "gay conversion" campaign—the success of Exodus International in having gay men and lesbian women return to heterosexuality, "by ongoing submission to the Lordship of Christ." At the same time, conservatives in the U.S. Congress sought to pass a harsh amendment reversing the federal ban on discrimination against gays. Senate Majority Leader Trent Lott said that homosexuality was a sin and compared it to alcoholism, kleptomania, and sexual addiction. A leading Protestant clergyman warned the city of Orlando that its support for a gay-pride celebration was inviting the "vengeance of God;" he later pointed to forest fires sweeping across Florida as an example of holy punishment.

Within numerous other areas of public life, homosexuals have made progress, but continue to suffer from overt or hidden discrimination. In the military, the Pentagon ousted over a thousand homosexuals following the Persian Gulf war, including a number of celebrated men and women with outstanding records. In June 1992, a congressional study conducted by the General Accounting Office estimated the cost of replacing such individuals as over $25 million in a single year, and concluded that there was no evidence to support the Pentagon's argument that the ban on gays was necessary to ensure "good order, morale, and discipline."

Despite such reports and the Defense Department's "Don't Ask, Don't Tell" policy, in April 1998 it was announced that discharges of homosexuals in the military had increased by 67 percent since 1994. *Time Magazine* concluded that "for gays and lesbians, life in the armed forces means unflagging vigilance and some tactical deception."

In the mid-1990s, gay activists and civil rights supporters struggled against legislative efforts in states such as Oregon and Colorado to limit the civil rights of homosexuals. In the business world, despite laws prohibiting discrimination based on sexual factors, many gay men and women hide their sexual preferences. The clearest evidence of homophobia, the fear and hatred of those who choose to have alternative lifestyles, may be found in the growing incidence of "gay bashing." Statistics indicate that deliberate, violent, and unprovoked attacks on homosexuals and lesbians have been steadily rising, as "skinheads" and other prejudiced groups carry out random assaults, often with the expectation that they will not be punished for such criminal acts.

For example, in the fall of 1998, national concern was aroused and huge protest rallies were held following the brutal murder of a young gay college student in Wyoming—described as a clearly homophobic hate crime.

Leisure Pursuits of Gay Men and Lesbians

One might ask, Why should the leisure interests of any special segment of the population, in terms of gender or sexual affiliation, be stressed in a general text on the role of leisure in society?

The answer obviously is that, given the size and growing visibility of this population, constituting an estimated 10 to 20 million Americans, the leisure involvements of its members represents an important sociological concern. Beyond this, as gay men and lesbian women take part more openly in community life, recreation, park, and leisure-service managers must consider whether their special needs or interests should be considered at all, or whether they should be treated simply as members of the overall population.

In the past, many gay individuals typically sought out their own bars, resorts, bathhouses, and neighborhoods where they might cluster together and seek each other's company. Gradually, this clustering tendency evolved into what researcher John Lee has called the "institutional completeness" of the gay community—a homosexual second society, a social world that has sprung up in every large city and many smaller ones, involving several million men and women, hundreds of organizations, and billions of dollars' worth of business. Lee writes:

our gay citizen can clothe himself at gay-oriented clothing stores, have his hair cut by a gay stylist, his spectacles made by a gay optician. He can buy food at a gay bakery, records at a gay phonograph shop, and arrange his travel plans through gay travel agents. . . . Naturally he can drink at gay bars and dance at gay discotheques.[57]

Beyond such services, large cities in particular are likely to offer a host of leisure pursuits specifically geared to serving homosexual individuals, including lesbian radio shows, antique stores and art galleries, motorcycle clubs, and numerous other groups, enterprises, or services. Increasingly, gay themes and characters have been sympathetically presented in television shows and motion pictures. As striking evidence of the invasion of popular culture by homosexuals, in the early 1990s, two comic book superheroes, Marvel Comics' *Northstar*, and DC Comics' *Pied Piper*, came out of the closet and revealed their homosexuality to the reader.

Brenda Pitts points out that the lesbian and gay community has over the past three decades established numerous support, informational, political, and health-oriented groups, but had relatively few leisure-linked organizations, apart from gay bars or clubs. However, she continues, in recent years homosexuals have broadened their leisure activity base by forming a host of recreation clubs, leagues, and centers that function on local, state, national, and even international levels—such as the Gay Olympic Games, which have involved several thousand participants from nineteen countries in seventeen different sports. Pitts conducted a study of over 130 organizations providing organized sports or outdoor recreation activities for primarily gay groups of participants. She found that these groups offered a total of fifty-seven different activities, including camping, bicycling, backpacking, snow skiing, volleyball, swimming, cruises, bowling, sailing, travel, running, mountaineering, and tennis. She concluded:

> that the lesbian and gay populations are hard at work developing a broad sport and leisure activity service base of their own [centering] around two influencing elements. First, the failure of the existing leisure-service industry to target and satisfactorily service this population [and] second, the lesbian and gay population's . . . desire to promote strong and healthy life-styles [and] positive role models for its own population.[58]

Given the relatively high income of many homosexuals and their ability to spend freely on leisure products and services, they are increasingly becoming the focus of both general and specialized marketing efforts. A growing number of travel agencies, cruise ships, and resort areas are now targeting gays with promotional efforts to attract their trade.

Gay Games.   Amsterdam, widely recognized as one of Europe's gay capitals, hosted an influx of over 200,000 people for its summer 1998 Gay Games, which included participation by 15,000 people from many lands in varied sports and arts events—with substantial subsidies from government, the European Commission, and thirty-eight private sponsors, including KLM Royal Dutch Airlines and Kodak.

Curiously, the sponsors of the Gay Games have themselves been accused of gender-based discrimination, based on their policy of excluding mixed-sex couples from participating in such events as ballroom dance competition. The goal of this event, sponsors say:

> . . . is to [provide] an international showcase for homosexual athletes—men dancing with men, women with women. What that means, however, is that a lesbian schoolteacher from Brooklyn and her gay male dance partner will not be allowed onto the floor. Gay or not, they are of the opposite sex, and that has been deemed inappropriate.[59]

In general, there has been steadily growing acceptance of gay men and lesbians in community settings. Even in cities and towns known for a high level of homophobia, like Colorado Springs, Colorado, which had passed an initiative curbing homosexual rights, gay-centered enterprises and recreational groups were thriving:

> For the athletic, there is a gay bowling league, a local lesbian group that bicycles in the Rockies and the Colorado Springs Gay Rodeo, the end-of-summer social highlight.
>
> Culture vultures have Bacchus, a gay wine tasting group; Diversity Chorus, a gay chorale, and Ground Zero, a gay community group, and its newspaper, *Ground Zero News*.[60]

Yet the struggle continues on many levels. In a number of states the rights of homosexual parents to keep custody of their children, or recognition of same-sex marriages continue to represent controversial legal issues, along with the use of textbooks presenting a balanced view of the subject. Recreation and park directors have been faced by such challenges as lawsuits by gay couples demanding the same kinds of fee discounts as those given to heterosexual couples or families.

Roles as Youth Leaders. Lawsuits also continue with respect to the right of nonprofit youth-serving organizations to bar homosexuals from membership or leadership roles. In New Jersey, for example, two such cases in the late 1990s involved Boy Scout policy in ousting an Eagle Scout because he was gay and banning an assistant scoutmaster for the same reason.

A number of religious denominations have taken the position that homosexual individuals should not be employed in youth leadership roles. However, recent studies have shown that the American public has increasingly accepted the principle that homosexual persons should not be barred from teaching in public schools. While strong concern was expressed about the disclosure that a prominent Canadian male ice-hockey coach had sexually abused young boys on his teams, there have obviously been numerous heterosexual sports leaders who have abused children and youth, as well. Few recreation, park, and leisure-service agencies have begun to deal with such issues in a serious way, although a number of schools and public recreation departments in large cities have established counseling, support groups, and social programs for homosexual youth.

Sex and Leisure

We now turn to a final issue that links the elements of gender and leisure—the growing recognition that sexual activity represents a form of play in contemporary society.

Attitudes toward sex have varied greatly through history. While many literary classics have portrayed sexual dalliance carried on for pleasure, in the early American colonies such pursuits as adultery or sodomy were punishable as capital offenses, and routine fornication was dealt with by public whipping. However, there is evidence that the colonists had a wide range of sexual interests. Historians point out that men settlers cohabited with their neighbors' wives, with Native American women, and with animals. In eighteenth century New England premarital pregnancy was common; nearly one-third of rural brides were already with child, and bundling (the custom that allowed unmarried couples to sleep on the same bed without undressing, and with a board separating them) was widely accepted.

During the nineteenth century in America, there were ambivalent attitudes about sex. Initially, it was accepted that within proper social confines, sexual activity was enjoyable and healthy, and that women as well as men had sex drives. However, with growing religious fervor in the nation, authorities began to preach that sexual "indulgence" produced nervous disorders, and that respectable women were above "carnal passion." While prostitution flourished, ministers and educators warned that sexual entanglements outside of marriage were dangerous to the health and well-being of young men. Toward the end of the nineteenth century, as the birthrate declined, the federal government and the states passed harsh new laws that banned

> the teaching of birth control techniques, the manufacture, sale or use of contraceptive devices, and which prohibited premarital and extramarital sex or "unnatural" sex by married couples. Within marriage or without, mouth-to-genital or anal sex became subject to criminal prosecution, under numerous harsh antisodomy measures . . . life in prison in Georgia, thirty years in Connecticut, and twenty years in [several other states] . . . As for the man or woman who turned to solitary and private masturbation, nineteenth- and early twentieth-century medical authorities [warned] them that they would get skin cancer and become imbeciles.[61]

Gradually, such strictures declined in the twentieth century. A major influence, according to D'Emilio and Freedman, was capitalism, in the sense that the ethic that promoted the purchase of consumer products and encouraged an acceptance of pleasure and self-gratification was easily transferred to the province of sex. Particularly in the middle decades of the century, as birth control methods became more widely available and parental authority declined, sex became perceived more widely as a potential business product.

In the 1950s, the Kinsey Report demonstrated the tremendous discrepancy that had developed between the moral preachments and laws that had supposedly governed the sexual behavior of Americans and their actual practices. During the 1960s and 1970s varied forms of "aberrant" sexual behavior, such as group sex and "swinging," living together out of marriage, legalized pornography, and other nontraditional pursuits constituted a virtual revolution in sexual morality and public behavior.

Scientific studies of erotic behavior through the emerging discipline of sexology gained momentum, and sexual techniques began to be openly taught in school and college courses of human sexuality. But books and college courses were only one evidence of the American interest in sex. It became a major part of popular entertainment, advertising, and product development, and pornography, with the introduction of videocameras, made it possible to view "adult" films within the safety of one's home.

Dangers of Promiscuity

In the early 1990s, the great basketball star, Wilt Chamberlain, reported in an autobiography that he had had sexual relations with over 20,000 women during his career. At first this was the subject of amusement and joking on talk shows and in the press, but then comments began to be heard about the risk of sexual disease, and specifically AIDS, in such a lifestyle.

Clearly, sexual activity—either as participant experience or as a form of spectatorship—has become a major element in contemporary leisure. In 1992, for example, the National Centers for Disease Control reported that seven of ten high school students have had sex by their senior year—with implications for three major public health epidemics: (1) the dramatic increase of pregnancy among teenagers; (2) the growth of sexually transmitted diseases, including newer ones like herpes, papilloma virus, and chlamydia; and (3) the spread of AIDS, the deadly disease that is now posing a worldwide threat.

Responsible commentators raised the question of athletes serving as role models, an issue that reappeared when another widely admired basketball star, Earvin "Magic" Johnson, reported that he had HIV, presumably as a result of heterosexual intercourse.

The danger of promiscuity and the damage done to society by having increasingly greater numbers of children born to single mothers—many of them still children themselves—underlined the need to develop a fuller sense of responsibility, more accurate knowledge, and sounder personal values among young people, with respect to sex. At one point, the federal government entered the picture with the so-called teenage chastity bill, an amendment to the Public Health Services Act that sought to discourage sexual relations among unmarried young people by urging them to exert self-discipline. However, such efforts have generally been ineffective. Richard Keeling, director of Student Health Services at the University of Virginia, reports that lessons like that of Magic Johnson do not translate into changes in their behavior. Students still think that they can get away with it. They think that they can tell who has HIV and say that they only sleep with "nice" people. Keeling comments that the reason why so many practice unsafe sex

> has to do with the very confusing world in which we live. We sell products with sex; we use sex in movies, TV, music. Then we tell students, "Just say no." This creates a kind of chaos for them about making their own decisions about sex. . . . Many campuses now run peer education groups to let students build their skills.[62]

The extent to which the mass media promote sexual interest is illustrated even in the pages of such popular and established women's magazines as *Redbook* or *Ladies Home Journal* that publish articles with titles like: "The Sex Skill Men Adore," "The Best Sex I

Ever Had," "More Foreplay Please," or "25 Hot Sex Tips Tonight—How to Make Him Want You Bad."

The reality is that, despite our long-standing tradition of promoting sexual morality, there is little public consensus about many sex-related issues. When the Lexington, Kentucky, school board denied admittance to the National Honor Society to two high school girls who had achieved outstanding records because they were pregnant, a storm of both protest and approval resulted. There was little shock or surprise when research at the University of Minnesota and the Commonwealth Fund disclosed that one in four teenaged girls has been sexually abused, often by family members or friends.

The institution of marriage itself has come under increasing scrutiny in recent years. On the one hand, the conservative state of Utah, dominated by the Church of Jesus Christ of Latter-Day Saints, has excommunicated polygamists for over a century; however, social scientists report that the number of Utahans living in polygamous families has increased tenfold in recent decades. In June 1997, the 2.7 million-member Presbyterian Church passed a so-called Fidelity and Chastity Amendment barring from leadership anyone— straight *or* gay—sexually active outside of marriage.

A Pennsylvania woman comments that the assumption that marriage is a timeless and sanctified institution that exists apart from culture and history is erroneous. She writes:

> It is precisely this assumption that prevents us from realizing that what we, at the end of the 20th century, call marriage is in fact an odd accumulation of historic precedent, human need, social regulation, economic imperative and religious sanction. That over 50 percent of marriages end in divorce is eloquent testimony that it is now time for marriage to reinvent itself.[63]

Given this trend, issues related to sex and gender have become increasingly critical on the national scene, affecting many corporations, the military, and political life.

Sex-Based Concerns

Concern about sexual harassment grew during the 1990s, as claims of women employees being sexually harassed in many job settings and suing their companies for redress became more widespread.

In the summer of 1992, the seriousness of sexual harassment in the U.S. Navy became evident, following the so-called Tailhook incident, when twenty-six women, many of them Navy officers themselves, reported that they had been forced to run a sexual "gauntlet" of naval aviators who fondled and tore the clothes from them at a convention of Navy officers in Las Vegas, Nevada.

A 1997 book, *Ground Zero: The Gender Wars in the Military,* documented continuing sexism in the armed forces, marked not only by harassment but by pervasive demeaning of women as inferior.[64] In several instances during the 1990s, charges of sexual harassment or extramarital affairs became part of the ongoing struggle between opposing political forces, showing how sex was no longer to be regarded as a private matter, but was a key element in public life. In the area of sport, for example, there have been growing numbers of cases of harassment of women athletes by male coaches, leading to nationally publicized lawsuits.[65]

Implications for Leisure-Service Field

What do the trends related to sexual and gender identity and behavior that have been discussed in this chapter mean for the organized recreation, park, and leisure-service field?

First, it is obvious that the growing demand of both men and women for leisure opportunities that fulfill their special needs and overcome the limitations or gender-based stereotypes of the past be met. This is particularly relevant in such areas as sports and adventure recreation for women, but also applies to the important role of diversified recreation that meets the needs of both sexes for personal growth, creative development, and healthy socialization.

Linked to this priority is the increased awareness of the segment of the American population characterized as having "alternative" sexual lifestyles—and the responsibility for serving this group with supportive and enriching leisure programs. This challenge is tempered by the reality that homosexuality continues to be a contentious issue in American society, with strong religious and political forces determined to resist its spread or popular acceptance.

Finally, it is important to recognize that sex represents a powerful drive on the part of most boys and girls, men and women, and that it enters into or influences many forms of active play and entertainment. Leisure-service professionals must be aware of its impact in their programs and should guard against possible sexual harassment or abuse among participants, or between leaders and those served. Their responsibility should be to ensure that constructive, community-wide standards and values are taught and reinforced in all program activities or group events. Beyond this, leisure-service professionals have an obligation to promote healthy and humanistic attitudes with respect to all gender relationships, including tolerance for the differences that exist among people.

Summary

Gender and sex, perceived both as categories of biological identity and as sets of cultural traits and values, have a powerful influence on one's leisure interests and opportunities. Historically, women were sharply restricted in their personal and social lives, and only in the second half of the twentieth century were they able to break free from past restraints and engage more fully in such pursuits as sports or active outdoor recreation.

Men also are stereotyped in their leisure behavior by the need to conform to traditional views of appropriate masculine pastimes. Both sexes today are able to engage more freely in a wider range of recreation, due in part to fuller acceptance of the idea of androgyny, which challenges past polarized views of gender. This chapter goes on to discuss the changing place of homosexuality in modern society, and a number of the issues confronting leisure-service leaders with respect to serving gays and lesbians in community programs.

Key Concepts

1. Historically, women have been subordinated to men in many areas of daily life, including leisure, where prudery and a double standard often limited their roles.

2. While many feminists urge a "unisex" view that held that males and females were fundamentally alike, with social, cognitive, or other differences largely due to environmental influences, science suggests that there are a number of built-in, genetic differences between the sexes. Nonetheless, many stereotypic views of the differences are false, and conditioning plays an important role in developing varied skills in daily life.

3. Historical studies show that women traditionally had far fewer leisure opportunities than men, that they often had less free time, and that leisure often meant for them an important means of affirming their own identities and gaining a sense of empowerment.

4. One of the most important forms of leisure expression for girls and women is sports. In the post–World War II years, due in part to federal legislation (Title IX) and court decisions, there have been major gains in school, college, and community athletic programs for females—although full equity is still to be reached.

5. In addition to fuller support for girls and women in sports, a development over the past three decades has involved women entering new career fields in the mass media, in refereeing, in outdoor pursuits, and in joining former closed-membership clubs or societies.

6. Despite the accepted view of men as the dominant sex, authorities suggest that they often are weaker in terms of health, life expectancy, being subject to job pressures, and lack of congruence between the image typically painted of "macho" male lifestyles, and their own real lives.

7. Many of the past masculine behaviors with respect to sexual exploitation or racial discrimination are challenged today, and many men are assuming more sensitive and respectful roles in these areas.

8. The concept of androgyny simply suggests that rather than being uniquely different in their traits, males and females share a number of common traits, with actual behaviors often being influenced by societal expectations and pressures.

9. During the period of the counterculture in American society (see Chapter 3), homosexuals, who had been widely persecuted and often were forced to hide their identities, gained a new sense of pride and visibility in American life. While still rejected by major religious denominations and other conservative forces, gays and lesbians today play a much wider role in terms of their involvement in sport, travel and tourism, and popular culture, and represent both an opportunity and a challenge for many community leisure-service agencies.

10. Finally, there is growing recognition that sex, rather than being a purely private, personal matter, has become a much more visible element in society and constitutes a

significant type of leisure activity. The role of public, nonprofit, and other leisure-service managers with respect to sex, however, still needs to be defined.

Endnotes

1. Bronner, E. 1997. Study of Sex Experiencing 2nd Revolution. *New York Times* (December 28): 1.
2. Schur, E. 1988. *The Americanization of Sex*. Philadelphia: Temple University Press, pp. 10–11.
3. Money, J. 1970. In *Sexuality and Man*, ed. M. Calderone. New York: Sex Information and Educational Council of United States, and Charles Scribner's Sons, p. 8.
4. De Beauvoir, S. 1965. *The Second Sex*. New York: Bantam, p. xxii.
5. Fine, R. 1987. *The Forgotten Man: Understanding the Male Psyche*. New York: Haworth, p. 98.
6. Schroedel, J. 1985. *Alone in a Crowd: Women in the Trades Tell Their Stories*. Philadelphia: Temple University Press, p. 5.
7. Gorman, C. 1992. Sizing up the Sexes. *Time Magazine* (January 20): 42.
8. Fisher, H. 1988. A Primitive Prescription for Equality. *U.S. News and World Report* (August 8): 57.
9. Gorman, *op. cit.*
10. Peiss, K. 1986. *Cheap Amusements: Working Women and Leisure in Turn-of-the-Century New York*. Philadelphia: Temple University Press, p. 22.
11. Henderson, K., and J. Rannells. 1988. Farm Women and the Meaning of Work and Leisure: An Oral History Perspective. *Leisure Sciences* (10): 46.
12. Dauncey, H. 1953. *Planning for Girls in the Community Recreation Program*. New York: National Recreation Association, pp. 8, 16, 20.
13. Shaw, S. 1985. Gender and Leisure: Inequality in the Distribution of Leisure Time. *Journal of Leisure Research* (17/4): 266–282.
14. Shank, J. 1986. An Exploration of Leisure in the Lives of Dual-Career Women. *Journal of Leisure Research* (19/4): 312.
15. Green, E. 1998. Women Doing Friendship: An Analysis of Women's Leisure as a Site of Identity Construction, Empowerment, and Resistance. *Leisure Studies* (17): 171–185.
16. Allison, M.T., and M.C. Duncan. 1987. Women, Work and Leisure: The Days of Our Lives. *Leisure Sciences* (9): 143–162.
17. Frisby, F., S. Crawford, and T. Dorer. 1997. Reflection on Participatory Action Research: The Case of Low-Income Women Accessing Local Physical Activity Services. *Journal of Sport Management* (11): 8–28.
18. Keane, C. 1998. Evaluating the Influence of Fear of Crime as an Environmental Mobility Restrictor on Women's Routine Activities. *Environment and Behavior* Jan. (30/1): 60–74. Whyte, L., and S. Shaw. 1994. Women's Leisure: An Exploratory Study of Fear and Violence as a Leisure Constraint. *Journal of Applied Recreation Research*. (19/1): 5–21.
19. Gruber, K.J. 1980. Sex-Typing of Leisure Activities: A Current Appraisal. *Psychological Reports* (46): 259–265.
20. Gentry, J., and M. Doering. 1979. Sex-Role Orientation and Leisure. *Journal of Leisure Research* (11/2): 102–111.
21. Bedini, L. 1995. The "Play Ladies"—The First Therapeutic Recreation Specialists. *Journal of Physical Education, Recreation and Dance—Leisure Today* (October): 32–35.
22. Henderson, K., and M.D. Bialeschki. 1995. Career Development and Women in the Leisure Services Profession. *Journal of Park and Recreation Administration* (13/1): 26–42.
23. Arnold, M., and K. Shinew. 1997. Preventing the Career Advancement of Professional Women. *Parks and Recreation* (September): 26–27.
24. Sabo, D., and J. Pantopinto. 1990. Football Ritual and the Social Reproduction of Masculinity. In *Sport, Men and the Gender Code: Critical Feminist Perspectives*, ed. M. Messner and D. Sabo. Champaign, IL: Human Kinetics Books, p. 124.
25. Connolly, O. Cited in Bialeschki, M.D. 1990. The Feminist Movement and Women's Participation in Physical Recreation. *Journal of Physical Education, Recreation and Dance* (January): 47.

26. Gilbert, B., and N. Williamson. 1973. Sport Is Unfair to Women. *Sports Illustrated* (May 28): 85.

27. Nelson, M.B. 1991. Review of Guttmann, A., *Women's Sport: A History.* New York: Columbia University Press. In *Philadelphia Inquirer* (October 27): 3-C.

28. Durrant, S.M. 1992. Title IX—Its Power and Its Limitations. *Journal of Physical Education, Recreation and Dance* (March): 60.

29. Grant, C. 1989. Recapturing the Vision. *Journal of Physical Education, Recreation and Dance* (March): 44.

30. Ellyot, J. 1978. The Weaker Sex? Hah! *Time Magazine* (June 26).

31. Felshin, J., and C. Oglesby. 1986. Transcending Tradition: Females and Males in Open Competition. *Journal of Physical Education, Recreation and Dance* (March): 45.

32. Girls Seek Level Field for Access to Facilities. 1998. *New York Times* (May 10): 26.

33. Ackmann, M. 1999. It's High Time for a Fair Shot. *New York Times* (March 7): 37.

34. Whitney, M. 1988. Playing to Win. *New York Times Magazine* (July 3): 8, 27.

35. O'Connor, K., and J. Webb. 1976. Investigation of Personality Traits of College Female Athletes and Non-Athletes. *Research Quarterly* (47/2): 206–208.

36. Duda, J. 1988. The Relationship Between Goal Perspectives, Persistence, and Behavioral Intensity Among Male and Female Recreational Sports Participants. *Leisure Sciences* (10): 95–106.

37. Wrisberg, C. 1990. Gender-Role Orientations of Male and Female Coaches of a Masculine-Typed Sport. *Research Quarterly for Exercise and Sport* (61/3): 296.

38. Defensi, J., and L. Koehler. 1989. Sport and Fitness Management: Opportunities for Women. *Journal of Physical Education, Recreation and Dance* (March): 55–56.

39. Rubarth, L. 1992. Twenty Years After Title IX: Women in Sports Media. *Journal of Physical Education, Recreation and Dance* (March): 53–55.

40. Paul, E. 1991. Bared Buttocks and Federal Cases: Sexual Harassment or Harassment of Sexuality? *Society* (May-June): 4.

41. Female Ex-Umpire Files Sex Discrimination Suit. 1991. *Philadelphia Inquirer* (December 20): 1-A.

42. Breaking Into the NBA. 1997. *U.S. News and World Report* (November 10): 18.

43. Kimbrell, A. 1991. A Time for Men to Pull Together. *Utne Reader* (May-June): 66.

44. Scott, J. 1999. Hunk, He-Man, Mensch, Milquetoast: The Masks of Masculinity. *New York Times* (February 2): A-19.

45. Woestendick, J. 1998. Where Manly Men Preen in Manliness. *Philadelphia Inquirer* (June 21): A-3.

46. Morrow, J. 1991. The Child Is Father of the Man. *Time Magazine* (August 19): 52–54.

47. Mannis, R. In Kimbrell, *op. cit.*, pp. 70–71.

48. Whitson, D. 1990. Sport in the Social Construct of Masculinity. In Messner and Sabo, *op. cit.* p. 21.

49. Mann, F. 1988. Fratricide. *Philadelphia Inquirer Magazine* (Sept. 18): 1.

50. Ecenbarger, W. 1988. The Rise and Fall of the Greek Empire. *Philadelphia Inquirer Magazine* (September 18): 24.

51. Sanday, P. 1991. *Fraternity Gang Rape: Sex, Brotherhood and Privilege.* New York: New York University Press.

52. Mechling, J. 1985. In Fine, G.A. *Meaningful Play, Playful Meaning.* Champaign, IL: Human Kinetics Press, p. 47.

53. Gillin, B. 1983. Ogling the Male Stripper as He Dances in All His Glory. *Time Magazine* (November 27): 12-R.

54. Arens, W. 1974. An Anthropologist Looks at the Rituals of Football. *New York Times* (November 16): 16.

55. Reynolds, D. 1993. Song of Himself. *Philadelphia Inquirer* (January 30): A-9.

56. Born or Bred? 1992. *Newsweek* (February 24): 46.

57. Lee, J., cited in Harris, M. 1981. *America Now: The Anthropology of a Changing Culture.* New York: Simon and Schuster, p. 101.

58. Pitts, B. 1988–1989. Beyond the Bars: The Development of Leisure Activity Management in the Lesbian and Gay Population in America. *Leisure Information Quarterly* (15): 3.

59. Johnson, K. 1998. Event Founded to Fight Bias Is Accused of It. *New York Times* (August 1): A-1.

60. Brooke, J. 1996. Gay Life Thrives Where Ballot Fight Began. *New York Times* (May 12): A-12.
61. Harris, *op. cit.* pp. 84–85.
62. Teen-Age Sex, after Magic. 1991. *U.S. News and World Report* (December 16): 90.
63. Saunders, N. 1998. Letter to Editor. *Philadelphia Inquirer* (August).
64. See Francke, L. 1997. In the Company of Wolves. *Time Magazine* (June 2): 38.
65. Finn, R. 1999. Growth in Women's Sports Stirs Harassment Issue. *New York Times* (March 7): 1.

9 Pastimes I: Sports in Contemporary Life

In the end, you always get back to this, back to the game itself. The extraordinary appeal of baseball, its astonishing hold on vast adult sections of this nation, may be disparaged, deplored, dismissed or accounted for with dozens of simple or intellectual explanations.

But in the last analysis, it is not the spectacle of the game, not its unplanned aesthetics, not the self-identification nor the hero-worship, not the capitalistic aspects of the sport nor the democratic aspects, not its pleasant summer setting nor home-town pride which make baseball so popular. It is the game itself.[1]

In what recreational pursuits do people take part in their free time? What motivations drive their participation, and what benefits do they seek to achieve? What are the most recent trends in popular play, within such major activity areas as sports and games, outdoor recreation, and travel and tourism?

This chapter and those that follow examine several major uses of leisure today, with emphasis on their role in organized programs presented by public, nonprofit, commercial, and other leisure-service agencies. Throughout, it will be evident that many of the traditional forms of sport and outdoor play have been transformed by technological change. Although many active pursuits continue in their original forms, increasingly they have become more complex and diversified, influenced by commercial factors, and designed to meet public demands for excitement, challenge, novelty, and risk.

Overview of Leisure Experiences

The pastimes that people enjoy in their leisure range widely from the most vigorous and demanding pursuits to others that are essentially passive and undemanding. Some are presented in a structured and highly organized form by varied community agencies, while others are enjoyed in a spontaneous self-directed way by individuals or families. When formally sponsored by a public, nonprofit, or commercial organization, leisure pursuits may fall within a variety of formats, such as free-play, instructional, competitive, special-event, or club settings.[2]

Motivations for Participation

As earlier chapters point out, the common understanding is that people engage in recreational activities chiefly to experience pleasure or fun or to find relaxation or escape. While these are certainly valuable outcomes of leisure involvement, research studies have shown that there are many other motivations that drive free-time participation. Such personal motivations include the following:

> The search for new experience, excitement, risk, or challenge
>
> The urge to explore new and different environments
>
> Health-related needs, such as the effort to improve one's health, fitness, or physique
>
> The need to gain a sense of personal accomplishment, growth, or significant achievement
>
> Competitive drives, not only in sports and games, but in other areas of personal performance
>
> The need for aesthetic involvement, creative expression, and intellectual growth
>
> Social urges related to friendship and group involvement
>
> Nostalgia for the past, as evidenced in collecting hobbies, interest in older forms of play, or reenactment of historical events
>
> Having a sense of purpose and contributing to community welfare, particularly in volunteer-service activities
>
> Being close to nature, as in outdoor recreation and environmental pursuits, often with a spiritual dimension

Given this broad range of leisure activities, experiences, and motivations, how *do* the bulk of Americans spend their free time? While there is obviously no single pattern of behavior, and leisure involvement is influenced by one's age, education, economic status, and similar factors, a number of studies have examined the free-time pursuits of the population at large. For example, Robinson and Godbey report the results of systematic time-use studies showing that:

> . . . of the almost 40 hours of free time per week which Americans average, only 2.2 are devoted to participation in outdoor recreation, active sports, hobbies, crafts, art, music, drama, games and other forms of recreation.
>
> Social activities such as attending sports events, going to the movies, parties, bars and lounges, and social visiting account for 6.7 hours per week. Religion and cultural events each take less than an hour per week. By far the largest time consumer

is television, with 15 hours per week (and another 5 hours per week as a secondary activity).[3]

Statistical reports of this type must be viewed with caution. Obviously, different groups within the population would yield markedly divergent reports of their leisure involvements, and regional, climatic, and seasonal factors would also influence the choice of activities. For example, the finding that free-time travel amounted to 3.1 hours per week would clearly be different during vacation periods of the year. It should also be emphasized that television—although it consumes a considerable amount of time—tends to have relatively little meaning or importance for many viewers. Instead, the experiences that affect people greatly, that linger in their memories, or that are truly important in their lives tend to be active, creative activities. Gray and Ibrahim write:

> Recreation is a cluster of human experiences of great range and subtlety. Among them are some fleeting impressions that fit the popular stereotype—pleasurable for the amount and soon gone. But we have found when people are asked to recount their most memorable recreation experiences [they often recall] events of extraordinary personal meaning. These experiences are so significant that they are often a part of the personal identity of the individual and so memorable they last a lifetime.[4]

With this in mind, we now examine several categories of leisure involvement that do have significant meaning for participants, and that are linked to other important elements in national life, such as educational and economic implications, racial and gender factors, and even international relationships. The first of these categories includes sports and games.

Sports as Leisure Pursuit

In a brief definition, Allen Guttmann suggests that there are three essential features that distinguish sports from other related activities, such as games or fitness pursuits. These are that sports are physical activities demanding exertion and skill; that they involve a contest or competition; and that they have both formal rules and informal standards of etiquette and fair play. The term *athletics* is often used synonymously with *sports*, but tends to be applied more often to organized team sports on school, college, and professional levels, than to individual lifetime sports like golf, tennis, and skiing.[5]

Although sports are obviously an important form of free-time activity, in many ways they do not conform to the traditional view of leisure. Rather than relaxed activity carried on within a context of casual free choice, sports are often highly structured, purposeful, and disciplined, with elaborate rules and rich rewards. At the same time, sports represent an important social institution, recognized as such not only in the United States but around the world.

From any perspective, it must be recognized that sports represent far more than trivial amusement or children's play in American society. Any enterprise that involves hundreds of billions of dollars in equipment and facilities, personnel costs, admissions charges, television fees, and other forms of expenditure must be based on more than superficial appeal. Of all types of leisure involvement, it seems likely that sports command the highest degree of personal interest and emotional involvement—both for those who participate actively in them and those who are part of a vast army of fans of school, college, and professional teams.

Sports represent almost a religion today, in terms of the public's worship of leading athletes as folk heroes. They are closely linked to such social phenomena as politics, warfare, and big business, and citizens see their cities' reputations rise or fall depending on the fortunes of their professional teams. Alumni of colleges and universities contribute to athletic support and follow their schools' teams avidly throughout their lifetimes.

Scope of Participation

Most recreational sports have gained steadily in participation over the past several decades. For example, amateur softball play increased from 16 million participants in 1970 to 42 million in 1996; golf play rose from 11.2 million in 1970 to 24.7 million in 1996. Tenpin bowling increased from 62.5 million participants in 1975 to 91 million in 1996.[6] In terms of attendance at college and professional sports events, the number of spectators has risen steadily as well (see Table 9.1).

In secondary schools, there are millions of boys and girls playing on intramural and intrascholastic teams. The most popular sports for boys are eleven-man football, basketball, outdoor track and field, and baseball—with between 13,000 and 17,000 schools sponsoring each of these sports. Among girls' teams, basketball, outdoor track and field, volleyball, and softball rank in popularity in that order.

In addition to school, college, and professional leagues, millions of sports participants are served by municipal, county, or special-district recreation and park departments, nonprofit youth organizations (many of which focus on a single sport, such as Little League or Biddy Basketball), industrial sports leagues, country clubs, and military recreation services. In general, the management of sports events, the setting of standards and rules for play, and similar functions are carried out by national organizations that govern competition and promote instructional programs for youth.

As a single example of the popularity of youth sports, in the mid-1990s, 196,000 teams competed in Little League games in ninety-one nations. With over three million players—chiefly boys—participating, the Little League World Series held in August in Williamsport, Pennsylvania was the climax of 16,000 tournament games played by 7000 all-star teams over a six-week period.

Among American youth 12 years and younger, the most popular team sports in the mid-1990s were basketball (9.7 million), soccer (7.7 million), softball (5.3 million), baseball (5.1 million), and volleyball (5 million).[7]

At every level, ranging from youth sports to major companies competing against each other in baseball, softball, flag football, or bowling, or Senior Olympics involving thousands of elderly men and women continuing to play in their seventies and eighties, sports represent a major preoccupation today (see Table 9.2). In Philadelphia, for example, in the closing hours of summer days, the city parks' grass and clay diamonds are crowded with

TABLE 9.1   Selected Spectator Sports Attendance: 1985 to 1996

Sport	Unit	1985	1990	1996
Baseball, major leagues	1000	47,742	55,512	61,565
Basketball				
NCAA—Men's college				
teams	Number	753	767	866
Attendance	1000	26,584	28,741	28,525
NCAA—Women's college				
teams	Number	746	782	874
Attendance	1000	2,072	3,397	5,234
Professional teams	Number	23	27	29
Attendance	1000	11,534	18,586	21,797
Players' salaries—				
average	$1000	325	817	2,100
Football				
NCAA college teams	Number	509	533	566
Attendance	1000	34,952	35,330	36,083
National Football				
League—attendance	1000	14,058	17,666	(NA)
National Hockey League				
Regular season attendance	1000	11,621	12,344	16,237
Horse-racing				
Attendance	1000	73,346	63,803	43,365
Parimutuel turnover	Mil.dol.	12,222	7,162	14,902

Sources: Statistical Abstract of the United States, 1997 and 1998. NA means Not Available.

company teams—throwbacks to the days when people who worked together played together regularly. Leagues for law offices, banks, insurance companies, and advertising agencies fill softball fields nightly, from Monday through Thursday:

> Executives, bigwigs, secretaries, technicians and clerks; men and women; the highly paid, the lowly paid and the overpaid—all brandish their leather gloves and back-turned ball caps, dig their cleats into the dirt, take their swings and make their plays. Shipping clerks cover the outfield alongside six-figure-salaried managers. . . .[8]

Beyond team sports, however, an immense range of individual and dual sports, as well as competitive activities linked to outdoor recreation and aquatics, also represent

TABLE 9.2   Participation in Selected Sports and Fitness Activities: 1994 (For persons 7 years of age or older, based on survey of 10,000 households. In thousands).

Activity	All Persons	Male	Female
Total	232,986	113,093	119,892
Aerobic exercising	23,200	4,435	18,764
Badminton	5,424	2,413	3,011
Baseball	15,096	12,254	2,842
Basketball	28,191	20,492	7,699
Bowling	37,356	19,544	17,812
Calisthenics	8,536	3,634	4,902
Exercise walking	70,794	25,491	45,344
Exercising with equipment	43,784	21,173	22,611
Football	15,574	13,203	2,371
Golf	24,551	18,662	5,889
Racqetball	5,340	3,971	1,369
Running/jogging	20,640	11,981	8,659
Soccer	12,508	8,223	4,284
Softball	18,143	10,162	7,982
Swimming	60,277	28,960	31,317
Table tennis	7,817	4,965	2,852
Tennis	11,590	6,535	5,055
Volleyball	17,383	8,492	8,891

Source: National Sporting Goods Association and *Statistical Abstract of the United States, 1997.* Reports participation at least once in preceding year. See also *Table 10.1*, p. 241.

important leisure pursuits, as shown in Figure 9.1, with examples of sponsorship roles of public and nonprofit organizations.

Historical Perspectives on Sport

William Baker points out that almost every sport in the modern world is a refinement of physical contests originating in ancient and medieval times. Evolved from primitive hunting and warring pursuits necessary for survival, competitive athletics took the form of religious rituals in early pre-Christian cultures. These societies, he writes, developed precise standards of status, age, and gender for participants in their various cultic games.[9]

In the Middle Ages, peasant games like bowls were taken from rough grounds and rainy outdoors into the homes of the nobility and transformed into new games like "shovel-board" (shuffleboard) and billiards, played on a tabletop. A number of different sports were traditionally played on religious holidays such as Christmas and Easter during the Middle Ages and the Renaissance. As evidence of the historical linkage of religion and sport, in Mexico and other Central American countries, ball games were played with specific ceremonial purposes in stone courtyards that were part of temple complexes.

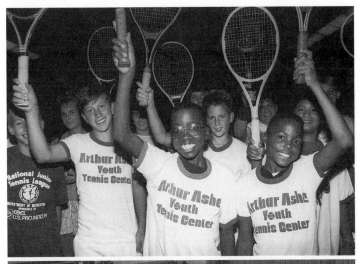

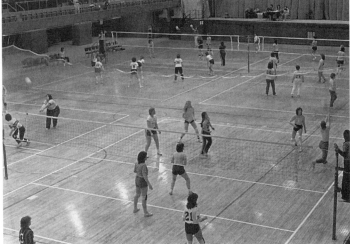

Sports appeal to participants of all ages and many backgrounds. Tennis is enjoyed by young players at Arthur Ashe Youth Tennis Center in Philadelphia. Women engage in volleyball competition in Westchester County, New York, and the Hershey corporation sponsors a national track and field youth program for thousands of young athletes.

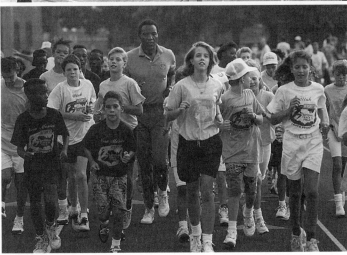

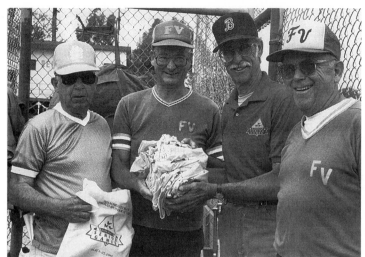

Older men enjoy softball competition in Long Beach, California Senior Olympics, while young soccer players compete in Orlando, Florida Morale, Welfare and Recreation program and in clinics sponsored by America Youth Soccer Association. Junior high school girls in Minnesota learn to officiate in Minnesota youth sports leagues.

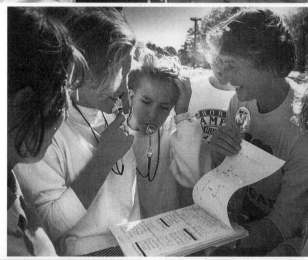

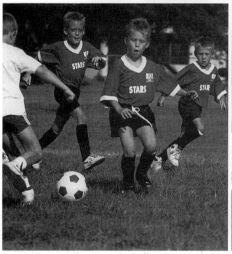

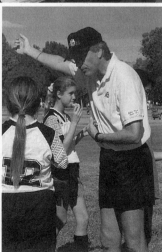

ADULT SPORTS

Aquatics and Sports Office, 4700 E. 10th St., 439-0213

The Aquatics and Sports Office offers a multitude of recreation team sport activities for all levels. Year-round play for participants 18 and older occurs throughout the city, weeknights and weekends. Enter your friends, neighborhood and co-workers into a league below. **CONTACT THE AQUATICS AND SPORTS OFFICE FOR REGISTRATION INFORMATION.**

The following information applies to the 6" and under, Men's Night and Advanced League for Women: Register by team only at the Aquatics & Sports Office: Long Beach resident teams, **$246,** *12/7-12/30; Long Beach business-sponsored teams,* **$276,** *12/14-12/30; Non-resident, non-Long Beach sponsored teams,* **$306,** *12/21-12/30. League begins in January.*

Basketball - 6" and Under League. Adult Men. Unclassified league. Teams consist of players 6" or shorter. Each team may have one player no taller than 6'3". Play on Saturdays at local High School gyms.

Basketball - Men's Night League. Adult Men. Consists of 5-12 players in four classifications. Recreational to former high school and collegiate. Two officials per game. Ten-game season, one night per week, M-Th, at local schools. A maximum of 48 teams can be accepted.

Basketball - Advanced League for Women. Adult Women. Recreational level players join former high school and collegiate players in this unique and highly skilled program. Teams play a ten-game league and playoff schedule. Games played Friday evenings at Pan Am gym. Two officials assigned to each game.

Basketball - Bayshore 3 on 3 Tournament. Adults. Men's Open 3 on 3 takes place on Sept. 12. Teams are guaranteed a minimum of five games. Call the Aquatics and Sports Office for registration information. **Cost is $51/team.**

PADDLE TENNIS (Beg)   **10yrs-adult**   **$42**
Basics of the forehand and backhand , volleys, serve and overhead, focusing primarily on the doubles game and the rules and regulations that apply. Must bring unopened can of tennis balls to first class. Instructor: Rexroad.
6497   Sa   9-10 am   9/26-11/14 Bayshore Playground

PADDLE TENNIS (Int)   **10yrs-adult**   **$42**
For those with experience or accomplished tennis players. Learn topspin,

Sunday Baseball Winter Mini League. Adult. Register by team only at the Aquatics & Sports Office: Long Beach resident teams, **$335,** 10/19-11/13; Long Beach business-sponsored teams, **$435,** 10/26-11/13; Non-resident, non-Long Beach sponsored teams, **$535,** 11/2-11/13. League runs Su, 11 a.m.-10 p.m. League begins in December.

Softball - Saturday Slowpitch League. Adult Men. 10-15 players in open classification. 10 games and playoffs. Register by team only at the Aquatics & Sports Office: Long Beach resident teams, **$263,** 11/30-12/18; Long Beach business-sponsored teams, **$303,** 12/7-12/18; and non-resident teams, **$343,** 12/14-12/18. League January 9, 1993.

Softball - Senior Saturday Slowpitch League. 55 and over. 10-15 players in Major and Minor Classifications. 16-game schedule. Register by team only at the Aquatics & Sports Office: Long Beach resident teams, **$184,** 10/12-10/30; Long Beach business-sponsored teams, **$224,** 10/19-10/30; and non-resident teams, **$264,** 10/26-10/30. League begins November 14, 1992.

Softball - Seniors Open. 55 and over. Slowpitch softball in recreational league structures year-round. Sunday play for all participants with informal teams. Wednesday batting and fielding practice. Play begins 9 a.m. at Joe Rodgers Field, corner of 10th St. and Park Ave. Register at the field or contact the Aquatics & Sports Office.

Softball - Senior Slowpitch Tournament. 55 and over. 10-15 players in this Senior Olympics event on Nov. 7-8. **Fee is $261/team.**

Volleyball - Bayshore Doubles Tournament. Ages 18 and up. Women's and Men's "A" Divisions. **Fee is $28/team** and tournament runs on Sept. 19 & 20. Call the Aquatics and Sports Office for more details.

The following information applies to Coed, Men's and Women's Volleyball Leagues: Register by team only at the Aquatics & Sports Office: Long Beach resident teams, **$202,** *10/26-11/13; Long Beach business-sponsored teams,* **$242,** *11/2-11/13; Non-resident, non-Long Beach sponsored teams,* **$282,** *11/9-11/13.*

Volleyball - Coed League. Adult. Indoor play at Pan Am gym and local middle schools. Beginner, advanced novice, intermediate, advanced intermediate and advanced leagues of 10 matches and playoffs. Each match has an official assigned.

Volleyball - Men's League. Adult Men. Indoor play on Tuesdays. Intermediate and advanced leagues of 10 matches and playoffs. Each match has an official assigned.

Volleyball - Women's League. Adult Women. Indoor play on Tuesdays. Intermediate and advance leagues of 10 matches and playoffs. Each match has an official assigned.

TENNIS (Int)   **16yrs-adult**   **$40**
Fee includes use of night lights. Participants must provide racquet and new can of unopened tennis balls. Instructors: Dennis/B.J. King, Delpino/El Dorado and Jenkins/Scherer.

6467	M/W	6:30-8 pm	9/28-10/28	B.J. King Tennis Ctr
6477	M/W	6:30-8 pm	11/4-12/4	B.J. King Tennis Ctr
6469	M/W	8-9:30 pm	9/28-10/28	Scherer Tennis Cts
6470	M/W	8-9:30 pm	11/4-12/4	Scherer Tennis Cts
6471	Tu/Th	8:30-10 pm	10/6-11/5	El Dorado Tennis Ctr
6472	Tu/Th	8:30-10 pm	11/10-12/22	El Dorado Tennis Ctr

The **American Youth Soccer Organization**'s mission is to develop and deliver quality youth soccer programs where everyone builds positive character through participation in a fun family environment based on the AYSO philosophies:

Everyone Plays
Every child, regardless of talent, plays at least half of every game.

Balanced Teams
Each AYSO program distributes skilled and less skilled players evenly throughout all teams.

Open Registration
AYSO has signups, not tryouts. Every child may register to play.

Positive Coaching
AYSO promotes coaching through encouragement rather than criticism.

Sportsmanship
AYSO has active programs aimed at creating good sports on the field and on the sidelines.

Coaching Program

Because "Positive Coaching" is one of AYSO's guiding philosophies, coach training is one of our highest priorities. AYSO also provides a wide range of courses to continue instructing its volunteer coaches.

No Experience? No Problem!
Our volunteer coaches receive complete training right from the beginning!

✔ *Certification and licensing* for all coaches.

✔ *Youth, Intermediate, and Advanced coaching courses* provide training for coaches of every level of experience.

✔ Complete with manuals, handouts and outlines that are continually reviewed and updated.

We Don't Stop There!
✔ Supplemental local instruction programs, *camps and clinics.*

✔ Held throughout the country, throughout the year.

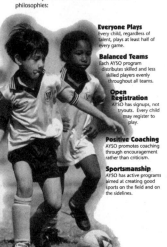
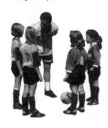

FIGURE 9.1 Many community groups sponsor sports for all ages. Public recreation and park agencies, as in Long Beach, California (above) offer instruction, leagues, and tournaments in varied individual and team sports. Organizations like AYSO (American Youth Soccer Organization) promote individual sports with coaching, officiating, administrative, and risk management services (left).

However, during much of this period sports were also condemned by religious authorities in Europe or had an unsavory reputation because of their linkage with gambling, drinking, and other forms of illicit play.

In time team sports gained respectability in England and America as the concept of "muscular Christianity" entered the literature and began to be heard in religious sermons. Churches, YMCAs, and educators all encouraged sports as a means of achieving physical fitness and self-discipline and as an alternative to other forms of dissipation in play. Gradually, sports became dominated by commercial interests, and the manufacture of sporting goods evolved into a successful industry. Hardy writes:

> Through their involvement with such nascent governing bodies as the National League, the Intercollegiate Football Association, and the United States Lawn Tennis Association, sporting goods firms helped turn informal activities into commodities of fun and spectacle. This collaboration set the foundation for an even larger sports industry; an interlocking network of the rules committees, trade associations, manufacturers, and professional groups that have heavily influenced both the range and styles of sports in America.[10]

The decade of the 1920s marked a spectacular growth of interest in sports in America, with the building of huge stadiums and expansion of college and professional competition. Star athletes became national heroes in baseball, boxing, golf, and football. Behind these public idols were shrewd promoters and managers, along with a host of sports journalists and broadcasters who helped to popularize them. In newspapers and magazines, on radio, and even in motion pictures, the heroic feats of athletes were celebrated.

Later, in the 1950s and 1960s, the widespread presentation of college, professional, and international sports events on television meant (1) that the enthusiastic audience for sports expanded tremendously, and (2) that the huge advertising revenues from television sponsors led to the growth of professional leagues and heightened the pressure to win on all levels.

Sport as Folk Religion.   Today, so popular are high school college and professional sports that many scholars have concluded that they have become America's newest folk religion. One such observer, Professor Charles Prebish of Pennsylvania State University's religious studies program states:

> For growing numbers of Americans, sport religion has become a more appropriate expression of personal religiosity than Christianity, Judaism or any of the traditional religions. [Prebish cited] terms that athletes and sportswriters regularly use: *faith, ritual, ultimate, dedicated, sacrifice, peace, commitment, spirit.*[11]

Similarly, James Mathiesen, professor of sociology at Wheaton College, an evangelical school in Illinois, comments that the collegiate bowl games and professional football's Super Bowl spectacular are "in fact, a ritual expression . . . communicating a secular religion of the American dream. If I were to show a visitor to the United States a single, recurring event which has come to characterize folk religion, the Super Bowl would be it."[12]

He goes on to point out that the Super Bowl is strategically located in the calendar year as part of a sequence of religious and lay holidays—Thanksgiving, Hanukkah, Christmas, New Year's Day, and others—along with an array of sports and games that provide entertainment and ritualistic celebration. "What is sacred and what is secular?" Mathiesen asks. "Does it matter for most Americans?"

The linkage of sport with religion was illustrated in a popular country music record that equated football with the game of life, in a religious allegory. Jesus was the head coach, and "Average Christian" was the quarterback. The idea was that if Christians followed their heavenly blockers they would make it safely to the big end zone in the sky. A later country singer recorded a hit song with the plea, "Drop kick me, Jesus, through the goal posts of life."

Numerous professional and college athletes are members of the Fellowship of Christian Athletes and similar associations, and other competitors. Teams hold prayer circles on the field, and sports evangelists are trained at a number of Bible colleges.

Although one may question the actual religious character of organized sport, it clearly represents a significant form of ritual in American life. Kendall Blanchard points out that collective rituals have six primary properties: repetition, acting, stylization, order, evocative presentational style or staging, and a collective dimension or social message.[13] Sports, with their singing of the national anthem, presentation of players and coaches, formal handshakes, organized cheering, and sacrificial moments (when players are injured and carried off the field), are clearly secular rituals.

Role of Spectators.   Historian Allen Guttmann tells how thousands of spectators cheered gladiatorial contests and chariot races in ancient Rome, and how different classes viewed sports events during the medieval and Renaissance periods in Europe. He points out that respectable middle-class members avoided most sporting events until the mid-nineteenth century, when private clubs, schools, and colleges began conducting rowing, track, and cricket and football matches, and safe and comfortable stands and stadiums began to be built.

A unique example of the emotional investment that many fans make in their favorite teams was cited several years ago when a group of physicians carried out an inquiry into the habits of British soccer crowds. They found that many middle-aged, industrious men who were normally models of behavior at work and at home turned into violent and abusive fans at soccer matches; there were numerous reported cases of husbands coming home after a losing game and beating their wives severely. So excited do many American sports fans become that heart attacks have become increasingly frequent at college and professional football games.

Beyond such traumatic outcomes, many fans become so involved with their teams that they visit them at spring practice, travel with them to distant games, wear special costumes, or adopt special cheers to root them to victory. An example was the Hogettes, a band of middle-aged, paunchy, bald businessmen and professionals who wore outrageous wigs, too-tight dresses, and molded rubber hog snouts over their noses while cheering wildly from seats behind the Washington Redskins professional football team's bench.

However, sports clearly represent more than entertainment or light amusement. Instead, they are played for heavy stakes—not only in financial terms, with top professional athletes making many millions of dollars each year, but also in terms of possible injury and even death. Each year, a number of major college or professional athletes are seriously crippled or paralyzed, and in sports such as auto racing deadly accidents are common.

Not surprisingly, sports have been an important element in terms of political ideology, competition among nations, and even as activities linked psychologically with warfare.

Sports and Nationalism

In several European nations during the period of growing nationalistic fervor and imperialist expansion during the latter half of the nineteenth century, sports were closely linked to military training and patriotic indoctrination. It was at this time that the first international sports contests were held between teams drawn from both bourgeois and aristocratic classes of European nations, while at the same time sports were used as a form of social control by channeling workers' energies and leisure time into sports imbued with such values as obedience, self-discipline, and teamwork.

In discussing the linkage of sports and political ideology, John Hoberman points out that in twentieth-century fascist and communist regimes, sports heroes were idealized, and political, military, and industrial workers all were depicted symbolically as athletic supermen. Grandiose and spectacular sports festivals were used for nationalistic purposes, with mass athletic demonstrations that displayed thousands of bodies in choreographed displays and athletic feats.[14] In Nazi Germany, the SS ideal of manhood was represented as a disciplined, perfectly formed, aggressive athlete, and the 1936 Olympics defeat in Berlin by the American black track star Jesse Owens was viewed as a major defeat.

In the Soviet Union, heroes of the Communist society were depicted as athletic supermen within a number of spheres: the Stakhanovites, or work-athletes, who accomplished brilliant feats in industry; the heroes of the stratosphere and Arctic expeditions; and workers driving underground shafts for the new Moscow subway.

For three decades, Iron Curtain countries like the Soviet Union, East Germany, and Romania subsidized their Olympic athletes generously, establishing elite schools (sometimes described as ruthless "sports factories") that selected children at an early age and groomed them intensively for world-class competition. The most advanced training methods, including both psychological conditioning and the use of steroids, were consistently employed.

In the late 1980s and early 1990s, the emphasis in international sport shifted from ideological and political goals to commercial ones. The United States Olympic effort became increasingly dominated by business sponsors of teams, lucrative television contracts, and star athletes making millions of dollars in advertising testimonials for running shoes, soft drinks, breakfast cereals, and other products. With the end of the Cold War, professional basketball and hockey teams in the United States began to sign star athletes from the former Soviet bloc, and basketball and football leagues were established in Europe. Commercial influence at the highest level was illustrated in 1999, when a major scandal of bribery and collusion surrounded the granting of the 2002 Winter Olympics to Salt Lake City, Utah, followed by similar charges regarding the selection of other cities for earlier Summer Games.

Role of Sports in American Education

When schools and colleges in the United States began to encourage team sports, it was assumed that sportsmanship, loyalty, unselfishness, integrity, and other desirable personal traits would be enhanced among student athletes.

In recent years, however, behavioral scientists have challenged these assumptions and found them wanting. Susan Greendorfer reviewed the literature on the outcomes of sport and found limited evidence supporting the view that sport helped athletes achieve upward mobility. She found that athletes tend to

> enter college with poorer academic background, receive lower grades, and have a relatively low probability of receiving an education or graduating compared to nonathletic peers. This is particularly true if they were on scholarship, were admitted with special consideration, or were in revenue-producing sports.[15]

She also summarized a number of recent studies showing that there was no proof that sports promote sharing, honesty, and altruism in children and youth. To the contrary, research suggested that competitive athletics tended to undermine prosocial behaviors, a finding reported by several studies of youth sports. Hellstedt acknowledges that many children gain from competitive sports play by having fun, making friends, and learning or improving skills. However, he cites three areas of negative outcomes, including low self-esteem, aggression, and excessive anxiety.[16] Similarly, Gelfand and Hartmann present data from several studies showing that in both laboratory and natural settings, strongly competitive athletic games lead to increased aggression and hostility in children.[17]

Despite such findings, there is a widely accepted belief that sports *do* contribute significantly to the lives of young athletes. In a discussion of the efforts being made to retain high school athletics in cities where school budgets had been cut sharply, Frank Lawlor points out that the vast majority of teenage competitors never get headlines, championships, or scholarships, but play simply for the love of the game. He continues:

> Surveys, in particular a broad 1989 study commissioned by the Women's Sports Foundation, show that high school athletes in almost every racial, social, and geographical category do better on standardized tests than nonathletes, achieve more in the classroom, and are more active in their communities when they leave school.[18]

As an example, he cites a study by the Minnesota State High School Athletic Association that showed that nonathletes in that state had an overall grade-point average of 2.39, while one-sport athletes had 2.61 and two-sport athletes had 2.82.

Wankel and Berger developed a four-part model of what are commonly considered to be the major areas of benefit from sports participation, including "personal enjoyment," "personal growth," "social harmony," and "social change."[19] However, within each of these categories, they concluded that it was not possible to assume that sport is automatically "good" or "bad," or that it routinely achieves certain outcomes. Instead, competitive athletics have the potential for achieving positive and negative outcomes, depending on the conditions under which they are carried on.

Frey and Massengale point out that the values associated with school and college sports reflect virtues that are generally approved in American society: striving for excellence, achievement, humility, loyalty, self-control, respect for authority, self-discipline, and deferred gratification. However, they conclude that, although athletic administrators profess to operate according to the goals and values of a participatory amateur sports model, in reality they are heavily influenced by professionalized sports practices.[20]

As a result, for decades there has been constant criticism of the leading team sports, ranging from the arrogant or lawless behavior of lavishly paid professional athletes to the violation of college athletic policies related to recruitment, eligibility, or academic performance. Charges that in schools and colleges today, the drive for sports victories and winning records has corrupted legitimate educational values are summed up by William Morgan:

> The signs of the degradation of sport are all around us. The mania for winning, the widespread cheating, the economic and political trivialization of sport, the thirst for crude sensationalism and eccentric spectacle, the manipulation by the mass media, the cult of athletic stars and celebrity, and the mindless bureaucratization are just some of the more ominous signs. These signs are too pervasive to deny, too steeped in our social milieu to pass off as anything other than social pathology . . .[21]

There are frequent charges that the negative elements in sport reach down into junior high and even elementary schools, in terms of the early recruitment of promising athletes at these levels, "coddling" them in terms of academic performance, or the growing practice of youth sports camps subsidized by major equipment manufacturers that serve as the first step in developing budding stars for college and professional careers.

Other attacks on youth sports criticize the high degree of pressure placed on young athletes in community sports leagues, with parents often driving their sons and daughters excessively and sometimes violently confronting rival coaches or officials. Given such pressures, recent studies have shown that many youngsters abandon organized sports at an early age because they fail to meet their true recreational needs for fun, positive group experience and a reasonable level of competition.

Promising Trends in Youth Sports Leadership

Yet, many parents and sports leaders are concerned with ensuring that the athletic experiences of their children contribute meaningfully to their overall development. Several national organizations have developed philosophy statements and guidelines for the constructive management of youth sports activities, including the principles of Child-Centered Coaching shown in Figure 9.2.

Philosophy of Sports

The functional and primary purpose of sports is to build positive self-worth, teach cooperative play, promote a sense of accomplishment through building athletic skills, engage children in spirited, fun, and friendly competitive play, and to foster the belief that trying one's best to succeed is as important in sports as it is in life. Hence, children are the center and the primary reason why the youth games are played.

Overemphasis on Winning

Winning is an attitude. The best athletes are the individuals who have developed a winning attitude to complement their athletic skills. A "winning at all costs" attitude puts performance as the primary concern, not children. While this attitude may reflect the state of sports at the professional level, placing a "winning at all costs" emphasis on youth sports has several major drawbacks.

Winning as Everything

1. Sets unrealistic expectations which lead to predictable feelings of failure.
2. Increases stress which reduces optimal performance.
3. Does not prepare athletes to deal with loss in a healthy way.
4. Stresses competition aimed at beating opponent—not at improving performance.
5. A focus on winning is also a focus on losing.
6. Takes the fun out of the game.
7. Only one winner—everyone else is a loser.

Winning as Secondary

1. Emotional and physical well being of the child is the main focus—not winning.
2. Optimal performance increases when trying one's best is stressed as the goal in sports.
3. Deemphasizing winning reduces stress to "have to win." Consequently, optimal performance is improved.
4. Winning is important as an attitude—not as the ultimate outcome.
5. Athletes, coaches, and parents can relax, enjoy the game, have fun, and applaud excellent performances of players on both teams.

FIGURE 9.2   *Guidelines for Youth Sports.* Published by National Institute for Child-Centered Coaching, Park City, Utah.

A number of examples of school systems or state educational authorities that sought to develop experimental approaches to managing youth sports were cited in the national press during the 1990s.

Plainfield, Indiana, Middle School.   In this unusual school, policies have been instituted that ensure that every child has a chance to participate in sport and other cocurricular activities, regardless of his or her ability. While all members of all teams and clubs are exposed to high expectations and a strong work ethic, with few exceptions no student is ever cut from a club or team:

The uncoordinated can be on the football team. The unmusical can be in the band. Anyone at all can be a cheerleader or serve on the student council . . . [While] the best football players get the most playing time, just as they do everywhere, hard-working scrubs get in for at least a few plays as a payback for effort.[22]

Anniston, Alabama. Often, such new policies are controversial. In Anniston, Alabama, where successful sports records had been linked to the failing performance of student athletes on standardized tests and the state accreditation bureau placed the Anniston High School on academic "caution" that might lead to a take-over by the state, a new "no pass/no play" rule was put into effect. While stricter grade standards that barred failing students from play led to mass protests by citizens, students walking out of school in protest, a skeletonized football team, and shorter basketball season, most students admitted that the policy was good for them in the long run.[23]

Massachusetts Youth Soccer Association. Similarly, when the Massachusetts Youth Soccer Association initiated a new policy—that all tournament games involving players under 10 would have no winners or losers, with trophies not allowed unless every player on a team received one—it was subjected to widespread criticism and even ridicule.

Nonetheless, on every level, efforts continue to reform youth sports. Realistically, it must be recognized that problems affecting such programs are part of a larger whole, with college sports competition influencing policy on all levels. Frey and Massengale argue that college sports are so entrenched, so "paranoid" about the edge in competition, so dependent on external constituencies, so enamored of their position of power and prestige that serious attempts to restructure the system would be vehemently resisted. How did this situation come about, and what are its implications?

Background of Intercollegiate Sports

As shown earlier, many American colleges and universities began to support sports clubs and intercollegiate competition in the second half of the nineteenth century. College deans and presidents felt that athletics, particularly football, were invaluable in building the visibility, enrollment, and reputation of their institutions. Rader writes:

Even the older, more prestigious institutions of the Northeast turned to football as a means of recruiting students. . . . [They] also found that football developed an alumni loyalty that was far more profound than fond memories of chapels, classrooms, pranks, or professors. "You do not remember whether Thorpwright was valedictorian or not," wrote a young college alumnus in 1890, "but you can never forget that glorious run of his in the football game."[24]

However, almost from the outset, there was severe criticism of the growing emphasis on collegiate sports, particularly football. In 1883 the Harvard Committee on Athletics declared that football was "no longer governed by a manly spirit of fair play" and had become dominated by "a spirit of sharpers and roughs." At the turn of the century,

Woodrow Wilson, then president of Princeton University, said, "So far as colleges go, the sideshows have swallowed up the circus, and we in the main tent do not know what is going on." In 1929, in a report entitled *American College Athletics*, the Carnegie Foundation for the Advancement of Teaching spoke of:

> demoralization of the college and of academic work, dishonesty, betting and gambling, professionalism, recruiting and subsidizing, the employment and payment of the wrong kind of men as coaches, the evil effects of college athletics upon school athletics, the roughness and brutality of football, extravagant expenditures of money and the general corruption of youth by the monster of athleticism.[25]

College basketball became the nation's most scandal-ridden sport when New York City became the hub of big-time college basketball during the 1930s and 1940s, with Madison Square Garden hosting major tournaments and bringing in the top teams from around the country. However, after a major point-fixing scandal involving players from seven colleges and the criminal prosecution of athletes and gamblers, New York's preeminence in college basketball declined, and state universities throughout the country began to fill the vacuum left by Madison Square Garden's discontinuance of big-time double-headers. In the 1960s and 1970s, they built over eighty huge new fieldhouses, many seating over 10,000 spectators, scheduled major intersectional tournaments, and intensified recruitment of star prospects. Basketball soon rivaled football for its flagrant violation of the rules of intercollegiate sport.

Through the 1970s and 1980s, the abuses of college sports continued to be widely publicized. A study conducted by the American Council on Education cited such practices of overzealous coaches, alumni, or athletic "boosters" as:

> Altering high school transcripts; threatening to bomb the home of a high school principal who refused to alter transcripts; changing admission test scores; offering jobs to parents or other relatives of a prospect; firing from a state job the father of a prospect who enrolled elsewhere than the state's university; promising one package of financial aid and delivering another; tipping or otherwise paying athletes who perform particularly well on a given occasion.[26]

There was little surprise or shock when the Washington Redskins' defensive end, Dexter Manley, was shown to have attended Oklahoma State University for four years without receiving a degree or having learned to read. One of the schools most frequently cited for its violations of athletic policy was the University of Nevada at Las Vegas, where it was almost impossible to control players' contact with professional gamblers. Their lives were not like those of other students:

> Like student athletes at many other schools, UNLV's players often arrive on campus with severe reading problems, poor study skills and swollen egos. They practice as much as four hours a day, seven days a week, and miss 30 to 40 days of classes

because of road games. During their absence, notetakers are hired to attend class for them. All players are required to attend a two-hour study hall after practice, but some are so exhausted they can barely keep their eyes open.[27]

In 1999, several University of Minnesota basketball players were suspended when it was found that course papers had been written for them by academic "advisors."

Policing College Sports.   The task of enforcing amateur athletic standards in colleges and universities is assigned to the National Collegiate Athletic Association (NCAA), which has sought for decades to crack down on recruitment and other athletic abuses. The NCAA has been described as an immensely wealthy organization with an operating budget of $168 million in a recent year, derived chiefly from television contracts, ticket sales, and government grants. Charged with enforcing amateur athletic policies at 847 institutions of higher learning, it has a small and poorly trained enforcement staff. Penalties are meted out by an NCAA panel, the "infractions committee," based on highly complicated rules and lacking in precise application.

In 1983, the NCAA voted at its national convention to adopt Proposition 48, requiring athletes to score a combined minimum of 700 out of a possible 1600 points on Scholastic Aptitude Tests—the equivalent of a generous D. Athletes who failed to reach the 700 mark might be "partial qualifiers"—eligible for a full athletic scholarship, but forbidden to practice with the team or suit up for a game until they had passed some eight courses. In 1985, the NCAA President's Commission urged a set of reforms to strengthen the role of the association, which had historically been dominated by athletic directors and coaches. At the instigation of 213 college presidents who attended the meeting, NCAA delegates voted overwhelmingly to apply more severe penalties to schools that chronically broke its rules and to give presidents more authority over athletic budgets. In 1989, NCAA rules governing academic eligibility were tightened with a new Proposition 42, and a number of college coaches denounced the association for its actions by claiming that the new, higher admission standards were aimed at black athletes, to prevent them from "dominating" college sports. Finally, in 1999, a federal court in Philadelphia discarded *all* NCAA minimum test score requirements for athletic scholarship eligibility, concluding that they discriminated against African Americans.[28]

What is ironic is that the public at large does not seem to care about the scandals and corruption that have afflicted school and college athletics. At the same time, it is also ironic that financial support is being increasingly withdrawn from the low-visibility sports, such as wrestling, fencing, or crew, which do not draw huge audiences or public interest, but which clearly represent amateur participation for its own sake. As an example, in February 1992, Cornell University announced over $600,000 in athletic department budget cuts, which would eliminate entirely four sports (men's and women's gymnastics and fencing), and would force four other non-revenue programs (nationally ranked men's and women's equestrian polo, men's lightweight football, and men's squash) to depend entirely on their own fund raising.

Yet, it is widely agreed that such sports are invaluable in terms of meeting the true educational goals of character development, fitness, preparation of lifetime leisure skills, and socialization. Beyond this, they are invariably far less expensive than the big-name sports. For example, a university professor did a study during the budget-cutting process that showed that Wisconsin spent an average of $45,000 a year on each football player, $30,000 on each women's basketball player, $17,000 on each tennis player and $400 on each rower. Only the men's rowers won a national championship.

With few exceptions—such as the colleges in the Ivy League, where athletics are administered within a framework of academic purpose and general scholarly restraint—college sports continue to be torn by morally conflicted values.

Many sports analysts suggest that underlying the problem today is the influence of television, which has sharply increased the revenues going to major colleges with winning records in football and basketball, particularly those playing in bowl games or key tournaments. With coaches' jobs depending on winning, many take the position that they are more likely to be fired for losing records than for violations of NCAA rules. The paradox is that the assumption that all colleges are getting rich from sports is a myth.

> Robert Atwell, president of the American Council on Education [states] "They are not." In fact, most universities lose money on their athletic programs. "Over 90 percent of the schools in [big-time college sports] are in deficit budgets," says Frank Windegger, athletic director at Texas Christian University.[29]

Realistically, major college football has become an important part of the national entertainment industry. Both its risks and potential earnings are high. For example, in the late 1990s, the University of Michigan, a member of the Big 10, earned $2.1 million in television revenue for the eleven or twelve games that it played each season, and nearly $1 million for radio rights, plus $13.5 million from gate receipts and varied smaller sums from food, program, and merchandise concessions.

However, with the costs of building and maintaining huge stadiums, along with groundskeeping, insurance, equipment, transportation, scholarships, and salaries for coaches, recruiters, trainers, and other employees amounting to many millions each year, a number of colleges and universities have abandoned football. For those who continue it or who initiate new programs, the goal often is more than purely financial. Instead, in the words of the chairman of the trustees at Ohio State University, football is used for "friend-raising and fund-raising." In the midst of an $850 million campaign, the entertainment value of football kept the university's name before the public.

Sport as Commercial Enterprise

Everything that has been discussed in this chapter—sport as popular pastime, international sports competition, and school and college athletics—is rooted in the fact that sports represent a universally popular form of diversion that is heavily marketed to the public at large.

Television's Role

As indicated, a major source of revenue for team owners and players comes from television and radio contracts for broadcasting games and fees for commercial advertising. Richard Zoglin points out that television coverage has contributed immensely to the popularity of sports by making it possible for the public to find some sort of athletic competition in progress at almost any hour of the day or night. At the same time, television has entailed a sort of Faustian bargain in its impact on the packaging of sports. Zoglin writes:

> TV is a double-edged sword for colleges. Media exposure brings attention and dollars into the coffers. But it also stretches out games and seasons, wreaks havoc with schedules and helps boost the importance of sports at the expense of academics. . . . The lure of lucrative TV contracts also contributes to a win-at-all-costs mentality that can lead to recruitment scandals and other abuses. . . .[30]

The initial coverage of sports by television was modest. Limited to the small screen, it tended to emphasize such indoor sports as wrestling, prizefighting, and the Roller Derby, which became highly theatricalized spectacles, rather than genuine sports contests. The later era of sports coverage, beginning in the 1970s, featured extensive television contracts for team sports, with new cable networks and superstations employing transmission satellites. With many more games and dramatically increased revenues, television influenced both the players and the audiences. Rader writes:

> The moguls of sports quickly began to package their games so that they would be even more appealing to television. To obtain a larger share of the new largesse, athletes organized unions, held strikes, and sought assistance in the court system. The battle of the networks expedited the professionalization of the amateur sports of college basketball and football, of track and field, and of school sports.[31]

At the same time, by overwhelming the viewer with excessive images and leading fans to expect only the best, television undermined the essential appeal of sports and their ability to truly release people from the boredom of daily life. Rader sums up its impact:

> With its enormous power to magnify and distort images, to reach every hamlet in the nation with events from anywhere in the world, and to pour millions of additional dollars into sports, television . . . has sacrificed much of the unique drama of sports to the requirements of entertainment. . . . [It] has swamped viewers with too many seasons, too many games, too many teams, and too many big plays. Such a flood of sensations has diluted the poignancy and potency of the sporting experience.[32]

Through the 1990s, advertising revenues continued to climb, with growing evidence that professional sports teams were heading for harder times, with new free-agent rulings permitting athletes to initiate bidding wars that result in multi-year contracts for several million dollars a year—in some cases for players who are little more than average.

In the early 1990s, McCarroll pointed out that baseball in particular was beginning to strike out financially:

> After years of booming ticket sales, record profits and lucrative television contracts, major league baseball has fallen into a slump. Stadium attendance is flat, payrolls are climbing, and revenues are on the decline. . . . There are even rumors of one or two franchises going bankrupt within the next few years.[33]

In the mid- and late-1990s, this prediction became a reality as in one major sport after another conflicts between players, players' unions, and team owners led to protracted negotiations over salary caps and free-agent contract policies. Baseball suffered from a painful strike that closed down a season and the World Series, and in 1998, basketball endured a lengthy lockout. With the building of elaborate new stadiums with skyboxes for wealthy patrons, and with escalating ticket prices, along with some team owners requiring spectators to pay costly license fees to be permitted to buy season tickets, many angry fans began to lose interest. In some cities, baseball enthusiasts turned to watching or attending minor league games that had much of the atmosphere and fun of old-time, traditional competition.

Despite such warning signs, it seems clear that college and professional teams will continue to represent a major form of sports enterprise in the years ahead. At the same time, there are numerous other examples of athletics being marketed to the public at large through innovative products and services. For example, while gambling on sports is illegal in most states, dispensing information on gambling is not. Thus, throughout the country, dozens of "tout" services that make use of the 900 lines for telephone advice on sports gambling (with names such as "Rolls-Royce selection" or "Diamond-studded play") have become a multi-million-dollar industry. In the late 1990s, the Internet began to be used more widely for betting on college and professional sports.

An immensely popular sideline for many athletes is selling their baseball-card rights to trading-card companies. In the 1950s, the value of baseball cards was in the dreams and visions of youth as they traded cards and completed collections of their favorite players and teams. By the late 1980s, baseball-card collecting had ballooned into a $50 million industry. Linked to card collecting are sports memorabilia shows, where fans and their children buy and sell autographs, publications, gloves, bats, and other baseball-connected items. Under the licensing agreements signed in the early 1990s by the Major League Baseball Players Association, every big-leaguer—from top stars to raw rookies—earned thousands of dollars from the sale of cards, figurines, and the like. Indeed, it was reported in 1993 that college merchandising of their names, insignia, and colors for sports equipment and clothing had been growing by 25 to 30 percent a year and had reached $1.5 billion in sales in 1992.

Trends in Recreational Sports Participation

Over the years, economists and sports analysts have monitored the growth or decline in interest and participation in varied types of recreational sports activities.

For example, Warnick and Howard have tracked the "market share" of such sports as tennis and golf in the 1980s and 1990s, including such dimensions as demographic factors in participation at municipal, country club, private, or daily-fee courses or courts. They found, for example, that:

> With respect to golf, private, daily fee and commercial sector providers have been the major beneficiaries of increased interest in the sport. . . . Thus, the future looks promising for public sector provision of golf playing opportunities. . . . [In contrast] the decade-long erosion of tennis' popularity has resulted in a deep decline in the public sector's share of tennis participation [while] the private sector, particularly resorts and condominiums, accounts for an increasingly sizable portion of the adult tennis market.[34]

Among the more striking trends of interest has been an expansion of participation in such diverse sports or outdoor recreation pastimes as skiing and snowboarding, in-line skating and in-line hockey, karate and other forms of martial arts, marathons, and triathlons. As an example of the meteoric rise in popularity of some sports, snowboarding is America's fastest-growing winter sport. Only a decade ago, "boarders" were considered the curse of the ski slopes—reckless, rude, and bad for business. In 1987, there were less than a half-million snowboarders in the United States. In 1998, about 50 percent of the world's 7 million snowboarders were American. With the admission of snowboarding to the Winter Olympics in 1998, it was estimated that within fifteen years snowboarders would outnumber skiers, with the global retail market for its equipment rising by 40 percent a year.

Statistics show that snowboarders are disproportionately male, in comparison to skiing, and that they are strikingly young—with 95 percent of snowboarders younger than 24. This trend reflects the nature of the activity itself, with competitive snowboarding events featuring spectacular aerial acrobatics and risky stunts similar to those developed by skateboarders. In skiing, ski jumping, and snowboarding today, performers risk their lives and spinal columns with spectacular flips and somersaults in the air, maneuvers over, around, and through moguls and chutes, and similar displays.

Extreme Forms of Play. One might speculate that these high-risk, daring stunts are a response to many of the action movies and television series of the last decade, which used computer-generated technology to create the illusion of people doing literally impossible airborne feats. Beyond this explanation, it is clear that the urge to take part in "extreme" forms of sport and outdoor recreation has been a dominant thrust in leisure participation over the past several years.

The Winter X Games held at Crested Butte, Colorado, as well as other televised winter sports competitions, have featured perilous ice climbing up sheer frozen cliffs, downhill snow biking, and snowboarding contests with aerial acrobatics. Other extreme physical pursuits today, many of which are televised, include skateboarding and bicycle contests on "half-pipe" structures or street courses with numerous man-made obstacles. Kayaking down turbulent mountain streams with precipitous falls or bungee-jumping from cliffs and radio towers have become commonplace. A few years ago, a California skydiver decided to try something new by jumping out of an airplane with a skateboard Velcroed to his feet—giving birth to the hobby of "sky surfing." In-line skating gave rise to "skitching," a city-streets pastime in which skaters cling to, and then launch themselves from the bumpers of speeding cars.

While such pursuits initially appealed to a small, semi-outlaw group of nonconformists and thrill seekers, with a much broader television audience for major competitions they have attracted major commercial sponsors, clothing and equipment designers, and other money-making outlets. Other variants of sport that gained popularity over the past two or three decades included American Gladiators, a colorful television promotion showing men and women teams competing against each other in a variety of newly devised stunts and games. Professional wrestling, classified as an exhibition rather than a legitimate contest, has gone beyond simply choreographing battles between "heroes" and "villains" to the point of becoming a soap-opera-like caricature of sport that nonetheless fills huge arenas and attracts a vast television audience—the most highly rated form of programming on cable networks. The traditional "good-guy" wrestler has been eliminated from the script, as

> . . . women with outsized physiques and leather bras stomp on stage and smack the men, as a heavy metal band rumbles from the side of the area. The imagery and music and pyrotechniques drawn heavily from the world of heavy metal rock music create a mood of apocalyptic darkness.[35]

Trend Toward Violence: "Extreme Fighting."   An example of newer sports spectacles that "push the limits" of legitimate competition involves extreme fighting, the most brutal contest of the modern age. One commentator writes:

> The rules are few, the spilling of blood is plentiful, and the violence has led to the banning of the sport in several states. In a typical match, two men combine techniques from boxing, wrestling, karate, and other forms to render opponents unconscious. There are no rounds, no timeouts, just all-out brawling.[36]

As indicated earlier, the trend toward violence has evidenced itself especially in the world of international soccer competition, with fans breaking down gates, climbing walls, assaulting players and officials, and stamping other spectators to death. In 1969, a disputed match between El Salvador and Honduras led to a brief war, known as the Soccer War, in which thousands were killed or injured.

Numerous learned papers and scholarly hypotheses have been offered to explain the causes that degrade friendly rivalry and turn it into confrontation. One group of sociologists suggests that sports violence is characteristic of social systems, with teams representing communities of subordinate ethnic minorities more likely to be violent than others. Others argue that sports violence has become a legitimate expression of masculine aggression among youthful peers—linked to a feeling of hopelessness stemming from poor economic prospects and limited job opportunities in drab housing environments. Sports riots are often stimulated by the media and the advance publicity that elevates simple sporting events into spectacles of intercity passions.

Reexamining Sports Values

Despite the commercialism, violence, and other negative aspects cited in this chapter, sports continue to represent a tremendously popular and appealing form of leisure pursuit for great numbers of Americans young and old. Why is this the case?

Sports clearly satisfy human urges to meet challenges, compete with others, master skills, release emotions, join with others in team efforts, and develop personal fitness. They may be experienced at any level of intensity, from relatively relaxed, informal play for the weekend golfer, bowler, or volleyball player, to highly skilled and strongly motivated competition by amateur or professional athletes.

Over the past three decades, a number of parents, teachers, coaches, and leading athletes have sought to change the face of youth sports, giving it a simpler, more inclusive, and psychologically positive character. Youth sports associations have striven to reform practices in youth sports, promoting more responsible coaching and stressing desirable values and outcomes.

In a major study of 10,000 students in eleven American cities that was sponsored by the Athletic Footware Association, it was found that even among the most dedicated athletes, winning took a back seat to self-improvement and competition. When asked to select the single most important reason for playing their best school sport, "to win" ranked in seventh place among boys and tenth place among girls. The five most important reasons cited by all youngsters were: (1) to have fun; (2) to improve my skills; (3) to stay in shape; (4) to do something I'm good at; and (5) for the excitement of competition. On the other hand, the reasons for stopping participation in a sport were: (1) I lost interest; (2) I was not having fun; (3) it took too much time; (4) coach was a poor teacher; and (5) too much pressure and worry.

Research studies have shown that it is possible to influence the values of young athletes in positive directions, in terms of fair play, honesty, and playing for fun, through changes in league formats and the screening and preparation of coaches. Increasing efforts are being made to ensure that all players receive fair amounts of playing time and that teams are balanced properly in terms of skilled players. Some community recreation departments and youth sports organizations today offer two kinds of leagues: one for highly motivated and skilled players and another for youngsters who wish simply to enjoy games and are not primarily motivated by the need to win.

The failure of many school athletic departments to teach and encourage positive social values was illustrated in a number of reports following the Littleton, Colorado,

Columbine High School massacre. These showed the degree to which sports team members tended to regard themselves and to be seen by other students as a social elite and—particularly in the case of football players—to be free to ridicule and in many cases even to persecute other, less popular students.

Role of Parents

In many communities, parents take the lead in conducting youth sports leagues and do an excellent job of volunteer coaching and officiating, fund-raising for equipment and maintenance, and giving other forms of supplementary program assistance to public recreation and park agencies. In Philadelphia, for example, dozens of athletic associations in the city's northeast area sponsor baseball, softball, basketball, soccer, and other leagues for thousands of children. In some cases, they design, build, and maintain fields, or remodel indoor facilities; in so doing, they help to maintain the character and stability of their neighborhoods. Infield writes:

> This kind of private enterprise on public property is a regular occurrence in Northeast Philadelphia. And that says a lot about the role of athletics in the community. . . . In many ways the clubs *are* the Northeast, the tie that binds in a region of 410,000 people, nearly the size of Pittsburgh. No other institution cuts across so many ethnic, religious and social boundaries, nor offers a comparable arena for people to meet each other.[37]

Beyond its contribution to neighborhood life, parental involvement in youth sports often becomes an important part of the tie between parents and children. Tom Brokaw, the NBC anchor, comments that, in his family's life, sports were not solely a father's province. His wife, liberated from her 1950s confinement to cheerleading, became a tennis player, skier, backpacker, and marathoner, and shared the role of family athletic model. He writes that, as parents, he and his wife sought to find the right balance between encouragement, perspective, and pride.

> It wasn't always easy. When one daughter's team won a volleyball championship, I wanted to cry. When the players kept their emotions in check, so did I. That same daughter set the school shot put record when she was 16. I was thrilled—my daughter the shot putter. . . . When another daughter won her school's award for the most inspirational athlete, she publicly thanked me for encouraging her. It was at once a proud, touching and embarrassing moment.[38]

Brokaw described another parent, a father who had dreams of his son—a better-than-average athlete but no star—breaking out of the pack and achieving glory. Going into the final lap of the two-mile relay, his team was about five yards behind. As the son took the baton for the anchor leg . . .

> his father came to his feet and began to shout, calmly at first, "Go, big boy, go!" The boy was running stronger than we had ever seen him. He took the lead. I stopped

watching the race, however, because I was transfixed by the sight of his father. By now he was standing on his seat, pumping his right hand in the air, his face a deep red, tears running down his cheek as he cried out, "Go, big boy, go!" over and over.[39]

Brokaw commented that the father's investment in the outcome seemed excessive. Yet it typified the emotional feelings that many Americans have about sports, and this, in the final analysis, must be what underlies their deep involvement in it.

Sport and Social Mobility

For many young athletes, sport may represent a powerful reason for staying in school or a potential means of social mobility. This is often particularly true for those who come from disadvantaged neighborhoods. An inspirational example may be found in the biography of Willie E. Gary, an African American youngster who was one of eleven children in a migrant farm worker family. Only five-feet-seven, he applied at several Florida colleges in the late 1960s, hoping to win a football scholarship—but found no takers until he used his last few dollars for a bus to Shaw University, a black institution in North Carolina. He found

> no spots there, but he hung around, sleeping on a couch, eating handout meals and voluntarily cleaning up the locker room. They made him water boy, until the day he subbed for an injured player and won a spot on the team—and an athletic scholarship. Now one of the most successful malpractice and personal injury lawyers in the South, the 44-year-old Mr. Gary announced . . . that he would give Shaw $10 million over the next five years. It is the largest gift ever for the historically black school. Mr. Gary, who is chairman of the university's board, called it "a very small payment on the very big debt I owe Shaw."[40]

Despite all the negatives then, sports somehow have a magical quality about them, tied to dreams of glory and fame.

William Allman writes of sporting events as a way of rising above life's ambiguities; sports represent an all-out assault on everyday life's compromises and uncertainties. In sports, there is always a final accounting, and there is the image of the hero. He describes the great basketball star, Michael Jordan, saying that in his miraculous leaps, Jordan typifies the willing suspension of disbelief that we bring to sports. It is a yearning to be removed from earthly complications and to experience a world made perfect and, in Jordan's case, played to perfection. Allman continues:

> Perhaps the best player in the history of the sport, he seems as reverent and respectful of his amazing abilities as we are. Jordan is precisely what we love about sports. He defies gravity as much as he defies the tyranny of everyday life. For the moment, he is flying. For the moment, we are transported to a world free of sticky ends, compromises and complications. We watch him leap, hoping he will never come down.[41]

Ultimately, the secret appeal of sports can never be measured by statistics of play or by empirical research that examines their economic, physical, or social outcomes. Instead, it is a matter of emotion, of being part of a game that has been passed down through the centuries, taking its shape from all those who have run the bases through the years. The distinguished philosopher Jacques Barzun comments that whoever wants to know the heart and soul of America should do it by learning about baseball and about

> the wonderful purging of the passions that we all experienced in the fall of 1951, the despair groaned out over the fate of the Dodgers, from whom the league pennant was snatched at the last minute [a loss that gives us] some idea of what Greek tragedy was like. . . .[42]

Finally, there is the tribute to baseball of A. Bartlett Giamatti, who left the presidency of Yale University to become the commissioner of major league baseball. Giamatti engaged in a protracted struggle to bar Pete Rose, a convicted tax evader and gambler on sports, from organized baseball. Shortly after this was accomplished, he died suddenly. Years before, he had written:

> It breaks your heart. It is designed to break your heart. The game begins in the spring, when everything else begins again, and it blossoms in the summer, filling the afternoons and evenings, and then as soon as the chill rains come, it stops and leaves you to face the fall alone. You count on it, rely on it to buffer the passage of time, to keep the memory of sunshine and high skies alive, and then just when the days are all twilight, when you need it most, it stops. . . . Of course, there are those who learn after the first few times. They grow out of sports. And there are others who were born with the wisdom to know that nothing lasts. They are the truly tough among us, the ones who can live without illusion, or without even the hope of illusion. I am not that grown-up or up-to-date. I am a simpler creature, tied to more primitive patterns and cycles. I need to think something lasts forever, and it might as well be that state of being that is a game; it might as well be that, in a green field, in the sun.[43]

Summary

This chapter begins with an overview of the varied motivations that impel people to take part in leisure pursuits, ranging from the simple desire for fun or pleasure to health-related, social, competitive, aesthetic, creative, and other drives.

It then examines the broad field of sports participation and entertainment—not just as a "children's game," as some athletes tend to minimize the sports they play, but as a major institution in modern life. Sport has obvious economic importance, but beyond this has almost religious meaning for many. It has historically had political and international implications and is closely linked to the educational system of the nation. The chapter examines children's sports involvement and goes on to review the history of college sport and the abuses that affect it. Television's role and the growing commercialization of sport are discussed. Finally, the chapter emphasizes the continuing appeal of recreational sports, their contributions to family and community life, and the positive values they hold for many Americans.

Key Concepts

1. Studies of the leisure pursuits of a cross-section of Americans reveal a surprisingly low percentage of time given to active, creative pursuits, and a major portion of leisure given to television. Nonetheless, the most meaningful and involving activities are pursuits such as sports, outdoor recreation, or creative pastimes.

2. Millions of Americans young and old take part in some form of sports, with the number growing decade by decades. Schools and national, organized sports leagues sponsor the bulk of team competition for children and youth. However, active play is also popular for adults and growing numbers of seniors.

3. So fervently are sports heroes admired, and so loyal are fans to their favorite college or professional teams, that sports have been described by theological scholars as a form of folk religion.

4. Similarly, many nations—particularly totalitarian ones—have used sports as a form of patriotic indoctrination and international image-building. Today, such motivations have largely shifted to commercial emphases.

5. The arguments that sports serve as a means of building positive character traits and behavior and enriching youth development are largely unproven, with numerous research studies reinforcing both "pro" and "con" positions.

6. From its early beginnings in the late nineteenth century, intercollegiate sports competition has been marked by various forms of corruption that include illegal recruitment and treatment of student athletes, violation of NCAA rules, involvement of athletes in gambling schemes, and general disregard of the appropriate goals of college sports.

7. With the advent of television, high-powered professional sports have been marked by escalating player contracts, rising ticket prices in expensive new stadiums and arenas, and player-management conflicts, along with a degree of fan disillusionment.

8. Despite such negative aspects of sports, including a growing tendency toward packaging synthetic or violent kinds of contests, they continue to provide important values for Americans of all ages. Sport as a source of economic or social mobility is illustrated in the chapter, along with its powerful emotional appeal for both players and spectators.

Endnotes

1. Angell, R. 1984. Baseball the Perfect Game. *New York Times* (April 1): 8-E.
2. Kraus, R. 1997. *Recreation Programming: A Benefits-Driven Approach.* Boston: Allyn & Bacon.
3. Godbey, G. 1997. *Leisure and Leisure Services in the 21st Century.* State College, PA: Venture Publishing, p. 170.

4. Gray, D., and H. Ibrahim. 1985. The Recreational Experience: A Source of Self-Discovery. *Journal of Physical Education, Recreation and Dance.* (October): 20.

5. Guttmann, A. 1988. *A Whole New Ball Game: An Interpretation of American Sports.* Chapel Hill, NC: University of North Carolina Press.

6. *Statistical Abstract of the United States,* 1998. Washington, DC: U.S. Government Printing Office, pp. 264–265.

7. Outlook: Data Base on Youth Sports. 1995. *U.S. News and World Report* (August 21): 8.

8. Smith, M. 1998. Batting for the Boss. *Philadelphia Inquirer Magazine.* (August 16): 10.

9. Baker, W.J. 1988. *Sports in the Western World.* Urbana, IL: University of Illinois Press, p. 1.

10. Hardy, S., 1990. In *For Fun and Profit: The Transformation of Leisure Into Consumption,* ed. R. Butsch. Philadelphia: Temple University Press, p. 72.

11. Prebish, C. 1987. In Chandler, R. Are Sports Becoming America's New Folk Religion? *Philadelphia Inquirer* (January 3): 1-C, 5-C.

12. Mathiesen, J. In Chandler, *op. cit.,* p. 5-C.

13. Blanchard, K. 1988. Sport and Ritual—A Conceptual Dilemma. *Journal of Physical Education, Recreation and Dance* (November–December): 48.

14. Hoberman, J. 1984. *Sports and Political Ideology.* Austin: University of Texas Press, p. 100.

15. Greendorfer, S. 1987. Psycho-Social Correlates of Organized Physical Activity. *Journal of Physical Education, Recreation and Dance* (September): 59.

16. Hellstedt, J. 1988. Kids, Parents, and Sport: Some Questions and Answers. *The Physician and Sportsmedicine* (16/4): 59–71.

17. Gelfand, D., and D. Hartmann. 1982. Some Detrimental Effects of Competitive Sports on Children's Behavior. In *Children in Sport,* ed. Magill et al. Champaign, IL: Human Kinetics Press, pp. 196–203.

18. Lawlor, F. 1993. Two Cities That Saved Sports. *Philadelphia Inquirer* (May 2): D-1, D-6.

19. Wankel, L., and B. Berger. 1990. The Psychological and Social Benefits of Sport and Physical Activity. *Journal of Leisure Research* (22/3): 167–182.

20. Frey, J., and J. Massengale. 1988. American School Sports: Enhancing Social Values Through Restructuring. *Journal of Physical Education, Recreation and Dance* (August): 40.

21. Morgan, W.J. 1994. *Leftist Theories of Sport: A Critique and Reconstruction.* Urbana: University of Illinois Press, p. 1.

22. Leo, J. 1991. On Society: Two Cheers for Plainfield. *U.S. News and World Report* (October 23): 19.

23. Cohen, A. 1997. Making the Grade. *Athletic Business* (May): 24.

24. Rader, B. 1983. *American Sports from the Age of Folk Games to the Age of Spectators.* Englewood Cliffs, NJ: Prentice-Hall, p. 76.

25. Maeroff, G. 1991. Big-Time Sports Don't Belong in College. *New York Times* (December 15): 14-E.

26. Chu, D. 1989. *The Character of American Higher Education and Intercollegiate Sports.* Buffalo: State University of New York Press, pp. 8–9.

27. Gup, T. 1989. Foul! *Time Magazine* (January 9): 43.

28. Drape, J. 1999. NCAA Rule Is Voided. *New York Times* (March 14): WK-2.

29. Myers, D.D. 1990. Why College Sport? *Commentary* (December): 48.

30. Zoglin, R. 1990. The Great TV Takeover: Billion-Dollar Fees and Ever-Expanding Coverage Are Re-Shaping American Sports. *Time Magazine* (March 26): 66.

31. Rader, B. 1984. *In Its Own Image: How Television Has Transformed Sports.* New York: Free Press, Macmillan, p. 5.

32. *Ibid.*

33. McCarroll, T. 1992. A Whole New Ball Game. *Time Magazine* (June 22): 63.

34. Warnick, R., and D. Howard. 1996. Market Share Analysis of Selected Sport and Recreation Activities: An Update—1979 to 1992. *Journal of Park and Recreation Administration* (Summer 14/2): 53–79.

35. Johnson, K. 1998. Professional Wrestling Cuts Good Guys From the Script. *New York Times* (March 30): A-1.

36. Marks, J. 1997. Whatever It Takes to Win. *U.S. News and World Report* (February 24): 46–49.

37. Infield, T. 1985. Where Sports Reign: Clubs Pinch-Hit for the City. *Philadelphia Inquirer* (May 1): B-1.

38. Brokaw, T. 1991. Of Fathers and Children and Sports. *New York Times* (June 16): S-9.
39. *Ibid.*
40. Mater Love. *New York Times* (Feb. 9,1992): E-7.
41. Allman, W. 1991. Liftoff: Rising Above the Ordinary Ambiguities. *U.S. News and World Report* (June 10): 10.
42. Barzun, J. 1984. Reveling in the Levels of the Game. *New York Times* (April 1): 8-1.
43. Giamatti, A.B. 1984. The Green Fields of the Mind. *New York Times* (April 1): 8-E.

10 Pastimes II: Outdoor Recreation, Travel and Tourism

Toward the close of a decade that has seen the mushrooming of cable television and the rise of the Internet, nearly 40 percent of United States adults are still answering the call of the wild. In a survey published at the end of last year [1997] the United States Fish and Wildlife Service found that 77 million Americans age 16 and older fished, hunted, and watched wildlife in 1996.[1]

Tourism is forecasted to be the largest business activity in the world by the turn of the century. It is the largest source of foreign exchange earnings for many countries of the world. . . . Yet, tourism is much more than a business. While many people travel to conduct business, sell services and products, and exchange information, most people travel to fulfill personal needs. They travel to refresh, revitalize, or enrich their lives. They travel to relax, learn and escape routine. . . . Today, many people perceive their vacation and leisure time as a necessity for a healthy, fulfilling life.[2]

Two of the most popular uses of leisure today are outdoor recreation and travel and tourism. In many ways, these pursuits overlap. Although outdoor recreation may be enjoyed close to home, it often requires travel to distant locations where skiing, whitewater rafting, hunting, and similar pastimes are available. Similarly, although tourism may involve trips to cities for cultural events or stays at luxurious resorts, it may also incorporate various outdoor pursuits or the exploration of unique natural environments or the observation of wildlife.

At the same time, both types of recreational activities are also intertwined with sports. As Table 10.1 shows, many compilations of leisure pursuits combine both outdoor recreation interests and sports involvements. This chapter will show their separate meanings and will show how both outdoor recreation and tourism may run the gamut from safe

TABLE 10.1   Participation in Selected Outdoor Recreation and Sports Activities: 1996

Activity	All Persons		Sex	
	Number	*Rank*	*Male*	*Female*
Total Participation	237,745	X	115,443	122,301
Aerobic exercising	24,119	11	5,314	18,805
Backpacking	11,469	22	7,240	4,229
Badminton	6,084	28	2,909	3,175
Baseball	14,823	18	11,610	3,213
Basketball	33,281	9	22,375	10,906
Bicycle riding	53,342	3	28,595	24,747
Billiards	34,477	8	21,841	12,636
Bowling	42,895	6	22,579	20,316
Calisthenics	10,064	25	5,023	5,041
Camping	44,695	5	24,102	20,593
Exercise walking	74,307	1	26,666	46,641
Exercising with equipment	47,823	4	22,200	25,622
Fishing, freshwater	40,208	7	27,160	13,048
Fishing, saltwater	11,045	23	7,926	3,119
Football, tackle	8,953	27	7,969	983
Football, touch/flag	11,645	20	9,603	2,042
Golf	23,082	12	18,219	4,863
Hiking	26,457	10	14,465	11,992
Hunting with firearms	19,251	15	16,317	2,933
Martial arts	4,673	30	3,286	1,387
Racquetball	5,582	29	3,768	1,814
Running/jogging	22,239	13	12,320	9,919
Skiing, alpine/downhill	10,466	24	6,277	4,188
Skiing, cross-country	3,385	31	1,820	1,566
Soccer	13,876	19	8,626	5,251
Softball	19,873	14	10,837	9,035
Swimming	60,223	2	29,145	31,078
Table tennis	9,542	26	5,907	3,635
Target shooting	15,695	17	11,097	4,598
Tennis	11,485	21	6,381	5,105
Volleyball	18,535	16	8,970	9,565

Source: Statistical Abstract of the United States, 1998, p. 266. In thousands; describes population 7 years of age or older who participated in activity at least once in preceding year.

and relatively passive forms of spectator activity to challenging and even high-risk pursuits. Taken together, they comprise a major, multibillion-dollar sector of the leisure market today, appealing to all age groups and socioeconomic classes.

How popular are such uses of leisure? The *Statistical Abstract of the United States* reported in 1997 that the number of visits to parks operated by such federal outdoor recreation agencies as the Forest Service, U.S. Army Corps of Engineers, Bureau of Land Management, or National Park Service had risen from 6.3 billion visitor hours in 1980 to almost 8 billion in the early 1990s.[3] Visitors to state park and recreation areas totaled 745 million in 1995, and comparable numbers enjoy outdoor recreation pursuits in municipal or county-operated parks, nature preserves, pools, beaches, and boating areas.

Meaning of Outdoor Recreation

On the face of it, the term *outdoor recreation* applies to any form of play or leisure activity that is carried on in the outdoors, such as strolling through a park, playing basketball in a school yard, or attending a band concert in a city square. However, a stricter definition would suggest that outdoor recreation consists primarily of activities that depend on the natural environment, such as camping, nature photography, scuba diving, and similar pursuits.

Although outdoor recreation may take many forms, its primary manifestation is found in such wildland activities as camping and backpacking, canoeing and wildwater rafting, mountain and rock climbing, fishing, and hunting. Such pursuits are uniquely linked to the history of the United States—both in terms of the lives of many hundreds of Native American tribes throughout the continent and the land's settlement by English and other European colonists.

From the time of the earliest settlements, Americans have enjoyed hunting and fishing in wilderness settings—partly for food, but also as a traditional form of play. In the mid-1980s, as growing numbers of well-to-do easterners began to engage in outdoor play in such regions as the remote Adirondack Mountains, the view was widely shared that nature was the "dwelling place of God," offering cures for both physical and spiritual woes.

Others have concluded that Americans' interest in the outdoors in the present day stems from our long and rich history of exploring the wilderness, and that it is linked to the nation's popular folklore about the exploits of loggers, hunters, cowboys, and pioneers crossing the land. La Page and Ranney describe this fascination with America's wilderness as an integral part of our common culture, writing:

> One of the most powerful sources of this country's essential cultural fiber clearly is in the land. The roots of the new nation and its people became the forests and rivers, the deserts and mountains, and the challenges and inspirations they presented, not the ruins of ancient civilizations most other cultures look to for ancestral continuity. Thus, America developed a different attitude and identity.[4]

It was to satisfy this interest that Congress created the National Wilderness Preservation System in 1964, with an initial nine million acres that provided places that were untrammeled and unmodified by the human hand, settings that were dangerous, unpredictable, and wild. McAvoy and Dustin point out that such areas offer us the opportunity to resurrect the feeling of the frontier, to live simply, and to meet challenges to our safety, through courage and self-reliance.[5]

While outdoor recreation in wilderness settings is a valuable personal experience linked to patriotic values and historical perspective, it also represents an important economic function. Greer points out that outdoor recreation involves a variety of leisure-oriented products

> such as camping paraphernalia, outdoor sports equipment, and clothing, as well as a bewildering array of trail bikes, four-wheel-drive vehicles, and snowmobiles. There are also transportation, tours, lodging, and dining intended for outdoor recreationists. The profitable production and sale of these recreational goods and services requires the existence of certain kinds of physical settings and an elaborate infrastructure of roads, trails, ski runs, and campsites.[6]

Realistically, much outdoor recreation does not take place in remote wilderness settings. Instead, it may be enjoyed in a neighborhood park, a nature center, or a heavily used beach or lake close to a crowded urban environment. A major conclusion of the Outdoor Recreation Resources Review Commission in 1962 was that many urban dwellers are at a distance from available wilderness areas, and that there is a continuing need to establish more parks and other areas close to the crowded metropolitan regions of the country. As a consequence, a number of National Seashores and Recreation Areas have been established close to large cities, particularly along the east and west coasts.

Overview of Major Pursuits: Hunting and Fishing

We now turn to a direct examination of several of the most popular types of outdoor recreation pursuits enjoyed by Americans, beginning with hunting and fishing. Table 10.2 shows the gradual increase in spending on participation in these two activities from 1980 to the mid-1990s. Additional surveys by the U.S. Fish and Wildlife Service report that over 35 million fresh- and saltwater fishing enthusiasts spent over $23.9 billion on their hobby in the early 1990s, while fourteen million big- and small-game hunters spent $12.3 billion.

Fishing as Outdoor Recreation

Of these two popular pursuits, fishing is more readily accessible; it can be carried on in many different settings—in local streams, ponds, and lakes, along ocean beaches, or from private or commercial fishing craft. In a study of urban youth who fish, Dargitz explored the influence of such factors as race, gender, residence, and angling socialization (family interest) among several hundred teenage students in a midwestern city. He found that

> gender appears to be a more important factor in angling socialization than either race or residence. . . . Children who have anglers in their households are more likely to engage in fishing more frequently and are more likely to enjoy angling as a leisure

TABLE 10.2   Sport Hunting and Fishing Licenses 1980–1995

Activity	1980	1985	1990	1995
Fishing licenses: Sales (in millions)	35.2	35.7	37.0	37.9
Paid license holders	28.0	29.7	30.7	30.3
Cost to anglers (mil. dol.)	196	282	363	449
Hunting licenses: Sales	27.0	27.7	30.2	32.1
Paid license holders	16.3	15.9	15.8	15.2
Cost to hunters (mil. dol.)	222	301	363	533

Source: U.S. Fish and Wildlife Service. Note slight decline in number of paid hunting license holders, but heavy increase in costs.

activity than are children who do not have anglers in their households. Because males are more likely to enjoy angling than are females, teenage boys are more active within the urban context.[7]

As a form of outdoor recreation, fishing varies greatly, often according to geographical or climate-based factors. For example, through much of the American midwest, ice fishing on frozen lakes represents a legendary part of the region's culture. Thousands of Minnesotans, for example, spend a sizable portion of the winter months holed up in 8-by-10-foot shanties in self-imposed exile, intermittently fishing, napping, snacking on fish and deer meat, and drinking beer. Greg McCullough writes:

> Each winter, the lure of big fish attracts tens of thousands of anglers to the ice that covers Minnesota's 10,000-plus lakes. . . . Some merely walk out, chisel a hole, and bait a hook. Most build or rent modest portable fishing houses for overnight stays [in temperatures that may go below 30 or 40 degrees below zero]. But a few participate in much more elaborate schemes, hauling mobile homes out onto the ice or mammoth, custom-built houses—complete with kitchens, entertainment centers and wet bars—to spend weeks at a time in icebound seclusion.[8]

At another level, growing numbers of fishermen and women enjoy their hobby at private trout- or bass-fishing preserves, paying flat fees for boat rentals and scaled fees for trophy fish based on a per-pound charge. Another example of fishing's popularity may be found in cable television fishing shows or huge bass-fishing competitions held today around the country. Major tournaments sponsored by organizations like the Bass Anglers Sportsman Society (B.A.S.S.) offers prizes amounting to hundreds of thousands of dollars. Taylor writes:

> For the consistent winners . . . the prize money is secondary to a wealth of sponsorship and endorsement deals from boat, motor and tackle manufacturers eager to reach a $2 billion-plus market of 20 million bass fishermen. Syndicated television shows

have given the best fishermen widespread recognition, along with six-figure incomes. Izaak Walton's "calm, quiet, innocent recreation" is no longer "a reward to itself."[9]

Big-money bass tournaments are complicated, tightly run affairs, with rules governing the boats, equipment, timing, and reporting of catches. High-powered bass boats are equipped with sophisticated gear: foot-controlled electric trolling motors, gauges to measure the acid-base balance of the water, its temperature, and clarity, and depth recorders and liquid crystal screens that help locate fish.

Hunting as Outdoor Recreation

A second popular form of outdoor recreation includes both big-game and small-game hunting. Originally a primary source of food for rural families, hunting is still enjoyed for this purpose in many regions today, although it is chiefly a recreational pursuit.

As in fishing, enthusiasts may range from those who take their rifles or shotguns out for a casual afternoon's hunt close to home to others who pay huge sums to bring home trophy heads or hides. For example, some commercial hunt outfitters package big-game excursions into northern Canada, flying hunters into remote regions, with varied amenities, guide services, and guaranteed bear or other big game "kills," at prices ranging from several hundred dollars to several thousand dollars per hunter (see Figure 10.1).

Hunting is a peer-group activity participated in primarily by males. O'Leary, Behrens-Tepper, McGuire, and Dottavio describe the nature of the young hunter's introduction to the sport as a form of socialization into masculine society:

> a parent, close relative, or other responsible adult [acts] in the role of teacher and, not incidentally, transmitter of the hunting culture. It is perhaps not only in this intimate interaction with an older hunting companion that causes hunting to persist into adult life, but also the implied rite of passage.[10]

Although city dwellers may think of hunters as simple country folk, demographically today's hunters are relatively well educated and drawn from a range of occupations and status levels. Hunting technology, like fishing technique, has become increasingly complex, with so-called prey acquisition systems that include scents and wildlife calls to attract game, infrared binoculars, "bionic earphones" to sharpen hearing, and trail monitors that record animals passing by in a particular location. A growing number of private clubs and lodges own or lease land—much of it from timber companies—for hunting preserves. In some western states like Montana and South Dakota, livestock ranchers have turned to operating shooting preserves for game ranging from geese and pheasants to antelope and bison.

Objections to Hunting. The most serious objections to hunting practices today come from animal-rights activists who condemn hunting as a cruel and barbaric "sport." They are outraged by the practice of allowing hunters to shoot animals—ranging from otters to grizzly bears, whistling swans to bighorn sheep—on national wildlife refuges, tracts of prime habitat maintained by the U.S. Fish and Wildlife Service.

```
┌─────────────────────────────────────────────────────────┐
│  DISCOUNTS AVAILABLE ON GROUPS OF FOUR OR MORE            │
└─────────────────────────────────────────────────────────┘
```

TROPHY BEAR HUNT (GOLD MEDAL HUNT)

8 DAY HUNT (GUARANTEED)   **$2495.** US

****

(An all inclusive price) 100% SUCCESS

This special hunt for trophy bear is for 8 full days or more. You stay until you shoot one. WE ONLY WORK AT THE MOST ACTIVE BAITS and will put you where the BIG BEARS are working. This includes bear licenses, cabin lodging, meals, guides, boots, motor, gas and much more. This is probably one of the best chances you will ever have of getting quality black bear in the Canadian far north.

P.S.: WHERE A GUARANTEED HUNT IS ASSURED, THE NUMBER OF AVAILABLE RESERVATIONS IS LIMITED TO 20 HUNTERS PER SEASON.

VIP BEAR HUNT

6 DAY HUNT   **$1695.** US

***

This hunt was made for the real hunter who wants the good life in his hunting camp along with all the modern conveniences. This hunt includes food, lodging, guide, boat, motor, gas, and more. This hunt is not guaranteed, but we had a 75%+ kill last year. (License extra).

ECONO BEAR HUNT

5 DAY HUNT   **$595.** US

**

This is the original do it yourself kit. You will have your own camp, boat, bait, cabin and territory, but the rest is up to you. You hunt and fish whenever you want. You must bring your own food, sheets, etc. We will show you the baits and the hunt is on.

N.B.: A wounded bear is considered the same way as a killed bear.

FIGURE 10.1   Bear-hunting brochure, Northern Quebec Guide Service.

Cleveland Amory, founder and president of the Fund for Animals, extends the case against hunting, pointing out that millions of animals and birds are crippled each year and die painful, lingering deaths. Beyond this, in a recent year, 177 people were killed and 1719 injured by hunters, including many innocent bystanders walking in the woods or on their own property. Responding to the argument that hunters are the prime revenue source for protecting nonendangered wildlife, because they pay over $500 million a year for licenses, duck stamps, and excise taxes, Amory calls them "bloodthirsty nuts" and characterizes hunting as "an antiquated expression of macho self-aggrandizement, with no place in a civilized society."

On the other hand, many hunters claim that hunting represents an important spiritual experience for them. Columnist Darrell Sifford encouraged readers to debate the views of a psychiatrist who had told him that hunting had significant meaning in his life. One reader wrote that the pressure of his work life made hunting both an escape and a reminder that there is "man's time and God's time," with:

> The ebb and flow of the seasons, of life and death, moved by a cosmic force that has nothing to do with taxes . . . politics or most things important to human beings. . . . Hunting reminds me of that. I must dig through the crust of civilization and recapture the basic skills of my ancestors. . . . I touch a world where we've all—or at least most of us—forgotten how to cope, where we survive by our ability to take our sustenance from the wild state. It helps me put my daily world in better perspective.[11]

Other Wilderness Pursuits

Beyond the major pastimes of fishing and hunting, outdoor recreation enthusiasts engage in a huge range of wilderness experiences, including camping and backpacking, trail rides, dogsled trips, cross-country skiing, orienteering, rock-climbing, and similar pastimes. For many, outdoor recreation interest is centered around observing nature and wildlife in a totally noninvasive way. The Fish and Wildlife Service reports that wildlife observation, both close-to-home and on special trips and tours, is a favorite hobby for millions:

> Bird feeding is the most popular residential activity. More than 52 million people fed birds at least once a week for an average of eight months in 1996. Among the 44 million people who observed wildlife around their homes, birds were the favorite class of animal [with many enthusiasts seeking to identify as many species as possible during the year]. . . . Nonresidential wildlife watchers are fond of birds, too, but they are equally fond of deer, bears and coyotes [with some 24 million people taking] wildlife-watching trips in 1996.[12]

Skiing, Biking, Boating, and Surfing

Numerous other activities contribute to the volume of outdoor recreation participation today, including skiing and snowboarding, mountain biking, boating in a variety of different kinds of craft, and beach surfing.

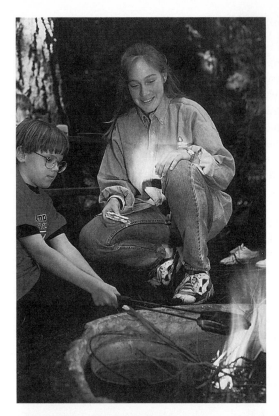

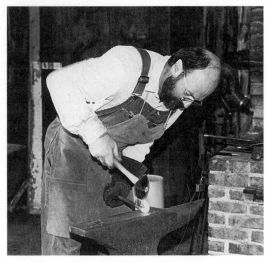

After World War II, millions of American families began to enjoy tent camping, often in state parks or lakeside outings sponsored by organizations such as Camp Fire. Today, commercial organizations such as Pocono Whitewater Adventures package varied river rafting and other outdoor pursuits for participants young and old. Often, state and county park agencies operate environmental centers or historical and heritage sites, featuring traditional crafts or folklore experiences.

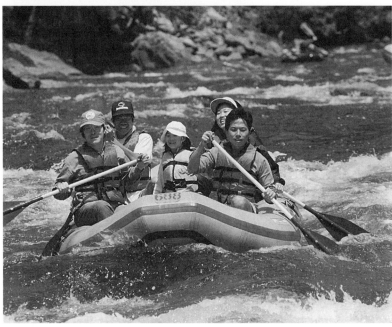

When it first became a popular pastime, skiing was a relatively simple sport, with close-to-home slopes, natural snow, inexpensive equipment, and simple rope tows. But as skiing became more popular in the 1960s and 1970s and hundreds of ski centers opened up around the United States, more elaborate and expensive equipment became necessary. Resorts from California to Maine, often with multi-million-dollar vacation-home complexes, conference centers, and upscale shopping and restaurant facilities, appealed to well-to-do singles and young families; in the 1980s, skiing became a $7 billion industry. However, changing demographics (with aging baby boomers and more young families unable to afford the cost of ski vacations), increased competition, concern about environmental problems, and disappointing weather conditions all led to a crisis in the industry, with many marginally profitable centers going out of business in the late 1980s.

Two factors have contributed to skiing's continued popularity. Snowboarding, as described earlier, has had an immense appeal, particularly for younger outdoor enthusiasts, and today comprises a major portion of the programs at winter sports centers. Today, it is often featured in community recreational sports offerings, particularly in Canada, where many municipal recreation and park departments offer varied instructional programs, camps, clinics, and competitions for all ages in skiing and snowboarding.

A second aspect of skiing's remaking itself has involved a number of entrepreneurs' having taken over independent ski centers—assembling them into major chains of centers and resorts, developing elaborate new facilities and year-round recreational activities and events appealing to a broad age range and using sophisticated marketing and promotional techniques.

Bicycling and Off-Road Adventure Travel

Another popular leisure pursuit that has been heavily commercialized in recent years is bicycling. In the mid-1970s, the A.C. Nielsen Company, a leading market-research firm, reported that bicycling was second only to swimming as a participant activity, with over sixty-five million participants each year. At that time and in the early 1980s, the lean touring cycles popularly known as 10-speeds accounted for 80 percent of United States bicycle sales. But in the late 1980s, a growing boom in biking interest—due in part to joggers who were frustrated with sore knees and ankles—led to a new kind of vehicle, the mountain bike. A crossbreed of rugged utility and European racing technology, these tough, practically maintenance-free cycles, also known as all-terrain bikes, make use of high-tech alloys, tubing, and lugs borrowed from the aerospace industry for lightweight strength. They feature flat handlebars for upright seating and thick tires that handle sand, gravel, and rough slopes as easily as pavement. It was reported in 1991 that sales of bikes had climbed by as much as 30 percent in one year, with mountain bikes representing over half of those sold.

As bicycling has become a more fashionable sport, as many as fourteen million Americans from 8 to 80 enjoy trail-riding in wilderness settings. But there is a dark side to this trend. Sandra Blakeslee writes:

> Many hikers and equestrians, who are being asked to share their favorite trails with
> mountain bikers, are putting up a stiff fight. They say that the bikers are eroding

mountain trails, shattering the peace and quiet of wilderness retreats and careening down hills at speed that endanger the safety of other trail users.[13]

This dispute is part of a much larger conflict between those who are concerned about protecting the natural environment and a diversified group of outdoor recreationists who are using off-road vehicles, as well as an ongoing conflict between different groups of recreationists themselves (see page 331).

Water-Based Outdoor Recreation

Another major form of outdoor recreation activity that has continued to grow in popularity involves various forms of water-based pastimes.

Boating as such—involving outboard- and inboard-powered craft, sailboats, canoes, rowboats, and competitive racing boats—is an immensely popular activity. The *Statistical Abstract of the United States* reports that the number of recreational boats owned by Americans increased from 9.7 million in 1975 to 17.1 million in 1995, with total boating expenditures rising from $4.8 billion to $17.2 billion over the same period.

Varied forms of water play have also expanded. For example, scuba diving has become a $1 billion industry, according to the Diving Equipment Manufacturers Association, which reports that there are about 2.5 million scuba divers in the United States, with several hundred thousand new divers being certified each year. Sailing and competitive rowing tend to be elite sports, often appealing to young men and women who encounter them in yacht clubs and colleges.

As another example of water-based recreation, surfing has long been a popular pastime of tanned, long-haired youth, particularly along the California coastline. Celebrated in movies and popular records, surfing represented a hedonistic lifestyle that flourished in the 1960s, when the quintessential surfer was a casual dude who lived for the moment. As surfing, like other leisure pursuits, has become increasingly commercialized, major beer, soft-drink, and other companies have used it as a focus of lifestyle marketing aimed at affluent young adults. Airlines and automobile companies today sponsor professional surfing tours and competitions, with television coverage and hundreds of thousands of dollars in prizes. In 1991, the Association of Surfing Professionals World Tour offered prizes totaling $2.2 million and packaged surfing with beach volleyball and waterskiing in popular television shows.

At another level, surfing has become available to millions of Americans who do not live near the ocean through the introduction of wave pools, which use one of several engineering methods to send a surge of water several feet high from one end of the pool to the other at regular intervals. In a number of cases, such pools have been made part of complex water-play parks that include diving platforms, waterfalls, body flumes, and slides that provide exciting fun for family groups.

A unique example of how water-based recreation may be adapted to different leisure needs consists of its growing use for special populations. Water aerobics and modified exercises are increasingly being used for persons with disabilities and the elderly. In some cases, varied programs of outdoor recreation activities for those with disabilities have been developed, as shown in Figure 10.2.

- **F.L.O.A.T., Forming Leisure Opportunities using Aquatic Techniques,** is an adaptive aquatic program that creates and provides leisure choices for people with and without disabilities through participation and education of aquatics.

Recreational Swimming Program

- **One-on-One Swim Lessons** are designed to provide basic swimming techniques and build confidence in and around the water.

- **Team F.L.O.A.T.** is a recreational swim team designed to teach people with disabilities competitive swimming with the hopes of eventually participating and competing in an integrated swim team.

- **H20 Hi-jinx Bus Camp** is a week long camp in which kids with and without disabilities engage in numerous aquatic activities and is designed to promote new friendships between disabled and non-disabled participants.

Outdoor Aquatics

- **Sailing** consists of a four hour excursion on Lake Mead in which participants of all ages and abilities can either learn the basics of sailing or just enjoy the ride.

- **Adaptive Water-skiing** teaches skiing fundamentals, whether it be standing or sitting, and has something for everyone from skiing to riding on tubes to kneeboarding.

- **Paddling Workshops** teaches the basic skills needed to paddle a canoe or raft.

- **Black Canyon Canoe Trips** are overnight canoe trips that emphasize teamwork and friendship building as they travel down one of the most popular canoe destinations in the country.

- **Kern River Raft Trips** are four day common adventure experiences that offer the ultimate in fun and excitement while teaching teamwork and stressing the independence of each individual.

FIGURE 10.2 Aquatic activities for persons with disabilities. F.L.O.A.T. program sponsored by Parks and Recreation Department's Adaptive Recreation Division, Las Vegas, Nevada.

Motivations for Aquatic Play. Water-based recreation meets a wide variety of interests and personal needs. Rivers, lakes, reservoirs, and beach areas all provide settings for diversified pastimes, many of which have been systematically studied.

For example, in the mid-1970s, Ditton, Goodale, and Johnsen studied a five-county area in Wisconsin in order to identify clusters of water-based recreationists to assist in government resource planning efforts. They examined participation frequencies for eight activities (fishing, sailing, waterskiing, motorboating, swimming, duck hunting, picnicking, and camping), and studied the interaction of these activity choices with such factors as age, level of education, and occupation. Based on their findings, they identified eight different clusters of participants who were attracted to different types of water-based environments—a useful tool in outdoor recreation planning.[14]

Similarly, John Heywood explored the relationships among different types of river recreation groups, in terms of their activity choices and the characteristics of their social groups. He identified a set of thirty-six different motivations for engaging in water-based recreation and found that these were linked to streams with different types of flow characteristics. Whitewater rafting, for example, at one level—that of relaxed floating down a gentle stream in inner tubes or on rubber inflatables—is likely to appeal to teenagers, family groups, or others seeking casual fun. On the other hand, whitewater rafting down powerful streams with turbulent rapids may attract individuals who seek excitement and adventure.[15]

Conflicts Between Environmentalists and Recreationists

The sheer volume of outdoor recreation activity has led to major conflicts and disagreements between groups of outdoor recreation enthusiasts. Many of these conflicts involve concern about the impact of recreational pursuits on the environment.

As an example, the use of off-road vehicles on Bureau of Land Management properties rose from 19.4 million visits in 1982 to 63 million in 1990. But by the mid-1980s, public opposition to the use of all-terrain vehicles had grown dramatically in many areas of the country. Many property owners in rural areas have been disturbed by the use of vehicles that destroy property, cause land erosion, create high noise levels, and are used for illegal hunting of deer. In some cases, booby traps have been placed in wooded rural areas, with hidden pits and pointed oak poles implanted in them, and with fishing line, chains, baling wire, and steel hooks hung at eye level to catch riders. Additionally, a number of state park and environmental departments have passed regulations to prohibit the use of ATVs on public roads or on state forest or game lands. This represents only one of the areas in which authorities are concerned about the impact of invasive vehicles on wildlife, the natural environment, and other outdoor recreationists. Riders of jet skis, for example, have been described as "motorcycle gangs on the water," as they race at speeds of over forty miles an hour, are involved in frequent accidents, and harass other recreationists on the nation's lakes and rivers.

Beyond such problems, there are numerous other examples of conflicts between different groups of outdoor recreationists. Jackson and Wong document several studies that show marked differences in leisure motivations and outdoor behaviors that pit cross-country skiers and snowmobilers against each other.

> Cross-country skiers prefer self-propelled, low-impact activities which reflect their desire for solitude, tranquility and a relatively undisturbed natural environment.

Snowmobilers prefer machine-oriented and extractive activities which provide an outlet for adventurousness and sociability.[16]

Similar disagreements have been found between adherents of motorboating and canoeing, trail-biking and hiking, boating and fishing, and other outdoor pastimes. In part, the frictions stem from overcrowding, with many natural attractions experiencing what has been called "greenlock."

Overcrowding of Parks and Wilderness Areas

Numerous examples of the overcrowding of campgrounds, scenic and historical sites, and other park and wilderness areas may be cited. Ticketron reservations for campsites at Yosemite go on sale eight weeks in advance, and are snapped up in less than five minutes. Even bicyclists planning to pedal Canyonlands National Park's Island in the Sky Trail in Utah must apply at least two weeks ahead. In part, the problem is one of commercial interests dominating the nation's natural resources. For example, most of the 22,000 slots for riding the Colorado River through the Grand Canyon go to commercial companies; individual applicants face a minimum waiting time of three to five years. Beyond this, some of the most valued national treasures, unique for their natural wonders, have been outfitted with overly civilized amenities. Yosemite's Ahwahnee Hotel offers guests cozy rooms equipped with television sets and minibars; visitors can patronize a pizza parlor, a gourmet deli, a one-hour photo service, an automatic bank machine, and a gift shop filled with items with the Yosemite logo.

Critics of such arrangements cite the warning of Horace Albright, first civilian superintendent of Yellowstone and second director of the Park Service:

> Oppose with all your strength and power all proposals to penetrate your wilderness regions with motorways and other symbols of modern mechanization. Keep large sections of primitive country free from the influence of destructive civilization. Keep those bits of primitive America for those who seek peace and rest in the silent place . . . remember, once opened, they can never be wholly restored to primeval charm and grandeur. . . . Park usefulness and popularity should not be measured in terms of mere numbers of visitors. Some precious park areas can easily be destroyed by the concentration of too many visitors. We should be interested in the quality of park patronage, not in the quantity.[17]

Such major federal agencies as the National Park Service and U.S. Forest Service have begun to address this problem by withdrawing "built-up" or overcommercialized facilities from a number of important parks and wilderness areas, as described in Chapter 13.

Outdoor Recreation Management Priorities

Within the spectrum of conflicting leisure pursuits in heavily crowded outdoor settings, what values should be given priority? Robert Manning points out that wilderness visitors are not homogeneous populations, but have value systems that cover a wide and often conflicting range. Often activity choices are dictated by age and family life-cycle factors, with camping activities shifting through each stage of the life cycle. For example, from a Pacific Northwest study, it was determined that

> combination campers (those who participated in both wilderness and automobile camping) were found to generally represent the early stages of the family life cycle, automobile campers represented the middle and postretirement stages, and wilderness camping families represented those just beginning their families and those in the contracting stage of the family life cycle.[18]

As a way of dealing with such diversified interests and needs, a number of classification or zoning systems for recreation areas have been proposed through the years. Typically, these suggest six or seven types of zones, ranging from "wilderness" to "intensive-use" areas. Ultimately, since they are responsible for administering major outdoor recreation resources and dealing with the public that uses them, Leo McAvoy argues that members of the park and recreation profession should assume fuller leadership for environmental stewardship. He points out that too often recreation managers wind up battling with environmental advocates, with whom they should be allied.[19]

McAvoy urges park and recreation professionals to adopt an environment ethic that will serve as the basis for making policy decisions and choices in source planning and program development. Such an ethic would not only establish a code of behavior, but would also assign priority to educating the public with respect to environmental stewardship, and to developing political advocacy for needed policies and practices.

The Role of Adventure Recreation

A related concern in the management of outdoor resources has to do with the increased public interest in varied forms of adventure recreation.

Much of outdoor recreation's appeal stems from risk factors, as participants face the challenges inherent in the wilderness environment. To control these, many national organizations, recreation and park agencies, colleges, and universities offer clinics and classes teaching outdoor skills and safety principles.

Such activities as mountain climbing, hang gliding, parachuting, scuba diving, or downhill skating are often categorized as "risk" recreation, although they may have sharply different emphases. Some adventure programs are concerned with character development and may be used, in the form of survival training, with such diverse groups as business executives, military personnel, and disturbed or delinquent adolescents to strengthen their positive self-concepts, leadership skills, and modes of interaction with others. Most adventure activities, however, are not undertaken as part of such educational or therapeutic programs, but are simply part of the spectrum of outdoor play. Activities such as mountain climbing, ski jumping, and hang gliding satisfy the craving that some people have to experience danger and challenge. Alan Ewert and Steve Hollenhorst describe adventure recreation as: "A variety of self-initiated activities utilizing an interaction with the natural

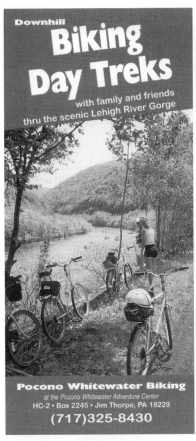

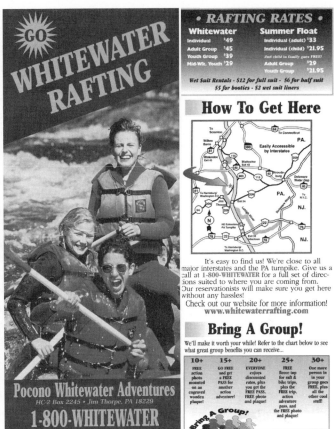

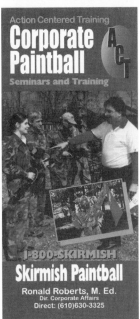

FIGURE 10.3 Leading example of commercially sponsored outdoor recreation activities. Pocono Whitewater Adventures in Jim Thorpe, Pennsylvania, offers wide range of year-round outdoor recreation activities for companies, families, and all age groups.

environment, that contain elements of real or apparent danger, in which the outcome, while uncertain, can be influenced by the participant and circumstances."[20]

Most forms of outdoor recreation involve a reasonable degree of risk, in which injury or death can be averted with common sense and caution. However, such pursuits as in-line skating, a typically urban pastime, regularly cause a considerable number of accidents. Others, like mountain or rock climbing, cause hundreds of fatalities over time. Often, accidents result from foolhardy behavior by sky divers or hang gliders, boaters who drink and race their craft wildly, tourists who ignore natural dangers such as bubbling hot springs or crocodiles in shallow rivers, and entrants in snake-sacking contests, who gather diamondback rattlesnakes as part of fund-raising drives.

Such forms of play, which involve deliberate flirting with danger, may in their most extreme forms become almost suicidal. Psychiatrist Paul Haun labeled them "pathological play," citing such pursuits as Russian Roulette as games that might have immediately fatal consequences. Regularly, brief items appear in newspapers giving details of children and youth who lose their lives playing chicken on the highway (two cars race toward each other, with the first to veer away labeled as "chicken"), riding on the underside of elevators in housing projects, or taking part in other daredevil stunts that appeal to youth gangs. Giant roller coasters, which are actually much less dangerous, but are designed to create fear, thrive on the element of danger and tragedy. When a major accident occurs at an amusement park, attendance climbs dramatically.

Risk-Seeking Drives

What accounts for this human fascination with risk, danger, and violence? One theory of play suggests that a common drive underlying much leisure activity consists of the personal need to experience competence or mastery in overcoming challenges that go beyond the sober realities of everyday life. Stainbrook writes: "So much of life has become sedentary, inhibiting action; thrill-seeking expresses an almost desperate need for assertive mastery of something."[21]

A psychology professor at Johns Hopkins University, Marvin Zuckerman, points out that boredom often leads people to engage in such thrill-seeking activities as risky forms of play, adulterous sex, the use of drugs or alcohol, and even physical aggression. Zuckerman has designed a "sensation-seeking" scale designed to show the extent to which different individuals need such forms of excitement and seek higher levels of stimulation in everything from commodities-market speculation to skydiving. University of Wisconsin psychologist Frank Farley suggests that the society itself promotes such behavior. He calls America a "type-T" nation—"the 'T' stands for thrill seekers—in which creative risk takers comprise as much as 20 percent of the general public. 'They are the great experimenters of life,' asserts Farley. 'They break the rules.'"

One researcher who examined a variety of different types of high-risk activities that he called "edgework" found that participants in these pursuits, such as sky diving, claimed that their experiences produced a sense of "self-realization" or "self-determination." Clearly, risk-takers were not suicidal; they experienced considerable fear in the early stages of an "adventure," but also felt that their experiences led to a sense of hyperreality—being much more vivid and real than other day-to-day activities. However, as in several tragic episodes in the late 1990s, fierce storms or avalanches have caused the death of numerous racing yachtsmen or Alpine skiers.[22]

No-Rescue Proposals

Some authorities have suggested that "no-rescue" areas should be established in remote wilderness regions, where those seeking adventure might come fully to grips with the possibility of life-or-death challenges.

In such remote and dangerous regions, with no trails, signs, or patrols, search-and-rescue operations would not be authorized. Despite support for such proposals—based both on the extreme expense and difficulty in carrying out many rescues and on the philosophical position that they would give risk-takers the ultimate degree of freedom and challenge that they seek, they have not been put into effect, for basically humanitarian reasons.

At the same time, many authorities are making increased efforts to control high-risk adventure activities. As an example, many arrests have been made of ice climbers ascending the Bridal Veil Falls, a 360-foot-high frozen falls in Telluride, Colorado, in the southern Rockies. In 1997, this dangerous challenge finally became legal through a pact negotiated with the landowners, the Iderado Mining Company, that exempted them of any liability for accidents or deaths of ice climbers.

It is worth noting that many girls and women have become involved in varied forms of risk recreation, including all-female rock-climbing groups, whitewater rafting trips, and wilderness exploration outings, partly because they perceive these as forms of self-empowerment. Indeed, Bialeschki points out that as long ago as the late 1800s, many women took part in dangerous expeditions and mountain-climbing adventures and were a large part of the membership of the Sierra Club and the Alpine Club of Canada.

Needs of Urban Residents

Although outdoor recreation is chiefly thought of in terms of wilderness areas and parks operated by federal or state agencies, over 80 percent of the nation's population lives in metropolitan areas. As described earlier, to meet their needs most cities and surrounding suburban communities today have park and recreation departments that operate sports facilities, pools, nature centers, marinas, and other leisure facilities.

A growing number of local recreation and park departments have established special facilities for skateboarding, in-line skating, and in-line hockey, despite relatively high insurance costs. Other communities have faced growing problems involving user conflicts on pathways and trails in local parks, where joggers, hikers, in-line skaters, bicyclists, and sometimes horseback riders cause crowding and frequent accidents. Establishing separate lanes for different uses, with better signage and more careful regulation and speed controls, has helped to solve such problems.

Even in ghetto areas of large cities, residents may engage in varied forms of nature-oriented play, including pigeon-raising on tenement rooftops, picnicking and even overnight camping in large urban parks, and visiting natural history museums, botanical gardens, and zoos that increasingly provide accurate replicas of natural settings. At the same time, it is a reality that many poorer urban residents are unable to afford more than the most limited exposure to such outdoor experiences.

For many years, poor and working-class children in the nation's central cities have been able to attend summer camps run by charities and nonprofit organizations, escaping crowded streets, subways, and tenements to become exposed to nature and learning important values and skills. However, in recent years that tradition declined as soaring operating costs and reduced government aid forced many nonprofit sleepaway camps for low-income families to close. In New York State, for example, Norimitsu Onishi writes:

> Between 1985 and 1996, more than a quarter of the state's nonprofit sleepaway camps were closed, dropping from 435 to 321, according to a study conducted last year by the New York State Camp Directors Association. About one-third of the city's 37 settlement houses once owned summer camps. . . . But only one still operates a traditional summer camp; Boys Harbor, which was founded during the Depression and is still supported by the Duke family.[23]

Given the fiscal restraints that have limited many public leisure-service agency operations and the growing gap between upper and lower socioeconomic classes, this trend illustrates the need to provide more adequate recreational and social opportunities—particularly for the urban poor.

Tourism: A Major Industry

Closely linked to outdoor recreation as a form of leisure activity is travel and tourism. The term *travel* usually describes trips extending over a minimum period of time, such as one day with an overnight stay, or trips covering a distance of 100 miles or more. *Tourism* represents that portion of travel that is carried on for personal reasons such as pleasure-seeking, visiting new environments, family reunions, or other leisure-related purposes, as opposed to purely practical functions. In the mid-1980s, John Hunt pointed out that tourism had become a major business enterprise in the United States and throughout the world:

> Tourism creates immense business activity. It accounts for 6 to 7 percent of the Gross National Product and ranks as the third largest retail industry in terms of sales and the second largest private employer in the United States. Estimates generated by the U.S. Travel Data Center indicate that Americans made total travel expenditures of $234 billion on trips of 100 miles or more from home in 1984. Nearly 93 percent of this was spent on travel in the United States. . . . [Expenditures] generated 4.7 million jobs with a payroll of $50.9 billion.[24]

The growth of travel and tourism through the 1980s and 1990s is shown in Table 10.3, which shows how trips taken for pleasure far outnumber those taken for business reasons.

As an indication of the economic value of tourism and travel, other reports show that expenditures by U.S. citizens in travel to foreign countries rose from $40.6 billion in 1988 to $50.7 billion in 1995, while expenditures by foreign travelers in the United States rose from $33.9 billion to $43.3 billion in the same period. Domestic expenditures are substantially higher.

There are five essential interrelated elements in tourism: the people who travel, transportation to and from destinations, accommodations and related facilities, information and travel arrangements, and attractions. The motivations for tourism are varied. Most people travel to meet personal needs—to revitalize or enrich their lives, to relax, to escape routine, or to learn about different environments. Based on these motivations, some authorities suggest that there are four different styles of tourism: (1) educational, cultural, and historical, involving cultural awareness and enrichment; (2) sightseeing, which focuses on spectacular, beautiful, or unusual scenery or natural phenomena; (3) relaxation and hedonism, which emphasizes simple pleasure as a focus of travel; and (4) adventure, in which the tourist seeks out experiences that provide challenges and often physical risks. A number of research studies have analyzed the personal reasons for engaging in tourism, in some cases using leisure motivation scales to study travel purposes and outcomes for such groups as British vacationers.

Given the commercial potential in tourism, a number of innovative entrepreneurs have packaged such unique offerings as tornado-tracking outings or, in one case, guided tours in war zones—with no guarantees of personal safety. A single leisure interest, such as sport, accounts for many trips each year, as millions of fans travel to major tournaments or other athletic events. For many, historical religious settings provide the appeal for individual or group tourism. Surprisingly, a growing motivation for much travel that combines pleasure-seeking and practical purposes involves discount shopping. In 1997, some 55 million Americans traveled 100 or more miles to shop at malls in destinations as varied as Connecticut, the California desert, and the Carolina coast, according to the Travel Industry Association of America.[25]

TABLE 10.3 Travel by U.S. Residents: 1985 to 1997 (in millions)

Type of Trip	1985	1990	1995	1997
All travel: total trips[1]	497.8	589.4	669.7	715.9
Business travel: total trips	156.6	182.8	207.8	207.8
Pleasure travel: total trips	301.2	361.1	413.0	443.2

[1]Includes other trips, not shown separately.

Source: U.S. Travel Data Center, reported in *Statistical Abstract of the United States*, 1998, p. 273.

Roughing It versus Luxury Tourism

Some tourist travel is rough and ready, with a minimum of personal comfort. Over 5000 guides, outfitters, and travel agents now offer or arrange packaged trips to locations that were almost impossible to reach in past years. It is possible to travel by horse, bicycle, dogsled, or one's own two feet, and to opt for primitive camping and total immersion in native cultures.

Hostelling International and the American Youth Hostels promote thousands of guided trips each year and millions of individual low-cost and low-environmental-impact tours by foot, bicycle, or other simple means, staying in basic hostel accommodations around the globe.

On the other hand, many travelers prefer the comfort of ocean cruises. During the 1980s, major cruise companies built huge new ocean liners that were far more than simply vehicles to get from one country to another, but instead evolved into floating amusement parks, health spas, nightclubs, and classrooms. The growth of ocean cruising has been spectacular, climbing from half a million Americans who took cruises in 1970, to 1.5 million in 1982, to a record four million in 1991. Booth writes:

> There's a cruise ship for virtually every taste and pocketbook—122 based in North America alone—from megalines with more than 2,600 passengers to small exploration-type vessels for fewer than 100. The 250 passengers now taking the full round-the-world cruise on Cunard's QE2 paid as much as $126,900 for their staterooms and luxurious lifestyle, but the rich aren't alone on the high seas. About 40 percent of today's cruise passengers earn $20,000 to $39,000 a year and a three-day cruise in the Bahamas can cost as little as $500 to $800 for two.[26]

Increasingly, cruise lines have redesigned their facilities and made other modifications to serve persons with disabilities, both as a marketing strategy and in response to the Americans With Disabilities Act. The U.S. Department of Justice has determined that this law applies to all places of public accommodation, including sightseeing boats, ferries, riverboats, and floating restaurants. Bathrooms, doorways, ramps, and other facilities must now be made wheelchair-accessible, and special provision must be made for the safety of persons with disabilities in the event of emergencies.

The same contrast between inexpensive, simple travel and more luxurious tourism may be found in the popularity both of basic forms of camping and the growing use of elaborate and expensive motor homes. Luscombe points out that there are nine million recreation vehicle owners in the United States, about one in every ten households:

> They own everything from huge 45-foot condo-on-wheels-type motor homes to the collapsible trailers that can be towed to a destination behind most any car and then cranked up to full size.[27]

RV ownership has been growing by about 100,000 a year and is expected to rise to an increase of 135,000 annually, influenced by the growing elderly population that enjoys this mode of travel. Campgrounds accommodating recreation vehicles are increasingly being built by theme parks and even casinos, as a means of attracting the public to these leisure destinations.

Educational and Cultural Tourism

In contrast to purely pleasure-oriented trips, many travelers today are shunning all-play vacations for archaeological digs, research expeditions, horticultural field trips, and other learning excursions concerned with finding out about the arts, history, science, and culture of different countries. In many cases, they are part of group tours—a popular phenomenon in modern-day tourism. Molly Schuchat analyzed such tours from an ethnographic perspective, pointing out that Americans often join such tours to be guided by experts, meet counterparts and unfold their own personal identities, and learn how to be travelers within an organized and relatively safe framework. Industry experts agree that people move in tour groups for safety and assistance, and to get more for their money—often within a limited period of time. Schuchat writes:

> Tour groups offer a delimited and defined testing ground for the resolution of identity crises. They are often used by individuals recently bereaved by death or divorce. Sometimes the group tour will provide support for a return to places previously visited with a loved one—or only known of through a loved one.[28]

Nostalgic tourism often is based on Americans who wish to explore or relive their personal past or interesting elements of the nation's history. This is made possible by the establishment of museums, restoration villages, or other tourist attractions that show buildings, occupations, ethnic customs, costumes, and lifestyles of earlier periods of history. Probably the best known example of historic preservation is Colonial Williamsburg—a depiction of what life was like in a colonial Virginia village. Recently, social critics have begun to challenge such reconstructions, claiming that they lack any sense of reality or historic continuity and instead are often detached, remote, and essentially lifeless.

Such criticism was stimulated by ferment in the historical museum field in the 1960s and 1970s, when grassroots museums sprang up around the United States to preserve and commemorate local heritage. In some cases, black community residents joined forces to save and maintain the slave cabins, "shotgun" houses, little frame churches, and one-room schoolhouses that tell the story of African Americans in the past. Museums and historical collections provide a broader perspective on blacks in America. Washington, DC, publishes an extensive list of tours and attractions highlighting African American history in the nation's capital, extending back in time to the role of Benjamin Banneker, a black mathematician who assisted Pierre L'Enfant in designing the city.

Native Americans represent a major element of tourist interest, with hundreds of attractions on Indian reservations that involve traditional ceremonies, rituals, and the display of dance and other customs, drawing many visitors.

Once discouraged and even forbidden by the federal Bureau of Indian Affairs, today these ceremonies, which blend religion, respect for nature, and community harmony, are increasingly finding their place as a national treasure. Due to concern that such religious rituals may be affected by the presence of too many tourists, tribal authorities try to regulate the number of spectators, although outsiders may attend most traditional events, provided that they maintain a respectful attitude. Authenticity is an important element in the appeal of Indian reservations that are visited each year by thousands of Germans, Italians, and other Europeans. Having grown up with stereotypical or superficial images of Native American life (in Germany, there are over 300 Indian "clubs," whose members who "adopt" a chief or tribe, and study its history), they are eager to experience the real thing. For example, visitors at the Blackfoot Reservation near Browning, Montana, take pictures of the bison herds that wander around the reservation, ride horses that are descendants of the mustangs brought to the Americas by Spanish conquistadores, and learn about the culture of Northern Plains Indians that have lived in this region for thousands of years.[29]

In general, the trend in museums, celebrations, festivals, and other cultural and historical tourist attractions is to provide a more accurate picture of America's past than textbooks and movies have traditionally done. For example, the familiar idea that heroic white males settlers brought civilization to a savage wilderness is now viewed as distorted and, in many cases, racist and sexist. Recent historical research shows that the early West was a place of pitiless struggle involving not only courageous white men but many other human types: Indian chiefs and black newspapermen, society women and prostitutes, fur trappers and squaws. More than half the people who traveled west to search for gold and silver found nothing and went home—if they went home at all—nearly destitute.

As part of cultural tourism, many museums have diversified their holdings and developed new appeals for the traveling public. For example, the famous federal penitentiary at San Quentin, California, has transformed an abandoned building into a museum designed to appeal to tourists. It features a rich and diverse history that makes use of old uniforms, photographs, a scale model of a gas chamber, a ball and chain, home-made weapons, depictions of a famous group escape, and other elements of life behind the bars.

Patriotic sites, military battlefields, buildings, and events provide the basis for other tourist attractions around the nation. Even the Vietnam Veterans Memorial, a long wall of black marble with the names of thousands of victims of this conflict, has proven to have such a powerful degree of public interest that four fiberglass replicas of its have been constructed and are touring the country, staying in different communities for set periods of time. People continue to have a strong reaction to these traveling walls. They leave flags, letters, poems, flowers, and Father's Day cards at them, and they touch the names lightly and cry.

While "cultural" tourism may provide valuable insights into the lives of other people, it may also represent a form of exploitation. When the countries that are visited are markedly poorer than the tourist-generating nation, leisure travel may involve callous indifference to the misery of the people who are being observed. Research in tourist settings in the Caribbean has shown that usually native residents hold only the most unskilled and poorly paid service jobs, with little income going directly to the local economies.

Sex-Oriented and "Sleaze" Tourism

One of the less savory aspects of international tourism involves travelers who seek forms of hedonistic play or entertainment that are not readily available in their own countries. For example, one of the most famous tourist attractions in India has traditionally been the Hindu temple complex at Khajuraho, a small, isolated town in the central Indian state of Madhya Pradesh. The temples are embellished with thousands of sculptures of gods and goddesses, spirits, men, women, and animals in an infinite number of sexual postures. In contemporary, puritanical India, where journals and movies are highly censored, this art is damned as pornography, but permitted to exist and to provide a major tourist attraction because of its legitimate religious origins and because its represents one of India's major cultural and economic resources.

In a more contemporary vein, tourism in present-day Thailand is heavily based on sex, with many thousands of visitors, particularly from other Asian nations, who come to the country because of its readily available prostitutes—particularly child prostitutes. As a consequence, Thailand is suffering from an epidemic of AIDS; in 1993 it was reported that 60 percent of Japanese men who had contracted AIDS through sex with women had caught it on overseas "junkets" in Southeast Asia. And in the late 1990s, growing numbers of traveling pedophiles began to prey on homeless children and youth in Central and Latin American countries that had been ravaged by destructive hurricanes.[30]

A related type of attraction involves so-called "sleaze" tourism—travel in search of more dubious aspects of American culture. Travelers by the millions seek out curious sites each year through "scandal tours" that visit such places as Bonnie and Clyde's death car; where JFK met Judith Campbell Exner; directions to Pete Rose's bookie's joint; where they ambushed John Dillinger; where Huey Long was shot; where Nixon's dog Checkers is buried. Prostitution as part of American frontier history is depicted in the restoration of Miss Laura's Social Club and other brothels in Fort Smith, Arkansas that have been entered in the National Register of Historic Places.[31]

Tourism and the Performing Arts

At another level, a major portion of domestic and international tourism is prompted by interest in the performing and visual arts. Recent studies in Great Britain by the English Tourist Board and the British Tourist Authority underline the importance of such attractions in providing economic support for major arts institutions. Gilbert and Lizotte write in *Travel and Tourism Analyst*:

> . . . once foreign tourists are actually in the United Kingdom (UK), roughly two-thirds of them (62%) visit museums, a third (34%) go to arts galleries and a third (32%) go to the theatre.[32]

In many cities, symphony orchestras, opera and ballet or modern dance companies, and drama serve as key elements that appeal to visitors, who, in turn, patronize hotels and restaurants, visit shops, and otherwise contribute to local economies. Often, regions that were known for a single major event or type of recreation have deliberately set out to diversify their appeal—as in Colorado, where Vail hosts two major orchestras during the summer months, and Aspen, where the Music Festival offers 150 events during a 63-day season. In Telluride, once a backwater silver-mining town, James Brooke writes:

> . . . there is a jazz festival, a blues festival, a bluegrass festival, a theater festival and two film festivals. Choking on culture, townspeople recently rebelled and created a guaranteed festival-free weekend in late July: The Nothing Festival.[33]

Economic Role of Tourism

Based on all the kinds of travel and tourism described in this chapter, pleasure travel represents a huge and growing source of income for many states, cities, and regions.

In the mid-1990s, annual travel industry revenues totaled $416 billion, with Americans taking 700 million vacations each year. According to the Travel Industry Association of America, tourism represents the nation's third highest retail or service industry, directly providing one job for every fifteen working adults, and contributing significantly to numerous other areas of the nation's economy.

While obviously the jobs generated by tourism are critically important in bolstering local economies, in some cases tourism has expanded so greatly that states have begun to discourage tourists, or at least to limit their impact on the lives of year-round residents. Similarly, growing concern about the effect of overuse and harmful forms of play on the natural environment has led many public officials and conservation and tourism organizations to promote "eco-tourism." This approach to protecting the environment and achieving constructive social outcomes through carefully directed tourism and outdoor recreation activities is described in Chapter 13.

Theme Parks: The Disney Phenomenon

No discussion of contemporary tourism would be complete without consideration of theme parks, which represent a key form of family-oriented travel attraction.

Theme parks had their origin in American amusement parks, which flourished in the late nineteenth century and the early decades of the twentieth. Often built in combination with transportation facilities, such as trolley-car lines or excursion boats, amusement parks usually combined several different types of entertainment—roller coasters and other "thrill" rides, midways with varied game booths, funhouses, "freak" shows, and restaurants and beer gardens.

Some of the more famous amusement parks, like New York's Coney Island, had large, impressive structures with fantastic or futuristic architecture similar to buildings designed for major world's fairs at the time. Others featured fire-and-rescue panoramas, pygmy tribe "villages," haunted houses, or rides through frightening environments.

During the years before and after World War II, amusement parks gradually became more tawdry and run-down, with forms of entertainment that were no longer family-oriented. As attendance declined and properties were sold for other real-estate uses, many parks were closed. Then, in the mid-1950s, a new kind of attraction—the theme park—

appeared on the American scene. The first major theme park was Disneyland, established in Anaheim, California, in 1955. Disney's formula was to provide a carefully designed, wholesome, and appealing environment geared to meet family values, with an astute combination of essentially passive recreational experiences—rides through imaginatively designed and technologically clever environments and entertainment featuring the Disney cast of characters.

During the 1960s and 1970s, numerous other theme parks appeared, usually with central themes or images drawn from children's literature, history, or exotic environments or forms of adventure. Among the most successful were the Bally Corporation's Six Flags chain, Busch Entertainment's Dark Continent, Olde Country, Silver Dollar City, and The Great Escape, and Marriott's Great America chain. Some parks, with a variety of rides, water-play facilities, and children's play areas, are participatory in nature; others provide essentially passive or spectator-type entertainment.

In some cases, such as Branson, Missouri, Bar Harbor, Maine, Jackson, Wyoming, or Sedona, Arizona, theme parks or other scenic outdoor recreation or tourist attractions have resulted in entire regions drawing millions of visitors each year. For example, the little town of Pigeon Forge, Tennessee, and its neighboring village of Gatlinburg in the foothills of the Great Smoky Mountains, are overrun by as many as 100,000 tourists each summer day. Hundreds of outlet and specialty stores and entertainment features such as folk museums and country music shows based on the region's culture are centered around Dollywood—an immensely popular theme park starring the singer and actress Dolly Parton.[34]

However, the leading influence in the theme park field has been the varied Walt Disney enterprises. Not content with the company's early success, Disney planners added the Disney World complex in Orlando, Florida, in the 1970s and then the Epcot Center (an acronym for Experimental Prototype Community of Tomorrow), an $800 million, 260-acre development consisting of two portions: (1) Future World, with corporate pavilions primarily concerned with technology; and (2) the World Showcase, with international pavilions showing tourist attractions of various nations around the world—all connected to Disney World's Magic Kingdom by a monorail. In the late 1980s, the Florida complex was expanded with the addition of Disney-MGM Studios, featuring the Great Movie Ride, a tram trip through cinematic wonders, a Backstage Studio Tour of Disney's television and movie-production facilities, and other inside looks at the world of movie "magic."

Disney's Continued Expansion. In the 1990s, the Disney entertainment operations continued to grow, with the 470-acre Disneyland Resort in California, a mega-project costing an estimated $3 billion, six times the size of the original Disneyland. Its new Westcot Center, modeled after the futuristic Epcot Center in Florida, is expected to create 27,900 jobs and generate about $2.4 billion annually. Beyond these domestic ventures, Disney has also expanded on the international scene, with new parks in Japan and France, built with cooperative planning and licensing arrangements with business groups in those nations. The Euro Disneyland, which opened near Paris in 1992, met angry criticism from French intellectuals and social critics, who saw it as evidence of American "cultural colonialism."

Despite such reactions and initially disappointing attendance, the spectacular Disney park, built on 4800 acres with six huge hotels and a championship golf course at a total cost of $4 billion, is expected to be a financial success—in part because it will facilitate the marketing of thousands of Disney-licensed products throughout Europe in the years ahead. The complex network of Disney entertainment ventures, of which tourism is only one part, clearly illustrates the domination of a major portion of American leisure by powerful conglomerates. The Disney empire, in addition to its theme parks (which include numerous hotels, restaurants, shops, and other profitable enterprises) encompasses a huge movie studio, which, in the late 1980s, ranked as the top American filmmaker, with a 30 percent share of all U.S. box-office revenues. The Disney television channel has been the fastest growing pay-TV service in the United States, and the company has expanded its Disney Store chain into a 100-shop operation, along with a successful direct-mail catalogue aimed at home buyers of Disney-related products.

These successes, along with Disney's innovative sports operations and role in totally reshaping New York City's Times Square—which had become a shabby, porn shop area— are described more fully in Chapter 12. Beyond their sheer financial impact, Disney operations have had a profound impact on American culture in other respects. Recognizing that the Disney parks draw more visitors annually than any other American attraction, and that they have become "total destination resorts" without rival, directors of museums of every kind are using their principles to attract, involve, and educate the public. Writing in *The Futurist*, Margaret King points out that the Disney-pioneered approach to theming has become

a standard and model for all large-scale exhibit installations. . . . Although often dismissed as mere entertainment, the theme park has generated an ever-widening circle of influence, ranging from town planning and historical preservation to building architecture, mall design and merchandising. Its impact extends further to video- and computer-assisted education, home and office decor, exhibit design, and crowd management.[35]

With their innovative applications of technology to design, construction, and entertainment, Disney's "Imagineers" have widely influenced the nation's cultural landscape, bridging the gap between art and science, in

the arts of audioanimatronics; applications of computers to problems in communication and exhibition; new uses of videodiscs, electronics and fiber optics; the remaking of historic artifacts as "surrogate objects" by advanced engineering; the melding of space-age with neotraditional forms and functions . . .[36]

Summary

Outdoor recreation and tourism represent two popular and closely linked forms of leisure involvement. Characterized as leisure activity that is heavily dependent on the natural environment, outdoor recreation includes such traditional pastimes as hunting and fishing, boating, camping, backpacking, and rock climbing, as well as such sports-connected pursuits as skiing, snowboarding, or biking. This chapter explores such issues as outdoor recreation's impact on the environment and the role of outdoor adventure and high-risk activities.

Tourism is examined in terms of its motivations and styles, along with its important impact on national and regional economies. Various tourist options include both "luxury" and "roughing" approaches to travel, educational and cultural tourism, "sleaze" and "eco-tourism," and others. The chapter concludes with a discussion of theme park trends, including the immensely diversified offerings of the Disney organization, which include not only travel destinations and entertainment centers, but films, theater, popular music, and a host of other leisure products.

Key Concepts

1. Outdoor recreation represents one of the most popular areas of leisure involvement for Americans, in part playing on our historic identity as pioneers who explored the wilderness and in part our traditional love of the land.

2. Hunting and fishing are two extremely popular outdoor activities. Hunting, as a primarily masculine activity, comes under increasing attack by "animal-rights" spokespersons; fishing takes many forms, often linked to the economic capability of its enthusiasts.

3. As an example of how demographic change influences leisure, skiing has undergone periods of extreme popularity and later declines in participation. In recent years, many skiing centers have become increasingly dependent on snowboarding, which appeals to a much younger, primarily male clientele.

4. Mountain biking and other forms of off-road travel represent another important trend in outdoor recreation, but often involve conflicts between participants and environmentalists because of potential damage to the natural surroundings.

5. Water-based recreation takes many forms, ranging from fishing, sailing, power boating, canoeing or kayaking, river rafting, swimming, fishing, lakeside camping, and other pursuits like water skiing, parasailing, or scuba diving. Again, participation is heavily affected by demographic factors like age or family circumstances, and by economic capability.

6. Adventure recreation fulfills important personal needs for challenge and risk in an increasingly urbanized and controlled society. At the same time, managers of parks, forests, and other outdoor resources must maintain policies to protect participants from excessive danger and, in many cases, to rescue them from injury or death.

7. Tourist motivations are complex, extending from the need to explore new environments, sightsee, relax, or enjoy hedonistic activities to serious educational and cultural drives.

8. As a uniquely American kind of phenomenon initiated in the 1950s by California's Disneyland, theme parks today are found around the world. Making use of varied approaches—centering on historical or fictional themes, natural wonders, daring high-tech rides, entertainment personalities, or virtual-reality settings—they have immense appeal for families and are heavily marketed to international travelers.

Endnotes

1. Winkler, R. 1998. Outdoors: Wildlife Participation Is Holding Steady. *New York Times* (February 8): SP-13.

2. Hunt, J.D. 1986. Tourism Comes of Age in the 1980s. *Parks and Recreation* (October): 31.

3. *Statistical Abstract of the United States*, 1997.

4. La Page, L.F., and S.R. Ranney, 1988. America's Wilderness: The Heart and Soul of Culture. *Parks and Recreation* (July): 24.

5. McAvoy, L., and D. Dustin, 1989. Resurrecting the Frontier. *Trends* (Third Quarter): 42.

6. Greer, L.S. 1990. In *For Fun and Profit: The Transformation of Leisure into Consumption*, ed. R. Butsch. Philadelphia: Temple University Press, p. 152.

7. Dargitz, R. 1988. Angling Activity of Urban Youth: Factors Associated with Fishing in a Metropolitan Context. *Journal of Leisure Research* (20/3): 192.

8. McCullough, G. 1996. Chilling Out. *Philadelphia Inquirer* (December 29): T-1.

9. Taylor, N. 1985. Fishing for Bass and Bucks. *New York Times Magazine* (July 28): 27.

10. O'Leary, J., J. Behrens-Tepper, F. McGuire, and F.D. Dottavio, 1987. Age of First Hunting Experiences: Results from a Nationwide Recreation Survey. *Leisure Sciences* (9): 225.

11. Sifford, D. 1983. It's Not the Quarry or the Trophy That Moves These Hunters. *Philadelphia Inquirer* (November 3): 3-D.

12. Winkler, *op. cit.*

13. Blakeslee, S. 1990. Mountain Biking High. *New York Times Magazine* (October 7): 15.

14. Ditton, R.B., T.L. Goodale, and P. Johnsen, 1975. A Cluster Analysis of Activity, Frequency and Environment Variables to Identify Water-Based Recreation Types. *Journal of Leisure Research* (7/4): 282–295.

15. Heywood, J.L. 1987. Experience Preferences of Participants in Various Types of River Recreation Groups. *Journal of Leisure Research* (10/1): 1–12.

16. Jackson, E.L., and R. Wong. 1982. Perceived Conflict Between Urban Cross-Country Skiers and Snowmobilers. *Journal of Leisure Research* (14/1): 47.

17. Albright, H., quoted in R. Reinhold. 1990. Environmentalists Seek to Run Yosemite Business. *New York Times* (September 23): 30.

18. Manning, R.E. 1985. Diversity in a Democracy: Expanding the Recreation Opportunity Spectrum. *Leisure Sciences* (7/4): 378.

19. McAvoy, L. 1990. An Environmental Ethic for Parks and Recreation. *Parks and Recreation* (September): 89–92.

20. Ewert, A., and S. Hollenhorst. 1989. Testing the Adventure Model. Empirical Support for a Model of Risk Recreation Participation. *Journal of Leisure Research* (21/2): 124–125.

21. Stainbrook, E., quoted in P. Axthelm, 1974. The Thrill-Seekers. *Reader's Digest* (November): 217.

22. Blank, J. 1999. Hell on High Water. *U.S. News and World Report* (January 11): 41.

23. Onishi, N. 1997. Great Outdoors Shrinks at Summer Camps for Urban Children. *New York Times* (August 16): NJ-23.

24. Hunt, J.D., *op. cit.*

25. Rozhon, T. 1998. The Outlet as Destination for Those Who Love a Sale. *New York Times* (April 5): TR-12.

26. Booth, C. 1992. Against the Tide. *Time Magazine* (February 17): 54.

27. Luscombe, B. 1997. RV Having Fun Yet? *Time Magazine* (June 2): 58.

28. Schuchat, M. 1983. Comforts of Group Tours. *Annals of Tourism Research* (10): 469.

29. Egan, T. 1998. Indian Reservations Bank on Authenticity to Draw Tourists. *New York Times* (September 21): A-1.

30. Roche, T. 1999. Tourist Who Prey on Kids. *Time Magazine* (February 15): 58.

31. Clines, F. 1997. An Ill Wind Is No Match for a House of Ill Repute. *New York Times* (November 27): F-8.

32. Gilbert, D., and M. Lizotte. 1998. Tourism and the Performing Arts. *Travel and Tourism Analyst* (1): 82–87.

33. Brooke, J. 1997. As Slopes Warm Up, the Sound of Festivals. *New York Times* (August 9): 1, 12.

34. McDowell, E. 1997. Nature Is Second Fiddle to Dolly's Theme Park. *New York Times* (August 14): B-1.

35. King, M. 1991. The Theme Park Experience: What Museums Can Learn from Mickey Mouse. *The Futurist* (November-December): 24.

36. *Ibid.*, p. 27.

11 Pastimes III: Popular Culture—Arts and Entertainment, Television, and Hobbies

Two studies, commissioned by the National Endowment for the Arts, conclude that despite higher incomes and better levels of education, younger Americans are unlikely ever to attend live performances of what one of the authors calls "highbrow culture"—especially classical music, opera, and musical and dramatic theater—in the same proportions or with the same intensity as the generations before them.[1]

Television has [for half a century] been gobbling up time the way a good running back gobbles up yardage. Regardless of income, education, or any major demographic indicator, Americans have made television the unrivaled consumer of their free time.

Until recently, when researchers began to record a drop in viewing among young people, nothing has remotely weakened its grip. Americans spend more time watching television than working out, reading, using the computer, working in the garden, and going to church—combined.[2]

We turn now to a third major sector of leisure involvement—what is commonly referred to as "popular culture." This term applies to a broad range of activities that include both active forms of participation and spectator involvement in the arts, television, video games and other computer-linked pastimes, movies and radio, and a host of hobbies and other home-based pursuits. Like sports and games or travel and tourism, popular culture has been transformed into a commodity in the sense that it now comprises an immense sector of economic activity and organized sponsorship. At the same time, it serves to communicate important societal beliefs and values and express the varied creative impulses of participants.

Meaning of Popular Culture

Typically, the term *culture* has been applied to such artistic pursuits as classical music, opera and ballet, drama, and serious literature, or the fine arts of painting, sculpture, and print making. However, this has been a narrow interpretation of the word, in the sense that culture really embraces a much broader range of values, customs, beliefs, and behaviors that characterize a people.

Social critics have often divided culture into two or three categories. For example, the distinction between the art of the common people and the upper classes is generally portrayed as a contrast between "elite" or "highbrow" forms of art and "vernacular" or "lowbrow" forms. The term *entertainment* usually implies that a play, movie, or book is not regarded as a serious piece of artistic expression, but is intended chiefly for easy, unsophisticated enjoyment. For example, symphonic music or classical opera would be considered elite musical forms, while rock and roll or country music would be seen as lowbrow forms. Dwight MacDonald describes the origin of popular or, as he calls it, "mass" culture:

> The historical reasons for the growth of Mass Culture since the early 1800s are well known. Political democracy and popular education broke down the old upper-class monopoly of culture. Business enterprise found a profitable market in the cultural demands of the newly awakened masses, and the advance of technology made possible the cheap production of books, periodicals, pictures, music, and furniture, in sufficient quantities to satisfy this market. Modern technology also created new media such as the movies and television, which are especially well adapted to mass manufacture and distribution.[3]

More recently, Shivers and DeLisle described a "two-tiered" system of culture:

> High culture, or the culture of the well-to-do, is concerned with music and literature and the support of the fine arts. Self-enrichment, education, travel, and an appreciation of nature are considered worthy of this class of individual. Popular culture describes the middle class way of life. This includes the knowledge, beliefs, art, morals, customs, and leisure pursuits of the most visible segment of society.[4]

Certainly, there is evidence to support this view. In the mid-1960s, an extensive research study on the arts sponsored by the Twentieth Century Fund showed that there was a highly limited audience for serious performing arts events in music, drama, and dance. This well-educated and affluent segment of society comprised no more than 5 million adults—about 4 percent of the overall population at that time. It is probable that the same situation prevails today, with a selective, elite audience for many serious cultural events or for fine arts or literature.

However, it should also be recognized that interest in the arts *has* grown steadily over the past century. In the early 1990s, the influential upper classes founded art museums and conservatories, symphony orchestras and ballet companies, and similar institutions. Growth in the arts was striking after World War II. At this time, the number of American symphony orchestras more than doubled, from about 600 to over 1400, and the sale of records and musical instruments increased by over 850 percent. Numerous community art centers were built to house the fine and performing arts, ranging from New York City's $142 million Lincoln Center for the Performing Arts to smaller centers in hundreds of other communities.

By the late 1980s, attendance at varied kinds of artistic events had grown dramatically throughout the United States. During the period between the mid-1970s and mid-1980s, attendance at live performances of plays, musical comedies, and other forms of theater rose from 53 percent of the adult population to 67 percent—up to 116 million people a year. Those attending live musical performances by popular singers, bands, and rock groups increased over the decade from 46 percent to 60 percent, a total of 104 million attendees. Attendance at live performances of classical or symphonic music, ballet, modern or ethnic dance, and opera and musical theater also rose sharply.

Other studies have shown widespread participation by the public in various types of crafts or creative activities, with the most popular pursuits being photography, needlepoint, or weaving; playing musical instruments; painting, drawing, or etching; writing stories or poems; doing ballet or modern dance, singing in a choral group; ceramics and sculpting.

As such forms of creative expression gain popularity and critical esteem, the historic separation of art into "high" art and "low" art, as described earlier—the one considered serious and worth of public support, and the other cheap and lacking in taste—is breaking down. Edward Sozanski writes:

> One could argue that the term "high art" is invalid, that art should not be defined as "high" or "low" but as either unique or mass-produced, and, within these categories, as good or bad. . . . The dichotomy between "high" and "low" developed with the rise of the mass media and the creation of elitist organizations such as symphony orchestras and art museums. Unique works such as paintings became the province of the moneyed class, while the working class made do with multiples and disposable images—prints, newspapers and magazines.[5]

Sozanski goes on to suggest that the distinction between "high" and "popular" art was sharpened by the development of movies, radio, and television, as "mass culture" forms. However, he writes, it is a distinction between the exclusive and the commonplace, between the expensive and the affordable, not between intrinsically superior and inferior ways of making art.

At the same time, popular culture includes many forms of entertainment or leisure participation that cross social class lines, including, particularly for the young, popular music and video games, television sitcoms, movies with broad appeal, or recreational reading. Many outdoor recreation pursuits or travel interests are shared by different levels of the population, with financial capability governing the specific forms they take. Given this background, it is helpful to examine the development of the arts in particular, in the American society.

The Arts in Leisure

First, there is growing awareness of the value of art as a form of personal leisure involvement. Both for those who engage directly in such activities and for those who are the audience for the arts, they have the following important benefits:

1. The arts provide beauty in our lives—not necessarily in the sense of attractive, harmonious, or beautifully designed objects or works, but rather in terms of their emotional impact and depth, and the vision they provide of the world.
2. In a world dominated by the mass media, marked by conformity of beliefs and behavior, the arts provide an opportunity for people to develop their individual talents and make unique personal statements in one or another area of aesthetic performance.
3. In a world that tends to value material accomplishment and competition for external goals, the arts provide an opportunity—not always realized—to be deeply immersed in an experience for its own sake.
4. Unlike very active sports or very vigorous outdoor recreation activities, the arts are easily adaptable to persons of all ages and at all levels of physical capability—including those who are physically or mentally disabled. From a therapeutic perspective, artistic expression often provides a valuable form of emotional release and may constitute a specific treatment modality.
5. Although audiences for the arts may be deeply affected by viewing paintings, sculpture, or theater pieces, or by hearing symphonies or chamber music, artistic involvement is particularly rewarding for those who participate actively and creatively.
6. Finally, art in all its forms represents a way of perceiving the world—either literally, as in a poem, short story, novel, or painting, or symbolically, as in the work of many modern artists or composers.

Tables 11.1 and 11.2 show attendance and participation rates in various arts activities by gender and race.

TABLE 11.1 Attendance Rates for Various Arts Activities

Activity	Jazz Performance	Classical Music Performance	Opera	Musical Play	Nonmusical Play	Ballet	Art Museum
Total	11	13	3	17	14	5	27
Sex: Male	12	12	3	15	12	4	27
Female	9	13	4	20	15	6	27
Race: White	10	13	3	18	14	5	28
Black	16	7	2	14	12	3	19
Other	6	12	5	11	10	6	29

In percent, for persons 18 years old and over, excluding elementary and high school performances. Reports attendance at least once in preceding 12 months.

Source: U.S. National Endowment for the Arts, *1997 Survey of Public Participation in the Arts*, in *Statistical Abstract of the United States, 1998*, p. 271

TABLE 11.2   Participation Rate in Various Arts Activities

Activity	Adult Population (mil.)	Playing Classical Music	Modern Dancing	Pottery Work	Needle-work	Photo-graphy	Painting	Creative Writing
Total	185.8	4	8	8	25	12	10	7
Sex: Male	89.0	3	8	8	5	13	9	7
Female	96.8	5	8	9	43	10	10	8

In percent, reports participation at least once during preceding 12 months.

Source: As in Table 11.1, National Endowment for the Arts.

Community Programs in the Arts

For all these reasons, the arts represent a major area of leisure activity and an important part of community recreation offerings. At the simplest level, they can represent a relaxing, "fun" kind of pastime, appealing at any age level. Working in a studio or at a play rehearsal is a social experience, involving cooperation and the blending of joint efforts, and the often leading to the excitement of an exhibit or performance before an audience. A strong case may be made that community recreation programs often provide more extensive opportunities in the arts than the public schools do. Since the 1950s, emphasis on science and mathematics and cost-cutting curriculum slashes have sharply reduced many school-based programs in the arts. Conn writes:

> Particularly in area where there had been major cutbacks in arts programs in schools, there was a real hunger for entry-level education in instrumental music, voice, dance, painting, ceramics, sculpture, and sometimes film and video. The early enrollees were children, but recreation departments soon got used to the long lines of adults waiting to sign up for classes for themselves *and* their children.[6]

In city after city, from Tulsa, Oklahoma, to Raleigh, North Carolina, and Miami, Florida, to Portland, Oregon, cities have established community arts centers with capable instructors, exhibitions, and performing groups that bring varied forms of art to the public at large. Community arts festivals including folk music, jazz, storytelling, ballet, modern, and ethnic dance, and theater productions have become popular across the country, and the field of arts administration has become a recognized discipline and area of special training today. In many cases, community arts programs are coordinated and promoted by arts councils, which assist them in obtaining funding and heighten the public's awareness of the arts.

A second important ingredient in arts sponsorship today consists of colleges and universities that have programs in their general curricula and specialized degree offerings in the various performing and visual arts. In many cases, universities have elaborate and well-equipped performing arts centers to serve both their own performing groups and touring professional companies.

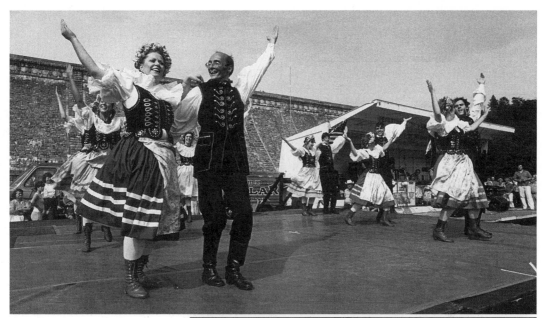

Millions of Americans enjoy varied forms of arts and crafts, music, dance and drama, and other creative pursuits. Here, Polish American folk dancers perform their traditional dances in Westchester County, New York. Older men and women take part in painting and drawing classes, while children enjoy a drama rehearsal in Vero Beach, Florida.

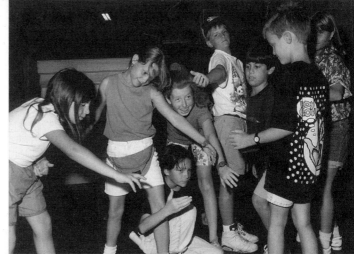

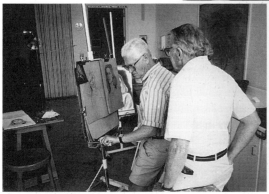

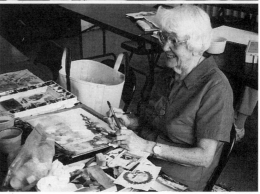

Several different types of artistic or creative activities may be enjoyed in leisure, including the visual and performing arts, electronic entertainment, and the literary arts.

Visual Arts.   This terms refers specifically to creative activities that yield actual products that are tangible and meant to be seen, such as graphic forms of expression like painting, drawing, or print making, or plastic arts like sculpture or ceramics. They may be approached at varied levels, from finger painting, simple crafts, and sketching for very young children to portrait and landscape painting for adults.

Public recreation departments usually offer arts and crafts as a staple of playground, day camp, or adult leisure programs—sometimes with an extensive battery of classes and clubs that use community-center or school facilities. Weaving, work with clay, nature crafts, jewelry, and metal working may be approached on different levels of expertise and may extend to such useful projects as dressmaking, sewing, and similar activities. Many public departments operate arts centers with workshops, exhibition galleries, and ties to community organizations concerned with the arts.

In addition, many private schools, summer camps, and arts organizations also sponsor extensive programs in the visual arts. Reflecting expanded interest in handmade crafts, dozens of huge craft fairs are held today around the United States, and the field itself, according to *Trade Show Week Magazine*, comprises a $3 billion retail industry.

Performing Arts.   The performing arts—music, drama, and dance—are important elements in the popular leisure. Just as in the visual arts, they may be approached on different levels of intensity or artistic quality. They may be enjoyed as leisure activity by young children in simple rhythmic or musical experiences, creative dramatics, or beginning ballet classes. On the other hand, adults may take classes in playing instruments, musical theory, or choral music, or may join performing groups on an amateur or professional basis. Each of the performing arts is linked to the mass media of entertainment—either in popular forms like soap opera, musical comedy, dance, or rock and roll or rap music, on the professional stage, or in television and motion pictures.

Audience involvement in the performing arts has generally risen over the past several decades, although in some cases there have been declines in attendance and financial pressures have constricted some forms of performing activity.

Music as Recreation.   Turning now to the separate forms of performing art, music represents a major leisure interest of millions of Americans, in terms of either making or listening to music. Music may be approached informally, as part of family recreation in the home, although the old tradition of families gathering around a piano and singing as a regular form of family "togetherness" clearly has declined through the years. However, in many other ways, music continues as a recreational experience. Children and youth join various types of musical groups, such as rock bands, marching bands, choral groups, church choirs, and similar aggregations; they enjoy Christmas caroling, singing around a camp fire, or playing guitars for folksinging.

Many public recreation departments sponsor varied forms of musical activity for children and youth, offering instrumental instruction, classes in musical theory, and different types of performing groups. Some sponsor summer music camps or schools, while others assist opera companies, chamber music societies, and similar organizations in finding facilities and promoting their performances with the public at large.

In addition to attendance at musical performances of all kinds, a key measure of music's popularity consists of the purchase of compact discs and prerecorded cassettes. Between 1975 and 1991, the number of unit shipments of various forms of recorded music rose from 531 million units to 801 million units annually, with total manufacturers' value that rose from $2.3 billion to $7.8 billion in the later year.

The immense sums of money involved in the public's enjoyment of music is further illustrated by the money earned by individual performers and groups within the popular music field, such as Michael Jackson, the Rolling Stones, and others. Madonna, the bleached-blonde pop star, is the president and sole owner of a multimillion-dollar corporate organization that in peak season has hundreds of employees and operates through half a dozen entities. Some performers, like Bruce Springsteen and Aerosmith, maintain popularity over a long period of time, while newer groups replace other entertainers in public appeal.

However, the popularity of youth-oriented musical products is accompanied by a number of critical abuses, which show how the public's leisure is often manipulated by commercial interests. For example, influencing disk jockeys to play albums on radio—which stimulates cassette or compact disc sales—has often been influenced by bribery or "payola." Beyond this, many social critics and parents are concerned about the content of much of the content of today's rock bands—often deliberately violent, crude, sexist, and racist. In Ice Cube's album, *Death Certificate*, Koreans are threatened: "Pay attention to the black fist, or we'll burn your store right down to a crisp."

In the early 1990s, rap music (a fast-talking, highly rhythmic form of pop entertainment) was identified by a large-scale research study in several major cities as the only form of communication that ghetto youth were really responsive to—the best way of reaching them with a social message. What was the message that rap groups were delivering to their most committed fans, African American youth? While some of it is simply light, entertaining, and amusing, much of it consists of an angry, racist, violent sermon. One critic writes that rap songs deliver a constant obscene onslaught about "bitches, whores and brutal sex." Women seem to exist merely to be picked up, used, abused, and quickly discarded.

As the society spends billions of dollars to produce and consume such tawdry and destructive forms of musical entertainment, other valuable forms of musical expression are being starved for financial support. For example, throughout the 1980s, a deepening economic crunch forced many orchestras to cut back on their seasons, reduce pay scales for musicians, and restrict their repertoire in other ways. In the early 1990s, twenty-eight of the nation's largest symphony orchestras reported serious budget crises; many were forced to reduce their operations significantly.

As reported earlier, public school programs in the arts have also been sharply curtailed; only nine states today mandate arts curricula for all high school students. In Los Angeles County, 30 percent fewer juniors and seniors take music courses than in the 1950s. Yet a College Entrance Board study

found that students who took more than four years of music and arts scored 34 points higher on verbal SATs and 18 points better on math SATs than those who took music for less than one year. At the University of California at Los Angeles, a study of students served by the . . . County's Artist-in-Residence program found improvement in reading, writing, and speaking skills, social studies, science and math.[7]

Drama as Leisure Activity.   The theater has had a long and rich tradition in American culture, ranging from the first struggling touring companies in the New England and Middle Atlantic colonies to a full blossoming of a native American theater in the twentieth century. Since World War II, in Broadway's Times Square district—traditionally the heart of American drama—many theaters have been abandoned because of rising costs of production, crime, and unstable real estate values.

However, the theater itself is far from dead in America. Many college and university towns have established cultural complexes with repertory companies that put on the works of Shakespeare, Ibsen, and other classical writers, along with new plays by native playwrights. In 1992, Barbara Janowitz, director of management services for the Theater Communications Group, the umbrella organization for the nation's nonprofit companies, commented:

> Despite all the negative implications of the recession, strong leadership and sophisticated management skills [in the nation's theaters] have been truly impressive. This, as well as an outstanding commitment on the part of theater trustees, will see the theaters through these difficult years.[8]

Many companies throughout the country are persuading the public that theatergoing is an exciting activity by presenting first-rate classical and modern plays in high-quality productions.

At the same time, there is growing evidence that in many performing arts centers around the country, serious drama, along with classical music and opera, is suffering from the competition of touring companies playing revivals of popular musical theater works. For example, "Phantom of the Opera," "Showboat," and the "The King and I" have played to full houses in regional theater settings in the late 1990s, while subscriptions to serious dramatic works have declined sharply.

However, studies of the theater in New York suggest that there has been a steady growth of young theatergoers, with those under 20 totaling 13.9 percent of the audience for Broadway performances, compared with 4.9 percent thirty years ago. In addition, research by the Theater Development Fund and the League of American Theaters has found that while audiences remain predominantly white, younger theatergoers are more ethnically diverse than older ones.[9]

Apart from professional forms of theater, a second important aspect of drama as a form of leisure is that it offers a major opportunity for creative self-expression in amateur theater performance. Among the programs that may be offered by public recreation and park departments, voluntary youth agencies, schools, and colleges are the following: (1) the use of dramatic play in regular recreation programs, including charades, pantomime, puppetry, storytelling, pantomime, dramatic games, and other unstructured and creative acting experiences; (2) amateur theatrical programs, including school plays for youth and one-act plays or drama festivals for local performing groups, in some cases linked to historical pageants or civic celebrations; (3) children's theater programs, in which they receive instruction in acting and stagecraft and put on formal drama productions; and (4) the specialized use of drama as a therapeutic technique with mentally or physically disabled persons.

Dance in Recreation.   Dance has two primary aspects as a form of leisure activity: as a *social pastime* and as a *stage art*. As a social activity it ranges from the more formal kinds of ballroom dance, such as the waltz, foxtrot, or Latin-American dances like the cha-cha, merengue or tango, to newer forms of disco, rock, or occasional "fad" dances that capture the public's imagination briefly. Social dances are enjoyed in many leisure settings, such as cruise ships, resorts, or clubs, and are supplemented by folk, square, country, and "line" dancing, which also have millions of adherents.

Beyond its social role in leisure, dance also is a concert art form. Its best-known form is ballet, originally a classical court dance in Renaissance Italy and France that was popularized in America by George Balanchine of the New York City Ballet. Today, there are a number of highly regarded companies in major cities such as Boston, Atlanta, Houston, and San Francisco, while numerous smaller companies enjoy public support in regional settings. An essentially aristocratic art form, ballet tends to be patronized by the well-to-do in American communities. Dance has traditionally had the aura of being a feminine art. Balanchine himself perpetuated this stereotype, speaking of ballet as ". . . a purely female thing; it is a woman—a garden of beautiful flowers, and the man is the gardener." Despite this reputation, many leading choreographers and performers are male, and ballet has come to be recognized as an androgynous art form—not to be labeled for one sex or the other.

A second important form of concert dance is modern dance, a movement that stemmed from the rebellion of Isadora Duncan, Ruth St. Denis, and Ted Shawn against the classical ballet during the early 1900s, and was brought to maturity by Martha Graham, Doris Humphrey, Merce Cunningham, and other choreographers and teachers during the middle decades of the twentieth century. Modern dance represents the more exploratory, avant-garde form of art dance that tends to be taught more widely than ballet in the schools and colleges of the nation.

At a much simpler level, dance may be approached in community recreation programs through the introduction of children's rhythms, singing games, simple folk and square dances, or through jazz dance, tap dance, or other ethnic dance forms. Often it is featured at community festivals presenting African American, Hispanic, or Asian cultural forms, or other traditional ethnic dances.

Mass Media of Entertainment

We now turn to a key element in America's popular culture—the electronic mass media of radio, television, and motion pictures. Unlike the visual or performing arts, in which many people participate as amateur hobbyists, the electronic media are almost totally professional forms of spectator entertainment. There are a few ways in which members of the public have been drawn in a participants: through radio and television talk shows, as contestants in television game shows or subjects of ridicule on programs like "Candid Camera" or taped episodes of family misadventures, or as protagonists in semifictitious televised courtroom trials. Essentially, however, the communication process in radio, television, and movies is in a one-way direction, with the public serving passively as members of the audience.

Radio

The first forms of electronic entertainment to capture great portions of American leisure were radio and motion pictures. Preceding television as home-based entertainment, radio was immensely popular from the 1920s to the 1950s, with a diverse array of programs. It contained news and sports broadcasts, popular variety shows, comedy hours, soap operas, discussion programs, quiz shows, classical music, and numerous other specialized kinds of programs.

With the onset of television, radio lost the bulk of its traditional audience to this new, richer form of entertainment and education. A major portion of daytime and evening radio was turned over to playing popular music—at first simply the top forty songs (as determined by national record sales), and in time more narrowly targeted programs focusing on rock oldies, hip-hop, and hard rock.

In addition to playing music, radio programmers also strive to reach other specific audiences: people in their cars who want to know about highway traffic conditions, sports fans who crave continuing discussion of their favorite teams, people who listen to music or talk shows while they work, people who seek religious consolation, and other fragmented groups in the population. A number of smaller radio stations have survived as independent community broadcasters serving local needs with call-in shows about controversial local issues, giving public-service announcements, offering offbeat folk entertainment, publicizing and sponsoring community festivals and other special events.

In opposition to the trend toward such individualized programming, in the early 1990s the Federal Communications Commission voted to turn the country's radio stations into a "homogenized" commodity controlled by large corporations. In arguable violation of the Communications Law of 1934, the FCC voted in 1992 to let a single corporation own as many as thirty AM and thirty FM stations, up from an earlier limit of seven stations in each category. Ben Bagdikian points out that the FCC policies allow joint ventures among giant station owners—arrangements that permit them to saturate the market with their offerings. He writes:

> By steadily relaxing limits on ownership and introducing other new provisions, the F.C.C. has done two things. It has fostered broadcasting that is a nationally homogenized mix of programs, indistinguishable from one market to another, and it has made licensing a game largely reserved for big corporations. More and more, local political, ethnic and social groups, women, minorities and unions are out of the picture.[10]

Finally, in the mid- and late-1990s, it was evident that talk-show radio had become an increasingly influential force in arousing interest in public affairs and in promoting heated controversies on matters of morality, political policy, and similar concerns. Federally assisted public radio has brought a valuable ingredient of classical music, human-interest or health-related themes, and other socially oriented programming to many communities around the country.

Motion Pictures

Beginning in the early twentieth century with crude black-and-white films that were viewed in tiny storefronts by spectators who paid a few pennies to see this miraculous new form of entertainment, motion pictures rapidly became a national craze. For several decades, the movies reigned unchallenged with a host of films of every type: comedies, dramas, romances, Western films, mysteries and crime films, war films and epics of history, biographies, and modern versions of old classics.

Controlled by several large studios, films nurtured male and female superstars who became idols of the American public and created an aura of glamour over Hollywood and the movie industry. With the onset of television in the 1950s, motion pictures had a marked decline, dropping from total attendance in 1948 (the year television networks got under way) of 3.4 billion admissions, to about 1.1 billion a year in the late 1960s. Since then, attendance has remained relatively stable, with revenues going up steadily because of increased admissions charges.

The power of the great film companies declined, with smaller, more flexible independent producers taking their place, and major performers and directors able to move more freely from project to project. Almost from the beginning, films were linked with their rivals for public interest—the television networks. Older films were regularly used to fill open time on television channels, and filmmakers moved back and forth from making feature movies to creating television specials and miniseries. Myron Marty sums up the trend at this time:

> Television did not bring about the demise of the motion picture industry, as some had predicted years earlier. The industry held its own partly by producing made-for-television films and selling broadcasting and videotaping rights of movies after they had run in theaters. Sales in foreign countries also helped. Most of the industry's revenue, however, poured in through box offices, as going to movies remained a popular social activity. People were still willing to pay more to see the film on a big screen and blockbuster films brought in much of the industry's revenue.[11]

A whole new opportunity for profit opened up when motion pictures began to be released for home viewing in the form of videocassettes after their profitability in movie house runs had declined. In 1997, the *Statistical Abstract of the United States* reported that total motion picture revenues from production, distribution, theater showings, and videotape rentals had risen from $39.9 billion in 1990 to $58.1 billion in 1995.

Films and Social Issues.   Motion pictures have both reflected the image that the nation had of itself and helped to shape its cultural values and behavior. In gangster films of the 1930s, for example, fascination with violence and big-city mobsters tended to be featured. American attitudes toward racial and ethnic minority groups under went a transition in the decades following World War II, as described in earlier chapters. Following this lead, the treatment of African Americans, Latinos, and other minorities shifted to more honest and sympathetic presentations of their lives.

The treatment of women in films reflected the influence of feminism, with women increasingly being shown in roles of strong career women, union organizers, detectives, and other powerful parts. At the same time, some critics suggest that current films paint a deliberately negative picture of independent women. Susan Faludi, for example, writes that in typical movies of the 1980s

> women were set against women; women's anger at their social circumstances was depoliticized and displayed as personal depression instead; and women's lives were framed as morality tales in which the "good mother" wins and the independent woman gets punished.[12]

Faludi concludes that Hollywood producers were deliberately reinforcing a backlash response to feminism; American women were depicted as unhappy because they were too free; their liberation had denied them marriage and motherhood. Opposed to this tendency, the early 1990s saw a number of successful women directors making films for the first time on a wide range of themes. Women directors are no longer limited by the notion that they are only capable of making delicate little films and are increasingly able to influence Hollywood moviemaking.

Gradually, films are dealing with the issue of homosexuality with more honesty and frankness. For years, homosexual characters in movies were portrayed as creepy misfits or campy caricatures—marginal, dubious people. However, in a number of films in the late 1980s and early 1990s, gay and lesbian relationships were portrayed more sympathetically.

At the same time, some of the controls on the portrayal of explicit sexual behavior on the screen have been relaxed. Since 1968 the Motion Picture Association of America had used a rating system that attached the X category to films that were in its view too overtly sexual. However, in the early 1990s, the Motion Picture Association removed the X category from its rating system, replacing it with an NC-17 (no children under 17 allowed).

In the 1980s and 1990s, a growing number of "blockbuster" films dealt with themes of mass destruction, science fiction projections of the future, bloody slaughters by synthetic heroes—many embodying computer-aided techniques to stimulate reality. Linked to this development was the growing domination of worldwide film, television, and home-video markets by American producers.

The box-office boom in Europe for U.S. entertainment products began in the early 1980s, when state-run television industries made room for private networks. Starved for programming content, these new channels began running American movies and language-dubbed television shows, which proved popular and created a larger audience for Hollywood products. Today, the export of entertainment yields an $8 billion trade surplus annually to the American economy. However, some critics wonder what Europeans must think of the America that is depicted: a relentlessly unfolding series of rapes, murders, shootings, and car chases. Media critic Ross Baker comments: "We have exported our culture quite successfully, but it is a culture that shows only the seamy underside of American society and offers little or no evidence that an alternative exists."

Television as Dominant Leisure Activity

The most powerful medium of popular entertainment in the United States is clearly television. The growth of this form of home-based leisure activity has been spectacular. By 1990, over 98 percent of American homes had television sets, and over 59 percent of these subscribed to cable television. In the mid-1980s television watching in the average home reached a new high of almost seven hours a day.

A study by United Media Enterprises concluded that television served chiefly as a backdrop for other family activities, and that it seemed not to erode basic family and community concerns as much as it coexisted with them. In effect, the report concluded that television had become "the new American hearth—a center for family activities, conversation and companionship." It explained:

> Far from creating a generation of television zombies, the tube showed almost no ability to deflect Americans from other favorite pursuits around the house. Frequent adult watchers seem to be as home-centered as those who watch very little TV. Avid TV viewers read to their children and engage in family chats, possibly because the prime evening viewing hours coincide with time usually set aside for family activities.[13]

Twenty years ago when students went to college, television sets were found chiefly in dormitory lounges, rather than in individual rooms. However, by the early 1990s, the new generation of college students—who had grown up on "Sesame Street," then moved on to MTV, the youth-oriented music video program—took television sets to college with them as a matter of course. Todd Gitlin, professor of sociology at the University of California at Berkeley, comments:

> TV is their collective dream machine, their temple, their sense of being members of a nation. It's as if they're carrying their pews with them. They've always watched "LA Law." They can't imagine a world without it. It's normal. College is one episode in this unfolding normality.[14]

A 1991 survey by Roper College Track, a market research service, found that college students watched television an average of eighteen hours a week, with the most popular programs including soap operas and late-night talk and comedy shows. At the same time, a number of students were critical of television's role in their lives. "TV's turning us into a mush nation," said one college senior. A freshman agreed, "Nothing's on, and they all sit around watching it. TV destroyed the American family. Adults come home from work and watch TV. It cuts off communication."

Impact on Children and Youth

Almost from the beginning, adults were concerned about the impact of television on children and youth. In the mid-1980s, it was argued that many of the educational programs for children, like "Captain Kangaroo," had disappeared, and that highly acclaimed programs offered by the Public Broadcasting System, such as "Sesame Street," were unavailable in many areas of the country. In May 1993, a former children's television executive for ABC reported that the number of educational programs offered by the three major networks, which had totaled eleven hours a week in 1980, now involved less than one hour a week. Instead, the major networks were offering chiefly vacuous cartoon programs in prime children's television time. The more serious criticism is that many children have become hooked on television and that it has been responsible for a wave of violence and delinquent behavior among the young.

A study by the National Institute of Mental Health concluded that "violence on television does lead to aggressive behavior by children and teenagers who watch the programs." The National Coalition on Television Violence, a citizens' group, reported "recent deluge of high-action, violent cartoon shows." The coalition's psychiatrist head concluded, "We can only pump so much violence into our people before we explode." In 1992, an article published in the *Journal of the American Medical Association* concluded that childhood exposure to television violence was at the heart of the nation's 100 percent increase in violent crime and the doubling of homicides since television was introduced. And, in 1993, despite assurances by the Motion Picture Association of America that video stores did not allow children to rent videos that contained clearly adult depictions of sex or violence, a field test conducted by *U.S. News and World Report* found that many children ages 10 to 14 *were* able to rent such films.

In response to such concerns, in the same year the three major television networks, ABC, CBS, and NBC, agreed on standards governing television violence that would result in toning down excessive or overly shocking scenes and use greater care when portraying children as the victims of violence, and in children's programming generally. However, some critics maintain that television is simply part of a total environment—including movies, rock music, and other media—that is drenched in sex and violence.

Concern about the violent content of much television today is only part of a broader set of criticisms of programming—which has increasingly been influenced by cable television networks, rather than the three major networks. While it is generally recognized that television offers many constructive and meaningful programs and sets the agenda for our national political, social, and cultural dialogue, critics argue that it too focuses on trivial, sensational, or pointless themes.

In part, television news and special-feature programming's emphasis on negative aspects of community life is seen as contributing to poor community morale and exaggerated fears of crime. Writing in *Commonweal*, Abigail McCarthy points out that, while major drops in overall crime and homicides are given little play in the popular media, the detailed daily reporting of murders, thefts, and muggings create an atmosphere of relentless danger.[15]

Another major concern has to do with television interview, talk, or confrontation programs featuring such hosts as Jerry Springer or Sally Jessy Raphael, who present individuals with severe personal problems, often in semi-contrived situations that lead to on-screen attacks. Sometimes called "freak shows," these distorted pictures of American life have been criticized by mental health authorities:

They exploit people who are deeply troubled and in need of more than an hour's worth of sound-bite advice. . . . By focusing on sexual abuse one day and transvestite weddings the next, they blur the line between major social problems and tangential or trivial issues. . . . Because these shows make a virtue of suffering, they glorify victimization but often fail to point out to victims ways of moving beyond their pain . . .[16]

At the same time, Alison Bass writes, such shows are also widely credited with being the first to illuminate the dark underbelly of our culture, such as the frequency of childhood sexual abuse and domestic violence.

Authorities differ regarding the responsibility of television networks and programmers as a key medium of mass communication. Many argue that they are justified in giving people what they want—as indicated by audience ratings—with limitations only on the deliberate instigation of public panic, extreme violence, or such elements as cannibalism or explicit pornography. They assume that television reflects but does not create or shape individual or collective attitudes, beliefs, or behaviors. Others believe that television, as a particularly powerful medium that enters the home for many hours a day, should have a social responsibility to contribute in a positive way to family and community values and relationships.

Video Games and Computer Pursuits

Another widely shared, related leisure pursuit among children and youth today is video games. *U.S. News and World Report* commented in the early 1980s that America had become a "stay-at-home society," with a flurry of electronic products—video games, video-cassette recorders, big-screen TVs, color cameras, and home computers—all filling the nation's leisure.

Through the late 1980s and early 1990s, the video game market proliferated, with companies like Nintendo and Sega designing a whole host of games with richer color, clearer sound, faster action, and more sophisticated play. By 1992, Nintendo controlled an estimated 85 percent of the almost $5-billion-a-year video-game market with thirty million families caught up in its successively more expensive and complex systems.

In the mid- and late-1990s, it became clear that video games had continued to expand in their appeal to include adults captured by their technologically sophisticated imagery. A 1996 study showed that a typical video-game devotee is male, in his twenties, with a comfortable income and a white-collar job, who enjoys violent action games (often on his office computer) and also is a fan of sitcoms and science fiction shows on television and of rock music.[17]

Don Steinberg points out that the technology used to produce today's virtual-reality and "fantasy" games is stunningly expensive. Arcades are no longer mere arcades, he writes—they are "location-based entertainment centers" with adults-only policies and microbreweries in the back. Computer games, he writes, have production budgets over $10 million, and new video games routinely make millions of dollars in days, putting Hollywood box office receipts to shame.[18]

As fantastically complicated and absorbing new video and on-line computer games with warfare, science fiction, sport, horror, adventure, and other action themes are introduced, obsolete video games are now being marketed as "classics." Earlier games like Space Invaders, Pac-Man, Centipede, and Asteroid are collected by enthusiasts and placed on exhibition in science museums.

Home Computer Uses

While hard data regarding the use of personal computers for leisure activities such as game playing, the Internet, or E-mail correspondence are difficult to find, varied national surveys suggest that as many as 70 percent of householders use computers at home for "enjoyment." In general, computer users also tend to be more active than nonusers in a wide range of leisure activities—attending arts events, museums, or galleries; playing sports; or reading.

Increasingly, evidence suggests that computer pastimes are not to be viewed as wastes of time or even "brain poison." Instead, researchers at the Microsoft Corporation have found that video games and other computer activities:

> . . . can help children develop their skills of visualization, concentration and problem-solving, as well as help them acquire a fluency in technology. . . . [They create] an "emotional rhythm" that moves a player across a psychic border, alternating a sense of achievement and loss, pleasure and disappointment [and bringing a moment] when curiosity turns to compulsion.[19]

At the same time, critics warn that addictive games and the Internet may also have negative outcomes that concern parents and child guidance experts—such as the surge of on-line child pornography. The growing use of the Internet by sexual predators has increasingly challenged legal authorities, along with the enforcement of new regulations against "indecent," "filthy," or "patently offensive" language and themes, authorized by the telecommunications deregulation bill approved by Congress in 1996.[20]

Finally, the growing use of computers as a form of study, research, and conversation on many campuses has resulted in both heightened levels of communication among students and faculty members and—for many—an intense degree of isolation. At Dartmouth College, where "Blitzmail," the campus E-mail system, delivers about 250,000 electronic messages a day to 5000 students and 3000 faculty and staff members, people may spend three or more hours a day sending and receiving messages. Some critics argue that the widely accepted assumption that personal computers are a necessary tool for higher education—with many colleges requiring students to own them, or placing high-speed Internet connections in every dormitory room—is a dubious one. Nate Shulman writes that many students:

> . . . are playing Tomb Raider instead of going to chemistry class, tweaking the configurations of their machines instead of writing the paper due tomorrow, collecting mostly useless information from the World Wide Web . . . [or engaging in] a host of other activity that has little or nothing to do with traditional academic work.[21]

Literary Forms of Leisure

We turn now to a fourth major category of leisure activity within the spectrum of arts and entertainment—literary and educational pursuits. While many informal kinds of play may deal with words as such—telling jokes, puzzles, storytelling, solving crossword puzzles and anagrams—literary leisure consists primarily of reading and writing in the full range of books, magazines, and newspapers that present fiction, nonfiction, criticism, and poetry to all age groups in the society.

Although it has been widely predicted that reading will disappear as a popular pastime under the impact of more visual, easy-to-comprehend communications media, over the past two decades the sale of books has continued to rise steadily. Total national expenditures on books and maps rose from $6.5 billion in 1985 to $20.9 billion in 1995, and on magazines, newspapers, and sheet music from $12 billion in 1985 to $25.6 billion in 1995.

The growing interest in reading is demonstrated by the growth of major book chains, with huge supermarkets offering every type of book. Companies like Waldenbooks, Dalton, and Crown have opened such outlets in suburban malls throughout the country; in many cases, they are designed to be everything a typical mall store is not, with gentle lighting, wooden shelves, armchairs, and even coffee bars, intended to make them "browser-friendly." Major chains like Barnes and Nobles often sponsor such book-centered programs as "meet-the-author" book signings, lectures, and other literary events with a strong social component.

Poetry is also an important part of the literary use of leisure and has undergone a period of unprecedented expansion in terms of publishing and reading habits. Never before have so many new books of poetry been published, so many anthologies or literary magazines or other forms of criticism of contemporary poetry. Congress and twenty-five states now have official poets laureate, and there are numerous grants for poets, including foundation fellowships, prizes, and subsidized retreats. However, the audience for poetry today is narrower than it was in the past, when a broader cross-section of public read verse as part of everyday cultural activity. It consists chiefly of teachers, students, editors, and publishers. An exception to this conclusion is the vogue of poetry readings, both in bookstores that feature authors of many different types and in neighborhood bars or coffeehouses. Open-microphone sessions and poetry competitions for cash prizes attract a young crowd, who enjoy hearing the spoken word, sometimes linked with projected videos.

Sometimes such readings have been transformed into colorful events attracting huge crowds of spectators, as in the annual Taos Poetry Circus at the foot of the Sangre de Cristo Mountains in New Mexico. Here, the attractions of round-table readings, open-mike "slams," and even lively "tag-team" poetry contests in a format adapted from professional wrestling bouts are judged by officials giving numerical scores.

As an extension of such literary competitions, some mass contests deal with other types of intellectual pursuits. In August, 1998, almost 3000 enthusiasts from around the world gathered in London for the second annual "Mind Sports Olympiad," a sort of Goodwill Games or mass spelling bee for people who would rather flex their brains than their muscles. In this unusual event, players competed in over thirty-five "mind sports," including varied card and table games and the Memoriad, involving the ability to memorize and regurgitate huge lists of facts and figures—all for cash prizes and medals.

Other literary leisure activities include a huge variety of magazines and newspapers. Although such popular weekly magazines as the *Saturday Evening Post, Colliers*, and *Liberty* went out of existence after World War II, the overall number of magazines of all types rose from about 9500 in 1970 to over 11,500 in the late 1980s. Each year, many new magazines start up, while others falter and cease publication. In an annual survey of new publications, it was reported that of 832 new magazines published in the United States, the journalism program at the University of Mississippi found that the two most popular themes were sports (67) and sex (44).

Ethnic-focused magazines have also become increasingly widespread, with print and television offerings aimed at blacks growing by 72 percent from 1985 to 1995, and those serving Hispanics and Asian Americans increasing by 160 percent and 173 percent respectively during the same period.

In terms of active participation, many public and nonprofit leisure service agencies offer courses and special events dealing with such diverse literary interests as Great Books classes, language and current events classes, creative writing clinics or seminars, computer skills, and similar themes.

Diversified Roles of Libraries and Museums

The expanded leisure services of other types of cultural institutions is reflected today in two other kinds of community-based organizations that have traditionally had rather limited educational functions: *libraries* and *museums*.

In the competition for higher levels of community support and in order to achieve better attendance and revenues to supplement tax-derived funds or charitable grants, both types of agencies have entered the field of providing diversified leisure-related programs. Instead of simply providing books, magazines, and research facilities or assistance, for example, many libraries today sponsor comfortable lounge and reading areas, coffee bars or other refreshment areas, storytelling hours, film series, lectures, concerts, and exhibitions.

Neal Peirce points out that for two decades libraries have been hit by budget reductions. To survive and grow, they've been obliged to become entrepreneurial and prove they are not simply hidebound relics. As part of this tradition, Peirce writes, many have entered the computer age wholeheartedly:

> A prime example is the Mecklenburg, North Carolina, Public Library, which now sponsors Charlotte's Web, one of the nation's leading community and Internet services. Another is the Flint, Michigan, Public Library with its KidsWebStation—library materials, programs, Internet access specially tailored for children.[22]

Museums have become even more innovative, in terms of assuming new identities, exploring new themes, and providing diversified social, educational, and environmental programs. There are now more than 200 major children's museums in the United States, with such features as huge water clocks, planetariums and "cinedomes," theaters, dinosaur "digs," mazes, log cabins and tree houses, geodesic domes, darkened crawling tunnels and climbing walls, and a host of scientific exhibits and sideshows.

Adult museums have become equally inventive in presenting provocative and entertaining exhibits and services. Beyond this, many new museums have been established centered around such themes as slavery and the historical Civil Rights movement, space exploration, science and industry, the lives of Native American tribes or tenement-dwelling immigrants from Eastern or Southern Europe at the turn of the century. Art museums have become equally inventive, featuring not only Van Gogh and Monet, but karaoke, poetry, disco, and social evenings.

Other Leisure Pursuits: Hobbies, Pets, and Sociability

Studies have shown that a major portion of leisure involves casual, inexpensive, and close-to-home activities, such as family interaction, reading, watching television, companionship with friends, parties, or going for a drive or walk. Beyond such activities, there are a number of other widely popular groups of leisure interests, described in the concluding section of this chapter. Sometimes these involve sudden fads like Pokémon, the Japanese trading-card craze in 1999 and 2000, that gave birth to a billion-dollar industry involving toys, video games, movies, and dozens of other consumer products.

Hobbies

Such pursuits cover a wide range of individual interests, including hobbies like collecting, model building, dressmaking, and home crafts. In some cases, special interests involve nostalgic pursuits or reenactment of past historical events. In 1997, almost 20,000 people in costume gathered to commemorate the 135th anniversary of the Battle of Gettysburg, and thousands of others in Confederate gray or Union blue uniforms celebrate other major Civil War battles.

Millions play card and table games regularly, including such favorites as chess, checkers, Monopoly, Scrabble, and Trivial Pursuit, or join clubs based on special interests such as astronomy or square dancing. It has been estimated that 80 percent of adults belong to such groups, with titles that range from "Aardvark Aficionados" to "The Diving Dentists Society" or "Sarcastics Anonymous."

Gardening is a tremendously popular leisure interest, carried on both for practical purposes, such as raising vegetables or maintaining the appearance of one's home, and purely aesthetic or pleasurable motives. In its various forms, including lawn care, flower gardening, or indoor houseplants, it is estimated that 72 percent of American households engaged in gardening in 1995, with a total expenditure of $22.2 billion in retail sales and substantially more in professional services.

Pet Ownership

Household pet ownership represents another major leisure interest, with 31.2 million families having dogs, 27.0 million cats, and other substantial numbers having birds, fish, horses, or other more exotic kinds of animal companions. Overall, there are 59 million cats and 53 million dogs in the United States, according to the American Veterinary Medical Association. Expenditures on pets are tremendous, with "doggie day care" growing steadily, and pet health care alone expanding to annual costs of $11.1 billion. Veterinary medicine has moved beyond routine rabies shots or heartworm pills to orthodontics for dogs, kidney dialysis for cats, Prozac and Valium for pets, and even emotional care by veterinary behaviorists for anxiety-ridden dogs or cats.

Americans as a whole spend over $20 billion a year for pets and pet care and, beyond this, make a substantial emotional investment in their nonhuman friends. In a 1997 research study, Cheryl Baldwin points out that animal care represents a "serious" form of leisure, involving intense, long-term attachment, responsibility, and, for many, membership in clubs and classes, competitive events, and other social interactions. Baldwin describes one pet owner:

> Her participation connected her with a network of friends and associations but was also an expression of her identity including her personal values and her need to "live a life connected to dogs." The leisure activity and club were "a place to go, something to do" but more than that also—participation represented a way to contribute, escape, and was a source of instrumental challenge and goal setting.[23]

Sociability as Leisure

Sociability represents a final important area of leisure involvement, and group acceptance. Such pursuits take many forms: (1) clubs based on shared interests, age groups, or special needs; (2) commercially provided settings for casual contacts and social fun; (3) mass events that bring people together for relatively anonymous participation; and (4) remote or distant relationships making use of technology.

Clubs related to common interests or needs may include school or college groups involved in the performing arts, publications, community service, or a host of other functions. They may also include church or synagogue youth or adult or family clubs linked to religious practice and social affiliation. Senior centers operated by public or nonprofit agencies serve millions of older Americans.

Millions of other individuals belong to support or therapy groups, such as Parents Without Partners, Alcoholics Anonymous, or other 12-step recovery groups. Still others linked to special interests may involve special forms of outdoor recreation, sports, hobbies, or political activity. But for all such clubs and membership groups, with their diverse themes and purposes, an underlying thrust is the need for friendship, social contact, and group acceptance.

Commercially provided settings for social contact obviously involve tens of thousands of bars, lounges, and nightclubs; resorts or membership clubs for singles; dating services; social recreation sessions on cruises or tours; and informal adult classes or continuing education offerings under profit-making sponsorship. At a quasi-legal level, they may also include massage parlors or escort services that, while they are often thinly veiled fronts for prostitution, are usually able to advertise legally in telephone yellow-page directories or in cities' tourist-welcoming brochures.

Mass events, such as the Million Man March or Million Woman March of the late 1990s or Promise Keepers and similar rallies that attract hundreds of thousands of participants, are nominally based on a shared theme, belief, or social purpose. At the same time, although they may emphasize spiritual revival and self-esteem, they also serve many individuals as a form of intense—though essentially anonymous—contact and group affiliation.

Another expression of such urges is found in traditional community celebrations that are often based on long-standing custom and may involve unusual forms of play. For example, in Southwest Louisiana, entire towns party from dawn to the wee hours in celebrations linked to Mardi Gras in New Orleans. In these areas, settled chiefly by centuries-past refugees from French Canada, it is the custom for "Les Courirs de Mardi Gras" to engage in a daylong rite of traveling about on horseback and flatbed trailer, on four-wheelers, and on foot. Shermakaye Bass writes:

> It is open season for buffoonery—a mandate for social anarchy when entire towns throw open their shutters and screen doors in a last ecstatic hurrah before Lent. During Mardi Gras, men become women and women men. Children grow up, adults regress. Strangers become friends.[24]

As in similar Easter-time celebrations in South America, the holiday season becomes a time for breaking free from the constraints of everyday life. Masked men roam the countryside, trailed by beer trucks, bandwagons, and lines of spectators, "raiding" farms of livestock and singing for their supper; making communal, spicy gumbo in church halls or veterans' posts; and dancing "fais do-dos," intergenerational two-steps through the night.

In another type of mass event—state fairs and agricultural expositions throughout the country—millions of people young and old see revivals of traditional folk arts and farming practices; compete at showing their crafts, livestock, or agricultural products; and share in a good-natured, informal gathering of people of varied social classes and backgrounds. Increasingly, such fairs and expositions, which are usually sponsored by a combination of governmental agencies and private sponsors through a special state authority or governing board, are being used to showcase local industries or commercial sponsors.

Electronic Sociability. Burgeoning technology is also used to help people form new relationships through electronic communication, such as the Internet, which permits people to search easily for others with common interests, values, or needs. Often correspondence begun through the Internet leads to direct social contact.

A variant of such computer-based sociability is found in electronic coffeehouses that combine computer bulletin boards with traditional coffeehouse culture. In one such enterprise in San Francisco, computer screens are installed into the tops of low tables, with keyboards just below them. By inserting two quarters, users purchase time to chat with others—either in the same coffeehouse or at

> . . . more than a dozen other cafes. Using handles they have concocted themselves, not their real names, they often talk to each other electronically for hours or months, before deciding whether to surrender their anonymity and actually meet.[25]

Clearly, in the years ahead, with new forms of electronic communication emerging, other innovative kinds of computer-based social contact are likely to emerge—with potential for both positive or negative outcomes.

The Leisure Activities Spectrum

Although this chapter has described several of the major areas of leisure involvement today, obviously it has not been able to deal with all of the varied leisure pursuits of Americans in detail. Millions of others enjoy cookery and winemaking, attend fitness centers regularly, join barbershop quartets, or engage in hundreds of other unique pastimes. They include:

> Retired individuals who live in travel trailers and go South in the winter and North in the summer, backpacking enthusiasts, scuba divers, antique collectors, swamp buggy racers, body builders, craftsmen and craftswomen, snowmobile racers, skydivers, folk music performers and fans, tailgating fans at professional football games, collectors, artifact searchers who use metal detectors, mummy dusters who volunteer in archaeological museums, hang gliders, performers in little theaters, people who practice "creative anachronism" (enacting lives of past or mythical cultures)—all illustrate such absorbing hobbies.[26]

Beyond such generally "respectable" pursuits, millions of others take part in leisure activities that represent morally marginal involvements—forms of play or pleasure-seeking activity that are legal in some settings but illegal or clearly destructive in others. Such activities, including narcotic drug involvement, drinking, commercialized or exploitative sex, or addictive gambling, are dealt with more fully in Chapter 12.

Summary

Leisure is closely intertwined with what has traditionally been called "mass" or "popular" culture. Social critics have suggested that culture exists on two or three levels of quality or taste, based on one's socioeconomic status, education, and lifestyle. Today, the distinction between "high" and "low" forms of culture tends to be breaking down, although it is clear that the audience for more elite forms of art, music, dance, or theater consists of a comparatively limited group.

This chapter describes the values of creative artistic experience, and discusses community programs in the arts, along with specific examples of creative and performing arts and varied literary pursuits carried on in leisure. It examines the role of radio, motion pictures, and television, emphasizing the concerns widely expressed about television's impact on the young. Video games and home computer activities are described, and the chapter concludes with an overview of varied hobbies, pet care, and sociability as examples of popular leisure pursuits.

Key Concepts

1. Culture is often thought of as meaning only artistic or intellectual pursuits. However, it really has the broader meaning of all the traditions, values, customs, and shared behaviors of a society.

2. Although so-called "high" or "elite" forms of culture tend to be patronized by a relatively small audience, American society has seen a striking growth of participation in varied forms of artistic activity—music, drama, dance, fine and literary arts—in post–World War II years.

3. While the most popular forms of creative expression, such as rock or rap music are immensely lucrative, other forms, such as orchestral music, opera, or ballet, receive much less support and have been forced to cut back in the 1980s and 1990s.

4. As examples of the mass media of entertainment, radio and motion pictures have reflected changing popular tastes and interests, with respect to public attitudes regarding gender and ethnicity. While American entertainment products are viewed around the world, often they present a limited and distorted picture of life in this country

5. Television continues to represent a major use of free time in family life today, although it tends not to involve a high degree of personal involvement among its spectators. There is considerable criticism of such elements as the proliferation of violence on TV or the many personal "problem" or "confrontation" shows.

6. Video games, which began as relatively simple pursuits chiefly for children and youth, today are much more complex and expensive and appeal also to an adult audience as well.

7. Despite predictions that the Internet and other electronic forms of entertainment or communication would displace the use of books, literary pastimes continue to consume a major portion of leisure.

8. Although libraries and museums continue to carry out their traditional functions of education or serving as repositories for scientific, historical, or other kinds of knowledge, they have increasingly been transformed as venues for innovative displays and entertaining leisure pursuits.

9. An immense variety of hobbies also consume the leisure time of many Americans, who express their creativity, personal interests, or need for sociability through individual or group pursuits.

Endnotes

1. In Today's Aging Audiences, Today Arts See a Cheerless Tomorrow. 1996. *New York Times* (February 12): C-12.

2. Seplow, S., and J. Storm. 1997. How TV Refined Our Lives. *Philadelphia Inquirer* (November 30): A-1.

3. MacDonald, D. In *Mass Culture*, eds. D.M. White and B. Rosenberg. Glencoe, IL: Free Press, p. 59.

4. Shivers, J.S., and L.J. deLisle. 1997. *The Story of Leisure*. Champaign, IL: Human Kinetics, p. 182.

5. Sozanski, E. 1990. Culture and Contemporary Art. *Philadelphia Inquirer* (October 21): 1-H.

6. Conn, B. 1988. Arts in the Mainstream: Recreation Give Arts New Focus. *Parks and Recreation* (June): 26.

7. Horn, M. 1992. Looking for a Renaissance: The Campaign to Revive Education in the Arts. *U.S. News and World Report* (March 30): 52.

8. Janowitz, B., quoted in Ridley, C.A. 1992. Beyond Present Gloom, Future Belongs to the Bold. *Philadelphia Inquirer* (April 6): C-3.

9. Pogrebin, R. 1998. Survey Finds an Upsurge in Theatergoers Under 30. *New York Times* (September 25): E-3.

10. Bagdikian, B. 1992. Pop Radio. *The Nation* (April 13): 473, 488.

11. Marty, M. 1997. *Daily Life in the United States, 1960–1990.* Westport, CT, p. 209.

12. Faludi, S. 1991. The Fatal Detractions by Hollywood. *Philadelphia Inquirer* (November 12): E-1.

13. Living: TV as the New Fireplace. 1982. *Time Magazine* (December 27): 70.

14. Gitlin, T., quoted in Rimer S. 1991. Television Becomes Basic Furniture in College Students' Ivory Towers. *New York Times* (October 27): 8.

15. McCarthy, A. 1998. Trivial Pursuits. *Commonweal* (June 5): 8

16. Bass, A. 1993. Talk: The Freak Shows of American Television. *Philadelphia Inquirer* (November 10): E-1.

17. Goodfellow, J. 1996. The Games People Play. *New York Times* (July 22): D-5.

18. Steinberg, D. 1997. The Quarter Century. *Philadelphia Inquirer Magazine* (July 22): 17–20.

19. Lohr, S. 1997. The Virtues of Addictive Games. *New York Times* (December 22): D-1.

20. Kaplan, D. 1997. New Cybercop Tricks to Fight Child Porn. *U.S. News and World Report* (May 26): 29.

21. Shulman, N. 1999. The Great Campus Goof-Off Machine. *New York Times* (March 15): A-25.

22. Peirce, N. 1996. Some Newfangled Notions for Hidebound Institutions. *Philadelphia Inquirer* (September 21): A-7.

23. Baldwin, C. 1997. A Case Study Examination of Leisure Meaning for the Serious Leisure Participant. *NRPA Research Symposium*: 48.

24. Bass, S. 1998. Cutting Loose in Cajun Country. *New York Times* (January 4): TR-8.

25. Lorant, R. 1995. A Coffee House Serving up the Hottest Technology. *Associated Press* (February)

26. Summarized from Jury, M. 1977. *Playtime: American at Leisure.* New York: Harcourt, Brace, Jovanovich.

12 The Commodification of Leisure

Two centuries ago Americans purchased few leisure goods or services; many made their own music and toys for their children and drank home-made cider. Today, most of our leisure activities depend upon some purchased commodity: a television set, a baseball, tickets to the theater. We spend much of our free (nonwork) time watching and listening to programmed entertainment distributed by large corporations; we use sports and recreation equipment supplied by oligopolistic industries. . . .[1]

In the final decades of the twentieth century, play has assumed a distinctly different identity in terms of its sponsorship, the forms it takes, and its implications for family life, the community, and the overall society. Increasingly, play has become a profit-seeking commodity—that is, a product or service controlled in a large measure by giant conglomerates that dictate public tastes through sophisticated marketing techniques and, in so doing, change the nature of the play experience.[2]

As earlier chapters have shown, recreation and leisure have increasingly been regarded as an industry—marked by the annual expenditure of several hundred billion dollars on play and by the field's adoption of business-based entrepreneurial principles and marketing methods. This chapter examines this important development more fully, showing how major social institutions like religion, health care, higher education, or the prison system have assumed many of the characteristics of profit-seeking businesses. Citing numerous examples of leisure pursuits being transformed into commercial enterprises, it shows how major corporations and conglomerates today dominate much of the nation's free time.

One area of such commercially driven leisure involves what the text calls morally marginal play—activities such as substance abuse, gambling, or commercialized sex, that are on the fringes of moral acceptability and legality. Describing the impact of such pursuits in detail, the chapter concludes with a discussion of the role of technology in creating new pastimes or facilitating their sponsorship.

Commodification and the Consumer Mentality

Taken altogether, the conversion of major forms of leisure involvement, such as sports and games or arts and entertainment, into a gigantic, profitable industry illuminates the extent to which we have abandoned the notion of leisure as a relaxed form of personal escape, creative development, or self-definition.

With high-powered, sophisticated marketing and advertising techniques, huge corporations play a major role in influencing our choice of leisure activities—the sports and games we play, the toys we give our children, the films and television we watch, the books we read, and the destinations we travel to. Several decades ago, the psychotherapist Erich Fromm pointed out that Americans had increasingly become dominated by a consumer mentality. As consumers, he wrote, we are manipulated and sold products we do not really need or understand. Marketing techniques have transformed ordinary people into passive alienated consumers of leisure goods and services that are thrust on us, and that we are brainwashed into accepting as necessary.

The term *commodification* has increasingly been applied to this process in modern society. Political scientist Sebastian de Grazia defined it several decades ago:

> Commodification of leisure is understood as a necessary element in the subordination of the entire social system to the reproduction of capitalism and its institutional structure. The consequence to the worker is surrendering to forms of leisure which turn away from self-defining, creative experience and instead, consume vast quantities of market-produced goods and services.[3]

This development is not necessarily bad. Adopting an entrepreneurial stance has permitted many public and nonprofit leisure-service organizations to flourish in a highly competitive economic and social environment. It has meant that leisure opportunities themselves have become far more diversified and challenging and that recreation has expanded immensely as a field of employment and organized service.

To better understand the impact of commodification of leisure, it is necessary to examine the growth of consumerism and a consumer mentality in contemporary life, and to recognize the increased support given to entrepreneurship in varied types of community organizations.

Consumerism as a Way of Life

In writing about the sociology of consumption, Peter Corrigan points out that only within the last century has consumption beyond the goods and services necessary to maintain life expanded on a mass scale, to make the production of "surplus" or "pleasure-based" goods widely available to all. Linked to this development, he recalls Thorstein Veblen's concept of conspicuous consumption, in which leisure offers a means of displaying one's own wealth and high social status. He points out that a key development in the growth of consumerism as a way of life was the creation of department stores in the mid-nineteenth century, which made shopping far more convenient for all classes.[4]

More recently, shopping has become not merely a practical act or casual leisure pursuit—but rather a significant part of self-identification. Sarah Boxer points out that many scholars view the admonition of "shop until you drop" as a form of "civic act." She writes that "how you shop is who you are."[5]

Extending this point, Ian Henry examines the difference between functional or practical kinds of goods or services and leisure-related purchases, which tend to have more expressive but less practical value. The latter type of purchase, he writes, enables buyers to

> . . . express something about themselves, to establish an identity they wish to portray. Thus, wearing sports-related leisure clothing may be taken as a symbol of a healthy lifestyle, of youth and exuberance. . . . Transport for many people is a necessity, but, for example, four-wheel drive recreational vehicles used predominantly in a suburban setting for domestic purpose and urban travel to and from work may be interpreted as expressing an attachment on the part of the owner to the image of an outdoor, activity-based lifestyle.[6]

Christopher Lasch characterizes much of contemporary life as a frantic consumer culture based on the ceaseless transformation of luxuries into necessities and evidence of the emergence of a society obsessed with the compulsion of "making it." John Kelly comments on the impact of such "commodity fetishism" on leisure and play in the contemporary world. Numerous social critics, he writes, argue that:

> Leisure has become so distorted by commodification that it is not a domain of freedom at all. A "good time" comes to be associated with spending and consumption. The "great vacation" is going to a place where opportunities to spend money and watch others perform dominate the time—Disney World or Las Vegas. Weekends are scheduled around events and the use of leisure "toys." Evening time is devoted to television, a medium for the direct and indirect promotion of the sale of things. Even in leisure, satisfaction is measured by spending.[7]

The creation of giant malls in the United States and Canada—including huge chain stores, specialty shops, and professional services, along with movie multiplexes, video-game arcades, and other attractions—illustrates the linkage of shopping and leisure. Today, the West Edmonton Mall in Alberta, Canada, and the Mall of America in Bloomington, Minnesota, offer an immense variety of places for play and diversified amusement activities (see page 66). The role of recreation attractions in such malls is twofold: (1) to appeal to patrons who come, often from considerable distances, drawn by the joint lures of shopping and fun; and (2) to serve as money-making ventures in their own right.

Commodification in the Larger Society

It should be understood that the trend toward entrepreneurial packaging of recreation elements is not unique in modern society. Numerous other types of human services or social functions have also been widely commodified, making use of businesslike methods to package, promote, and profit from their ongoing operations.

Commercialism in Religion

Numerous religious denominations have adopted sophisticated marketing methods to appeal to new and greater audiences and to raise funding support. Many churches today sponsor television evangelism programs; events, camps, and resorts; schools and colleges; and the sale of books, records, and video products. Some churches today offer "user-friendly" drive-in 22-minute services in suburban shopping malls. An increasing number of huge "mega-churches" present professionally choreographed services that are almost indistinguishable from popular rock-and-roll concerts.

Charles Trueheart describes the dramatic changes that such innovative churches—which represent the fastest-growing Protestant sects in the country—have adopted:

> No spires. No crosses. No robes. No clerical collars. No hard pews. No kneelers. No biblical gobbledygook. No prayerly rote. No fire, no brimstone. No pipe organs. No dreary eighteenth-century hymns. No forced solemnity. No Sunday finery. No collection plates.[8]

While all such mega-churches have not adopted all of these practices, many have. In addition to developing new images of religion, they tend to be "full-service," "twenty-four hour," "seeker-sensitive" institutions, with low staff-to-congregant ratios and many volunteers. Their varied functions include seminars and workshops on single-parenting, 12-step recovery meetings; grief-support ministries; women in the workplace; discovering divorce dynamics; men's retreats and women's Bible studies; worship music, drama, and dance; and other recreational activities.

Gospel music is increasingly popular, outselling other musical genres, and successful roadshows that combine religious messages with inspirational career or business themes today draw thousands of spectators and participants. Religious advertising today is often composed by Madison Avenue account executives and is far slicker and more persuasive than the traditional church announcements found on the religious pages of newspapers; often it appears on airborne streamers, telephone booths, and Web pages.

Health-Care Industry

One illustration of the degree to which health has become commodified less in the huge national chains of managed-care companies that combine hospitals, insurance companies, doctors, and other medical professionals in powerful alliances that dominate the health-care field.

Beyond this, major chains of nursing homes have frozen out or taken over many independent, smaller long-term care facilities. In a growing number of cases, both hospitals and nursing homes have now gone into a host of other health-related enterprises, such as sponsoring massage and "bodywork" therapy; hypnosis and meditation classes and lectures; weight-management support groups; Yoga, Tai Chi; land- and water-aerobic classes; nutrition assessment and counseling; arthritis clubs; and numerous other individual or group services. While all such activities normally involve fees and many clear a significant profit, often the health-care institution itself is nonprofit and tax-exempt.

A vivid example of how commercialism has become accepted in the health-care field came in 1997, when the American Medical Association announced that it planned to grant the Sunbeam Corporation exclusive rights to display its seal on products such as heating pads, thermometers, and scales—in return for a cut of profits of several million dollars a year. Public protest led the AMA to withdraw from the deal.

Commodification in Education

Major universities compete vigorously through advertising, offering scholarships, and raiding each others' star faculty members. Increasingly, they are now creating and shepherding new technologies to the marketplace by making deals with commercial companies for licensing inventions or research findings by their professors. Typically, such processes as computer software that maps investment strategies, new treatments for cancer, or cardiopulmonary resuscitation devices are helping to make universities into sleek new profit machines. Numerous other universities are developing for-profit subsidiaries that develop and sell online courses to other colleges, corporate training centers, or students to attend class at home.

The growing influence of commercialism is most evident in intercollegiate athletics, where many institutions have sought funding for new stadiums and other facilities from major corporations and have named their facilities after them. When Rutgers University in New Jersey sought a new athletic director to administer its sports programs, it did not hire an individual with a background in higher education or intercollegiate athletics. Instead, it recruited the head of the New Jersey Sports and Exposition Authority, who had been most familiar with administering professional sports stadiums, race tracks, and the state aquarium and convention center.

On elementary and secondary school levels, many public school systems have developed close ties with major commercial concerns, as shown in a recently published math text with numerous references to Nike, Gatorade, and Sony Play Stations as teaching examples. Based on the principle that school children are consumers in training, dozens of large corporations such as Exxon and McDonald's now sponsor varied in-school marketing projects. Typically, companies pay school districts to get posters promoting their products on school buses or in cafeterias, or create curricular materials that "huckster" candy or other products. Steven Manning writes:

> Coca Cola and Pepsi have turned some schools into virtual sales agents for their products. Districts across the country have signed multimillion-dollar "pouring rights"

contracts, which give soft-drink company exclusive permission to distribute its products in schools.

The rush to get computers into classrooms has opened up new commercial possibilities. Zap Me, a Silicon Valley company, gives schools free personal computers and Internet access in exchange for the right to display a constant stream of on-screen advertisements.[9]

Numerous other school districts have negotiated similar contracts with commercial concerns, usually without public notice or hearings, a trend that has caused concern, particularly in such West Coast states as California and Washington.

Prison Industry

As Chapter 3 indicates, the rapid growth of those imprisoned in the United States has led states to immense pressure to build and staff more prisons. Increasing, rural areas and high-unemployment regions are campaigning to have prisons built locally to assist their economies. The mayor of Canon City, Colorado, which proclaims itself "Corrections Capital of the World," boasts:

> We have a nice, nonpolluting, recession-proof industry here. With local coal mines closing and ranches limping, the prisons of Fremont County filled the vacuum, employing 3,100 men and women. Here, prisons are simply called "the industry."[10]

More and more, so-called "bed brokers" find prisoners from overcrowded jails and prisons and arrange their transfer to institutions—often out-of-state—with empty cells and a need for cash. Specialists in this field maintain listing services to match prisoners with institutions and ship hundreds of prisoners around the country each month. In the mid-1990s, more and more prisons instituted revenue programs, through which room and board fees have been collected from inmates, or inmates must pay utility bills for television or other electrical appliances, or share payment for money earned through work programs. Hundreds of companies in twenty-nine states now contract the use of prisoners in tasks ranging from manufacturing clothing or electronic circuit boards to taking airline reservations over the phone.[11]

Examples of Commodification in Leisure

For-profit recreation businesses today comprise a major sector of the overall leisure-service field. Such companies have become increasingly innovative in their marketing efforts. For example, Crossley and Ellis describe new sales approaches in sports stores, where a weak link in the retail process has traditionally been the customer's inability to test a product before deciding to buy it. A Denver-based chain of sports equipment stores has created so-called Sports Castles that have basketball courts, tennis courts, golf putting greens, fly casting areas, archery ranges, and treadmill ski machines for testing equipment and learning skills. Crossley and Ellis continue:

They also have a large multipurpose classroom where they teach fly tying, hunter safety and other classes related to the equipment sold. In addition [they offer] a full service travel agency, sell tickets to concerts and ski areas, and sponsor a variety of community sports events. In sum, [the company] sells a total recreation experience, not just sports equipment.[12]

Similarly, many health and fitness clubs offer a growing range of services. The New York Health and Racquet Club, with eight flourishing centers in the Borough of Manhattan, offers its members the following facilities or program elements: one-on-one fitness training; nutritional counseling; over 600 free classes weekly; swimming pools and spa facilities; racquetball, squash, and tennis courts; strength training and free weights; an indoor golf and "country club;" a beach and tennis club; basketball and other team games; baby-sitting services; corporate memberships; and use of a club-owned yacht.

A number of restaurant chains today have diversified their appeal by offering, in addition to food and drink, such varied forms of play as video games, karaoke sessions, mystery dinner theater, basketball hoops and shuffleboard courts, billiards, and interactive virtual reality games that simulate race-car driving, space combat, or other adventure themes.

Product Licensing

This offers another illustration of how play has been commodified in America. Today, hundreds of sports heroes, popular entertainers, and cartoon characters as diverse as Michael Jordan and Garfield the Cat are used to sell sporting goods, toys and games, health and beauty aids, food, beverages, apparel, and accessories. Overall, the licensing industry has grown from $11 billion in retail sales in the early 1980s to over $66 billion in the early 1990s, with over 10,000 licensed names and images in the United States.

Beyond such licensing arrangements, many entrepreneurs have seized the opportunity to create timely new products. For example, when Princess Diana died in a tragic accident in August 1997, a wave of television documentaries, docudramas, quiz shows, and other specials was produced dealing with her life and death in the months that followed. Within a few months, the Diana, Princes of Wales, Memorial Fund authorized the use of her name and image for products that amassed sales of an estimated $200 million. Elliott writes:

> The deluge of Dianabilia, as the goods generated by the phenomenon are described in Britain, includes dolls, coins, stamps, collector plates, books, jewelry, candles, music boxes, videotapes, flowers and compact disks. Still more collectibles— exploitive or commemorative, authorized or otherwise—are on the way.[13]

Holidays like Mother's Day, Christmas, or Thanksgiving become the basis for promoting products, sales events, and entertainment programs. Hallowe'en, once a relatively minor holiday based on the Christian All Hallow's Eve, has become a multimillion dollar secular event—often extending over weeks of parades, haunted houses, purchase of costumes, parties, property decorations, horror nights, and theme park programs that draw millions of spectators overall.

Within many other areas of public life, the money-making potential of leisure is exploited today. Many farmers today supplement their incomes by offering family-friendly tours and hayrides; pick-em-yourself fruit, berry, or other produce arrangements; petting zoos with farm animals; cornfield "mazes" and similar attractions. Rock and roll concert merchandise tapes and posters, T-shirts, sweat pants, and other forms of "swag"—including, in some cases, imprinted condoms—amount to a billion-dollar-a-year industry.

Growth of Leisure Conglomerates

More and more, play and entertainment have become the domain of huge companies and multinational business organizations that combine new technologies and promotional techniques to create new fads and leisure pursuits or capture a lion's share of the market.

An example of such leisure-directed conglomerates was found in the 1994 merger of Viacom, Blockbuster, and Paramount, which resulted in a $21 billion empire. This new organization controls major cable networks and systems, television and radio broadcasting stations, over 3000 home video stores, music and film producing and distributing companies, family fun centers, popular television programs, leading book publishers, sports stadiums and professional teams, and five regional theme parks.

Other major corporations include Rupert Murdoch's communications and entertainment empire, which spans six continents and includes books, magazines, newspapers, broadcasting, satellite television, and a movie studio. In 1996, Time Warner and Turner Broadcasting System merged, to create a massive company with over $18.7 billion in annual revenues, from sports, publishing, music, film, records, and other entertainment media. Similarly, numerous other television and communications companies have taken over ownership of major professional sports teams.

Walt Disney Operations.   Of all such ventures, none can compare with the Disney worldwide leisure operations, for sheer scope, creativity, and financial success. As described earlier, the Disney theme parks and animated films have been leading attractions for several decades. In the 1980s and 1990s, under the leadership of Michael Eisner, Disney continued to develop new enterprises, including two major theme parks in France and Japan, as well as a host of new attractions in Florida: Disney-MGM Studios, Pleasure Island, Typhoon Lagoon, Sports Complex and Wide World of Sports, Disney's Animal Kingdom, and a major new cruise line.

These striking new attractions blend the real and the virtual, as in the case of the Animal Kingdom, where some displays are technologically advanced animatronic creatures and others real beasts roaming the "African" savannah in central Florida. Nor do they all provide only passive entertainment. Instead, attractions like the Wide World of Sports involve cooperative tie-ins with a number of major sports organizations, sponsoring national tournaments and offering the opportunity to play in varied competitions. The company's 1997 promotional brochure boasted:

> . . . Rookies in the sports world we're not. This 200-acre, world-class sports complex [Wide World of Sports] is already the 1998 spring training home of the Atlanta

Braves, training center for the Harlem Globetrotters, and headquarters for the Amateur Athletic Union. Walt Disney World hosts major sporting events like PGA Golf and the Indy 200. Choose to have Disney host your event and we instantly field an all-star team of event planners and management teams to take you from start to finish . . .[14]

By July 1997, a variety of competitive sports events for athletes of varied ages, genders, and skills were under way. At the same time, the AAU's 13-and-under girls national basketball championship was ending, while a national "super showcase" for thirty-two teams of high-school-age male basketball players was beginning, with college recruiters attending by the hundreds. Other Disney-hosted events included a USA Track and Field developmental meet for young decathletes and a state tennis association tournament for 30- to 50-year-olds. Overall, Disney's thirty-year agreement with the AAU gives it access to some 450,000 amateur athletes of all ages, involved in 221 national championships in thirty-two different sports.

Beyond such innovative ventures, the Disney Company has also continued to produce successful animated films, develop highly acclaimed musical theater works, such as "Beauty and the Beast" and "The Lion King" (several of which have merchandising side ventures, such as tapes, toys, and similar products), and commission operas and major choral works. In the mid-1990s, Disney spearheaded the revival of New York City's Times Square and built an unusual planned community, Celebration, in Florida's Osceola County, designed to portray the architecture and lifestyles of Walt Disney's small-town roots.

Finally, Disney planners have developed training courses in recreation management for public and private leisure-service professionals. In cooperation with the National Recreation and Park Association, Walt Disney's World Seminar Productions began to offer *The Disney Approach: A Management Seminar*, in 1992.

Commodification in Public Leisure-Service Agencies

The trend toward regarding leisure as an "industry" has led to the aggressive marketing of recreational activities on a fee basis by public recreation and park departments and other nonprofit agencies. Typically, in many agencies, annual and seasonal program brochures contain hundreds of listings of classes, events, and trips under such headings as Arts and Crafts, Aquatics, Sports and Games, or Performing Arts. Illustrations of sample activities are shown in Figure 12.1, program offerings of the San Mateo, California, Department of Parks and Recreation, and Figure 12.2, summer trip programs and outings sponsored by the Morale, Welfare and Recreation unit at the Orlando, Florida, Naval Training Center.

Similarly, as Chapter 3 points out, public departments have also sharply increased charges for admission to pools, city-operated rinks or bowling centers, nature museums, or for golf or tennis permits. While some public recreation and park departments establish special group rates for disadvantaged groups or even fee discounts or waivers for families on welfare, inevitably many poorer individuals are excluded from large segments of program activities offered by public, tax-supported government agencies.

**GOLF FEES CITY OF
SAN MATEO GOLF COURSE
1700 Coyote Point Drive,
U.S. 101 at Peninsula Avenue**

Pro Shop 347-1461
First Tee Restaurant 343-6295
Sand Bar Lounge 347-2717
Maintenance 377-4750

GREEN FEES
(effective 1/1/96)

General or Non-resident

Weekday	$20.00
Weekend/holiday	$24.00
Evening and early morning back nine (weekdays)	$12.50
Evening and early morning back nine (weekends)	$13.50
Senior (over 60) 10 Play Card	$175.00

**City of San Mateo Residents
with Golf I.D. Card**

Weekday	$13.00
Weekend/holiday	$15.00
Senior (over 60) Weekdays	$12.00
Senior 10 Play Card	$100.00

Junior

Jr. Weekdays	$8.00
Jr. Weekends	$24.00
Jr. Weekends (after 12:00 N)	$8.00
Jr. Playcard Weekdays	$75.00
Jr. Playcard Weekends (after 12:00 N)	$75.00

Private Piano Lessons: age 6 yrs. and up.
In PRIVATE lessons, learning to play can be fun and easy! Instructors, Walter Asvolinsque, Judi Lozada, Newton Colburn and Jennifer Hsiung are outstanding piano teachers, with years of experience. Lessons are structured to each individual's ability from beginning to advanced. Space is limited to one student per half hour. Fee is $142/177 for 9 lessons. Music books are extra. A piano or keyboard at home is required for practicing. We are currently filling our summer openings and fall wait list. If you are interested, please leave your name and a day and evening phone number at 377-4775.

Private Voice Lessons: age 7 yrs. and up.
Do you want to learn to sing better, louder, and with more confidence? In PRIVATE lessons, Instructor Judi Lozada will show you how using the famous Garcia-Marchesi method. With emphasis on giving the singer the tools of voice building and basis for belcanto singing, performance and musicianship, the Garcia-Marchesi method provides the singer agility, endurance and a sensitivity to their own individual vocal apparatus. Lessons are structured to each individual's ability from beginning to advanced, child or adult. Space is limited to one student per half hour for nine lessons. Fee is $142/177. Music books are extra. We are currently filling our summer openings and fall wait list. If you are interested, please leave your name and a day and evening phone number at 377-4775.

Beginning Folk Guitar (Teen/Adult)
Dust off that guitar in your closet and with our new instructor, Matt Mattei, learn the basic chords and strumming techniques to begin playing traditional and contemporary folk guitar in just a few lessons. Great for campfire sing-a-longs! Come enter the wonderful world of music. It's never too late to start! Your own guitar is required. Music books are not included and are purchased separately. Instructor will inform at the first class meeting what you will need. (8 mtgs)

CP260-111 Tu   5:30–6:30 pm $39/49   6/24–8/12   Beres

FIGURE 12.1   Examples of program activities and fees from San Mateo, California, program brochure.

Implications of Commodification Trend

Beyond the issue of excluding those unable to pay fees or charges, a broader question concerning the commercialization of leisure centers around its role in community life—its image and the nature of the experience that people share.

First, as pointed out earlier, there is a growing tendency to regard leisure—or recreation—simply as a product or service that one buys, like items off a supermarket shelf. As

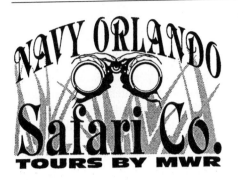

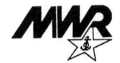

6 July	**Silver Spurs Rodeo** Enjoy ropin' and ridin' the cowboy way. Ye-ha! Leave ITT at 1300 and return by 1830. $16.00 includes transportation and admission. Sign-up at ITT by noon, 3 July.
11 July	**Paintball at Night** Experience 60 acres of outdoor war games complete with sandbag bunkers, forts, trenches, and fire bases at Paintball World. $20.00 includes 100 rounds of paint, gun, mask, and four hours of play time. Transportation is available for $3.00 extra. Depart at 1700 and return by 2300. Sign-up by 1200, 9 July.
19 July	**Wet-n-Wild** Enjoy an exciting day at the water park! Complete with slides, flumes, a wave pool much, much more. $20.00 includes transportation and admission to the park. Depart ITT at 0830 and return by 1800. Sign-up at ITT by 1200, 17 July.
26 & 27 July	**Daytona Beach Overnight Trip** Spend the weekend at the world's most famous beach! Stay at the Daytona Inn, located on the beach within walking distance to many shops, restaurants, clubs, and the boardwalk. Cost: $20.00 (quad); $23.00 (triple); $29.00 (double); $47.00 (single). Cost includes transportation and lodging. Depart ITT at 1000 Saturday and return by 1700 on Sunday. Deadline to sign-up at ITT is 1200, 23 July.
2 Aug.	**Canoe Trip to Katie's Wekiva River Landing** Take a relaxing three to five hour canoe run down the Wekiva River. Cost is $25.00 and includes transportation, lunch and the canoe rental. Sign-up at ITT by 30 July. Departs ITT at 0830 and return by 1800.

FIGURE 12.2 Examples of trip programs and fees in armed forces recreation from Orlando, Florida, Naval Training Center.

such, it often lacks meaning, compared to the kind of active free-time pursuit that one chooses, shapes, and is shaped by. Obviously, not all commercially sponsored leisure experiences involve being a spectator in a passive way. However, many do, and in this sense recreation becomes far less valuable in terms of meeting one's physical, social, or emotional needs.

The influence of huge corporations or conglomerates in controlling vast spheres of leisure offerings means that essentially they are programming the free time of millions of Americans. By offering unusual or spectacular settings and technologically sophisticated play or entertainment, and by advertising them skillfully or packaging them so as to create the powerful impulse to buy (both with one's money and with one's time), huge corporations make the leisure attraction or product difficult to resist.

Ultimately, the effect is to create virtual brainwashing of the public in its leisure choices, with the growth of mass cultural patterns that inhibit personal growth and spontaneity and lessen the potential value of the free-time experience. Extending this criticism, the harsh reality is that the commodification of leisure becomes most destructive when it is used as a means of profiting from human weakness, by systematically promoting forms of play that, while financially profitable, are socially or morally destructive.

The Shady Side of Leisure: Morally Marginal Play

What is not generally acknowledged in scholarly studies of leisure and its effects is that many of the most widely engaged in forms of play in American society have potentially negative outcomes.

As earlier chapters have shown, leisure has historically been viewed from two sharply contrasting perspectives. On the one hand, it has been seen as socially desirable, contributing to cultural enrichment and the quality of life, and even linked to spiritual goals and personal self-actualization. On the other hand, throughout history, the work ethic has been sharply opposed to idleness and play; in successive eras societies have sought to control gambling, sexual activity, drinking, drug use, and other forms of morally marginal play. The term *marginal* is used here because most of these forms of leisure activity are on the fringe of social acceptability. In some cases, they are widely engaged in, legally permitted, and even sponsored by government and by religious authorities. In other cases, they are viewed as immoral, illegal, and to be resisted at all costs.

Many morally marginal leisure pursuits are carried on for reasons similar to the motivations prompting other forms of recreational participation. They may involve socialization with others, relaxing or escaping from tensions and pressures, the lures of excitement and challenge, risk, and reward. At the same time, each of these pursuits may lead to feelings of guilt and failure, to physical and economic self-destruction, to alienation from one's family, and even to criminal prosecution.

Marginal Play as Addictive Behavior

What makes such forms of leisure behavior so appealing? Anthropologist Lionel Tiger suggests that the search for primitive "sensory pleasures" has deep roots in humankind's past and that there is a significant relationship among power, pleasure, reproduction, and human nature. Indeed, he writes, a nation's success in providing an array of legitimately enjoyed pleasures may have much to do with its ability to survive in the modern world.

A unique aspect of morally marginal forms of play is that they often take the form of addictions. Why do some persons become addicted and others not, despite similar family backgrounds or environmental circumstances? Research suggests that addicts resemble each other in certain ways. They tend to have difficulty in recognizing and expressing their feelings, in relating to other people, and in forming long-range goals because they focus too much on short-term, immediate gratification. They do not anticipate or respect possible harmful outcomes of risky behavior and are consequently unable to create a safe, healthy lifestyle. Many of them have been raised in dysfunctional families where parents or other siblings may be substance or physical abusers, where too little love has been expressed, and where there has been too much early discipline or too little.

Gambling as Leisure Pursuit

We now turn to an examination of several forms of play about which society is ambivalent. The first of these is gambling, defined as any sort of game or contest in which individuals wager money in the hope of financial gain.

In the early New England colonies, some forms of gambling, such as lotteries, were regarded as socially acceptable and in fact were used to finance worthwhile community projects. Others, like racetrack betting, cards, and dice, were regarded as a vice; the Puritans condemned them as akin to taking the Lord's name in vain, because they "prostituted the divine providence to unworthy ends."

Throughout the nineteenth and much of the twentieth century, efforts both to legalize and to control gambling followed a piecemeal pattern. The only state to permit legalized casino gambling was Nevada; however, numerous other states encouraged parimutuel betting on horse and dog races, allowed nonprofit organizations to operate bingo games, and permitted other forms of gambling to exist.

In the decades after World War II, gambling became more popular as a recognized form of recreation, as a number of the legal restraints on it were withdrawn. In states like New York, Florida, Pennsylvania, and California, advocates were pushing for more casinos, slot machines, race betting, and other games. By the early 1980s, doubts and fears about games of chance were falling by the wayside, as gambling became increasingly perceived both as a direct economic benefit to the states and communities that initiated it through taxes and employment and as a boost to tourism. In 1985, Americans legally wagered more than $177 billion at casinos, parimutuels, and state-owned lotteries, with another huge amount of illegal gambling that could only be guessed at. As an organized activity, this took the form chiefly of betting on major sports such as basketball or football, or horse racing, through "wire rooms" run by illegal bookmakers.

Growth of Legalized Gambling

In city after city and state after state, citizen referendums were held to approve various forms of gambling—usually justified to gain revenue and provide a boost to employment.

Giant new casinos were built in both Atlantic City and Las Vegas, capped by Donald Trump's billion-dollar Taj Mahal and his rival Steve Wynn's $600 million Mirage. In the early 1990s, a number of states, beginning with Iowa, approved riverboat gambling along the Mississippi River, in the hope that floating casinos would not only bring new revenues but would also raise the image and stimulate the economy of depressed riverfront towns.

By 1991, every state except Utah and Hawaii had legalized lotteries or some other form of gambling or betting, and *Gaming and Wagering Business Magazine* reported that

Americans had legally wagered $286 billion in the most recent year—more than $1000 per capita and 6.2 percent of U.S. total personal income. A number of states had instituted off-track betting parlors for horse racing. In the same year, gross revenues from legalized gambling were more than five times the box office of the domestic movie industry.

By the mid-1990s, it was reported that people were spending over $480 billion a year legally on all forms of gambling, 85 percent of which was bet in casinos in twenty-seven states—most of them having been built within the last five years. In no state was gambling as diversified as in Iowa, a state generally viewed as morally conservative, in America's heartland. In addition to craps, blackjack, roulette, and slot machines on its floating casinos (gambling having been legalized on riverboats), Iowa offered a state lottery, horse and dog racing, bingo, and Las Vegas nights for charities.

Beyond simply *legalizing* gambling enterprises, state governments have vigorously *promoted* them. For example, thirty-six states and the District of Columbia spent over $370 million annually in advertising their lotteries in the mid-1990s. As a result, total lottery sales rose from $9 billion in 1985 to $31.9 billion in 1995.[15]

It was persuasively argued that gambling would provide employment for economically impacted cities and regions, and that it would provide funding for education, programs for the elderly, and similar services. In Gary, Indiana, for example, an economically depressed community, 200 church leaders opposed a proposal to legalize casino gambling in 1991. For nearly its entire history, Indiana had a constitutional ruling against lotteries, but a proposition passed in 1990 to permit lotteries encouraged the legislature to consider other proposals for horse and dog track racing and casinos. Opponents of the proposal cited both moral and practical arguments against it, while Gary's major argued that gambling would bring tourism from Chicago and throughout the Midwest.

In East St. Louis, Illinois, Biloxi, Mississippi, and dozens of other cities with high unemployment rates, heavy pressure was exerted on civic leaders to approve new gambling enterprises. At the same time, new venues for gambling were explored to circumvent state or federal laws limiting its spread. In some cases, "river" boats were placed in fixed locations in newly constructed "lakes" along the Mississippi, with channels out to the river itself. In the mid-1990s, gambling over the Internet, allowing people to use personal computers and credit cards, began to receive major political and media attention. Gambling promoters initiated electronic gambling on international airline flights in the late 1990s, with lotto, keno, and video slots on Swissair flights, and blackjack, slots, and poker on Singapore planes.

Social and Economic Impact of Gambling

While there has generally been widespread support for new forms of legalized gambling, many civic groups opposed its spread and pointed out some of the negative outcomes of the new trend. In some cases, bingo or Las Vegas nights that were sponsored by religious or charitable organizations were shown to be run by professional gambling groups linked to organized crime.

When New Jersey's legislature first considered legalizing casino gambling in Atlantic City, it was argued that the move would curb illegal gambling activity. However, in the late 1980s, the state's highest-ranking police officer concluded that instead it had helped organized crime augment and expand its illegal gambling operations. New Jersey State Police Superintendent Clinton Pagano pointed out that gambling continued to be the primary consistent source of revenue for traditional organized crime enterprises. William Safire explains the continuing appeal of illegal bookmakers to sports bettors:

> State-advertised lotteries and state-approved casinos add to, rather than replace gamblers' operations. An illicit bookie, with no cut to give the state, can give higher odds than those offered by the tax-paying "gambling industry"; moreover, high rollers [who win] don't share their winnings with the tax collector. State-sponsored gambling gives moral sanction and fresh impetus to bookies, numbers racketeers—and the Mafia.[16]

Numerous other studies testify to the negative social effects of legalized gambling. In a number of small cities that have established casinos, the result has been an increase in crime, traffic, and noise, a change in the community's social fabric, and the loss of a number of businesses. Bad checks, felonies, physical assaults, and forgeries have all proliferated. According to the National Council on Compulsive Gambling, at least half of the nation's pathological gamblers eventually turn to illegal means of obtaining funds, from bad checks or phony insurance claims to embezzlement. Studies at two New Jersey prisons showed that over 30 percent of the prisoners were pathological gamblers.

It is estimated that 2 million Americans are compulsive gamblers, an illness defined by the American Psychiatric Association as a serious addictive disease. There is growing awareness of its appeal for young people. A 1990 study of 2700 high school students in New Jersey, Virginia, California, and Connecticut showed that half the students gambled occasionally, 13 percent financed their gambling with crimes, and 5 percent were classified as pathological gamblers, using American Psychiatric Association criteria. Finally, new reports indicate that a growing number of elderly persons are becoming compulsive gamblers and confirm that the suicide rate in major gambling cities in the United States was up to four times higher than in cities of comparable size that did not have legalized gambling.[17]

Economic Impact of Gambling.   While gambling has undoubtedly provided a healthy boost to the local economy of a number of cities or disadvantaged regions—and to a number of Indian tribes (see page 162)—its overall economic impact has been far more dubious.

First, it is apparent that all forms of gambling—and particularly lotteries—prey heavily on the poor, who seek miraculous solutions to their economic problems. One authority, who has studied gambling for over twenty years, points out that the lottery system is "a fraud that preys on the lower classes." The reality is that players have a six times greater chance of being hit by lightning than of winning major prizes. Essentially, the lottery, which pays only a 50 percent return to betters, compared to bookies who skim less than 5 percent from their customers, is a tax on the poor. Seven of the nine biggest state lotteries are in states with a large number of urban poor, such as Pennsylvania, Ohio, and Massachusetts, with California having the highest volume of ticket sales.

Beyond such criticisms, there is evidence that legalized gambling is now taking so many forms and becoming so available that it has reached a saturation point and has drawn customers away from other forms of entertainment, including nightclubs and taverns, shows, racetracks, and other competitors for the sophisticated leisure dollar.

In the early 1990s, Atlantic City's boardwalk casinos reported combined losses of over $260 million and two of Donald Trump's financially troubled casinos filed for bankruptcy in an effort to restructure their debts. Even casino owners in Las Vegas began to fear that they were chasing a dwindling number of high rollers during the recession, although the industry began to make a recovery in the following years.

Religious, civic, and other organizations note the bittersweet experience of Atlantic City where gamblers stay in the casinos while the surrounding city remains a devastated ghetto. Although the casinos brought in millions in taxes and created thousands of new jobs, economic spinoffs never developed for the resort city. There are fewer restaurants today in Atlantic City, for example, than there were before casinos were legalized. The risk factor for host communities as well as gambling patrons was vividly illustrated when a number of the riverboat casinos that had begun operations in Iowa were moved down the Mississippi to the Gulf Coast after only a year or two, in search of fewer restrictions and higher profits.

In some cases, the expectation that gambling would bring immense revenues to save the economy of a troubled city has proven false. Instead, revenues have been heavily diverted to the operators of major casinos and yielded comparatively little to civic services. Writing in *State and Local Government Review* in 1997, Miller and Pierce concluded, on the basis of fiscal analysis of education funding in twelve states that had lotteries intended to support educational funding, that exactly the opposite had taken place:

> In the years following the initial use of the lottery, the rate of growth in education spending declines. . . . States *without* lotteries actually maintain and increase their education spending more so than states *with* lotteries.[18]

In January 1990, the governor of South Carolina waged a campaign to combat the proliferation of video poker machines in restaurants, bars, and truck stops that had, he said, "caused collective misery, spawned a new generation of addicted gamblers and destroyed families." His effort was part of a larger movement throughout the United States, in which church leaders, civic officials, and organized community groups battled gambling interests to defeat legislation designed to promote gambling. Increasingly, referenda and constitutional amendments to legalize new forms of gambling have met stern taxpayer resistance, despite high-pressure advertising campaigns.[19]

In some cases, organized gambling has begun to crumble, based on unrealistic expectations and an increasingly high level of competition from other gambling communities or types of attractions. In New Orleans, for example, during a three-year period in the mid- and late 1990s, three downtown riverboat casinos

> . . . foundered on economic, regulatory and legal difficulties. . . . Worse, the city's only land-based casino has folded too, and a gambling pleasure dome that was to replace it, a blocksquare structure designed to compete with anything in Las Vegas or Atlantic City, sits half completed on the edge of the French Quarter, mired in bankruptcy, its developers desperately searching for a way to head off liquidation.[20]

In the major gambling cities of Las Vegas and Atlantic City, however, gambling continues to flourish, with casino owners building huge, new, impressive structures to attract fresh crowds of high rollers. At the same time, the gambling industry has sought to broaden its market among all socioeconomic markets, with particular emphasis on cultivating the family and youth market. For example, in Las Vegas a number of major casinos are offering such attractions as continuous trapeze acts, nightly jousting tournaments, dolphins on display, a man-made volcano, and white tigers to draw sightseers of all ages, including a "no-nudes" policy. Some observers suggest that gambling companies anticipate good times ahead as baby boomers, raised on a credo of "sex, drugs, and rock 'n' roll" grow older and turn to gambling to meet their need for sensational forms of recreation.

Substance Abuse and Leisure

We turn now to a second important form of morally marginal leisure activity: substance abuse, or more specifically, alcohol and drug abuse. Both are similar in that they involve ingesting substances to reach a "high," or a state of excitement or euphoria. Both are usually carried on in social situations, and both may be pursued over a lengthy period of time in a moderate, controlled way. However, addiction-prone individuals often become obsessively dependent on alcohol or drugs, using mind-altering substances more and more frequently to the point that they suffer extreme psychological, physical, and economic injury and can no longer function in healthy, autonomous ways.

Both kinds of substance use are often referred to as leisure pursuits. The term *social drinking* is commonly heard, and the press frequently describes such substances as marijuana as "recreational drugs." Indeed, during the Vietnam War, *Time* characterized heroin as a "plaything" of returning American service personnel.

Despite their similarities, the use of alcohol and of narcotic drugs differ in two respects: (1) alcoholic beverages are legally sold, while narcotic drugs are illegal and have become the driving force behind an immense network of criminal activity, both domestic and international; and (2) while drinking is a recognized part of many community and family-centered occasions, narcotic drug use is, with relatively few exceptions, perceived negatively by Western society and is carried on furtively. Although alcohol is generally regarded as less harmful and dangerous than drug use, there are many more alcoholics in American society than there are drug addicts, and the cost of drinking in physical, psychological, and economic terms is vastly greater than that of narcotic drug use.

Drinking as a Social Problem

When drinking alcohol becomes a habit, a necessity for the individual in his or her daily life, it represents an addiction. The American Medical Association declared alcoholism a disease in 1957, reversing the long-held view that alcoholics were not sick, but sinful. Later, the AMA defined it more precisely: "Alcoholism is an illness characterized by preoccupation with alcohol and loss of control over its consumption such as to lead usually to intoxication if drinking is begun, by chronicity, by progression, and by tendency to relapse."

Some authorities have recently contended that alcoholism is essentially a behavioral rather than a medical problem, and that the disease concept blurs the issue of moral responsibility. Most medical authorities, however, do not accept this position; there are growing evidences of biological as well as psychosocial causes of this form of addiction. One researcher, a professor psychiatry at New York's Downstate Medical Center, has found abnormalities in brain-wave patterns of alcoholics that suggest physical rather than environmental influences in alcoholism. Other scientists have discovered a gene that governs a part of the brain called the dopamine receptor, which plays a crucial role in Parkinson's disease, schizophrenia, and pleasure-seeking behavior such as drinking alcohol, suggesting a possible inherited tendency to alcoholism.[21]

Whatever the causes, there is no doubt that problem drinking represents a major source of concern in the United States. Fully 55 percent of the public report knowing someone who "drinks too much," and Louis Harris reports that 32 percent of the nation's households have someone at home with a drinking problem. Depending on the criteria used, national surveys indicate that there are between ten and eighteen million problem drinkers in the United States. By income, excessive drinking is found most frequently among those earning $35,000 to $50,000 a year—very much a middle-income affliction. There is evidence that the national consumption of alcoholic beverages has declined over the past two decades. However, the number of persons seeking treatment for problem drinking has continued to rise and the physical and social fallout from drinking is tremendous. Drunkenness is involved in 30 to 50 percent of traffic deaths, 45 percent of all fatal falls, and 50 to 70 percent of homicides. A 1998 report by Dr. Joseph Califano, of the National Center on Addiction and Substance Abuse, shows that alcohol and drugs are now involved in the crimes and incarceration of 80 percent of the men and women in prison, with alcohol being more closely associated with crimes of violence than any other drug.[22]

In particular, alcohol represents a growing problem for America's youth. Although their use of other "recreational" drugs has diminished since the end of the 1970s, alcohol's staying power as the intoxicant of choice among the young has made it the nation's most persistent problem drug. According to the *New York Times* in the early 1990s:

> Even as alcohol use has diminished over the last decade, a federal survey of students in eight states shows that 10.6 million of 29.7 million seventh through twelfth graders drink, though all states now prohibit drinking before the age of 21. Eight million of them drink at least once a week, and 450,000 drink at least five or more drinks at a sitting.[23]

In the 1990s, attention was focused on the problem of binge drinking, defined as having consumed five drinks in a single session for men, or four drinks for women, within the past two weeks. While the percentage of college students who were binge drinkers declined slightly during the mid-1990s, the number who binged often rose. With the highest frequency among residents of fraternity and sorority houses, the incidence of deaths as a result of alcohol poisoning or accidents stemming from drunkenness shocked the nation.[24]

For many young people, drinking is a matter of wanting to belong and to be accepted by others. For others, as in the case of high school seniors who take class trips to Mexican resorts or other southern seaside vacation spots, it is also a symbol of their freedom from parental supervision and linked to the determination to engage in sex—with "all-you-can-drink" parties lowering their inhibitions.

Alcohol Advertising.   The Surgeon General of the United States points out that alcohol advertising frequently shows people racing cars or surfing, ignoring the fact that drinking would make these activities perilous. She comments:

> It is no coincidence that sports such as boating, swimming, skiing, surfing, car racing and mountain climbing—which have strong links to alcohol-related injuries—are the very activities glamorized in alcohol beverage ads and promotions. I have asked them to stop using ads that lead our youth to think they can ski, swim, scuba drive or race cars better if they drink.[25]

Timothy Dwyer points out that from locker rooms to grandstands, from the postgame interview to the player-of-the-game award, alcohol and sports are as intertwined as the seams on a baseball. Anheuser-Busch, the largest brewer and advertiser, is a major sponsor for twenty-three of twenty-four domestic major-league baseball games, twenty-five National Basketball Association teams, thirteen of fourteen domestic National Hockey League teams, and other sports—paying hundreds of millions of dollars annually for broadcast ads and stadium billboards.[26]

There have been relatively few research studies of the relationship between alcohol abuse and leisure values and behavior. One such study was conducted by Sessoms and Oakley, who examined a select group of adult male alcoholics at a state rehabilitation center in North Carolina.

> The alcoholics' [time-use] patterns seem to be filled with additional work [including a high rate of moonlighting], spectator activities, and drinking. . . . The sample displayed a minimum of concern in current affairs, the performing arts, social dancing, and civic club activities.[27]

In general, the individuals studied showed little interest in activities that did not lend themselves to drinking, whereas they did participate in activities like bowling or billiards that did. As a rule they tended not to be joiners, but if they did join a club or organization, it was usually one in which alcoholic beverages were readily available as part of the group activity.

One factor in controlling liquor abuse is that public policies regarding the use of alcohol in the United States are inconsistent and ambiguous. Five states and the District of Columbia, while outlawing the sale of alcohol to minors, do not specifically make its purchase by minors a crime. And in forty-four states, minors are allowed to sell and serve alcoholic beverages without adult supervision.

One of the key problems is that government itself has assumed the role of liquor entrepreneur in eighteen states, through state agencies that distribute and sell alcoholic beverages. The claim that state-run liquor stores help to reduce alcohol abuse and drinking-related auto accidents does not appear to be valid; Pennsylvania, which has a state-controlled system, has a higher rate of alcohol-related fatalities than nineteen states that do not have state liquor monopolies.

At the same time, drinking to excess is more widely condemned today than in the past. Corporate office parties are more likely to get along without alcohol, and there is a greater consciousness of the dangers of liquor in the workplace. The days of the "three-martini lunch" appear to be over.

While major attention has been focused on the 5 percent of the population that is technically considered to be alcoholic, some authorities point out that problem drinkers, whose liquor dependency causes major economic, health-related, or family problems, comprise 20 percent of adults. While one group of experts suggest that fuller emphasis should be placed on helping this group deal with the problem by learning to *control* their drinking, organizations like Alcoholics Anonymous preach *total* abstinence from liquor. Beyond this, in their 12-step treatment approach, they argue that it is essential to incorporate a moral or spiritual dimension in one's recovery efforts—and that a total change in one's values and lifestyle is needed—rather than simply ending drinking behavior.

Drug Abuse as Play

We turn now to the second major area of substance abuse that represents a morally marginal form of leisure activity—the use of narcotic drugs that initially create a sense of euphoria and escape, but then become powerful controlling agents in the lives of their users. For years, the use of drugs was regarded as a semi-respectable act; many doctors made personal use of heroin or cocaine, and women's patent medicines often contained narcotics.

Particularly during the era of the youth rebellion in the late 1960s and early 1970s, young people dismissed the possible health hazards of narcotics and argued that smoking pot was no worse than their parents' daily quota of cocktails. Realistically, the sensations gained from drug use provided—at least at the outset—pleasure that was more satisfying than other leisure activities could offer. One leading researcher commented:

> The simple fact is, marijuana is fun to smoke. . . . In my own study of marijuana users, pleasure emerged as the dominant motive for continued use. Almost 70 percent said that sex was more enjoyable high. Almost 90 percent said that the simple act of eating became more fun. . . . Marijuana has become, and will continue to be, increasingly a *recreational* drug, and for larger and larger numbers of young (and not so young) people. This will not disappear, and it will not abate; drug "education" campaigns are doomed to failure. . . . Outlawing fun has always been a tough job.[28]

Documented Danger of Drugs.   Despite such views and the widely expressed conviction that recreational drugs did little harm to their users, through the 1980s a series of studies documented their negative effects. In 1987, a study financed by the National Institute on Drug Abuse found that heavy users of marijuana had suffered decreases in concentration and short-term memory and had gravitated to less mentally demanding jobs. In a 1988 study published by a UCLA psychologist, it was reported that heavy drug use as a teenager severely disrupted a person's emotional and social growth during the transition to adulthood, although occasional drug use of hashish and marijuana did not appear to have significant effects.[29] The unpredictable effects of drugs like cocaine, heroin, LSD, and other synthetic substances clearly involved major health risks, as evidenced by the deaths of numerous popular music stars over the past two decades.

In 1997, research studies reported in scientific journals indicated that persons who regularly smoke large amounts of marijuana may experience harmful changes in their brain chemistry similar to those found in persons who abuse heroin, cocaine, and other "hard" drugs. Scientists concluded that:

> . . . all addictive drugs corrupt the same brain circuits, although to varying degrees and . . . that chronic marijuana use may literally prime the brain for other drugs of abuse, a notion known as the "gateway effect."[30]

Scale of Drug Use.   Until the post–World War II era, drug abuse tended to be thought of as a relatively minor social problem. In the 1970s, in addition to the great numbers of affluent white college and high school youth who began to experiment with drugs, it became apparent that millions of middle-class Americans were using narcotics in one form or another, including employees in large corporations, successful professionals, and members of highly respected families. Indeed, a 1986 study directed by the Harvard University School of Public Health revealed that a high proportion of doctors and medical students had used illegal drugs.

> More than half the physicians and three-quarters of the medical students who participated in a Harvard University survey said they had used drugs at least once for self-treatment, to get high, or to help them stay awake. Nearly 40 percent of doctors under age 40 reported in the survey that they had used marijuana or cocaine to get high with friends, and a quarter of doctors of all ages said they had recently treated themselves with mind-affecting drugs.[31]

In the same year, it was reported that Americans consumed 60 percent of the world's production of illegal drugs. An estimated twenty million persons were regular users of marijuana, four to eight million more were cocaine abusers, and 500,000 were heroin addicts.

By the mid-1990s, reports by the United Nations International Drug Control Program indicated that drug trafficking had become a $500-billion-a-year business worldwide. Marijuana is used by 140 million persons, with high levels of use of cocaine and heroin, and a striking growth in addiction to synthetic drugs, such as amphetamines. It concluded that the drug industry represented a sophisticated international criminal enterprise.[32]

Involvement of Youth.   In the United States, concern about the involvement of youth in narcotic drug use has grown steadily. Surprisingly, despite constant media images of black youths being arrested for drug-related crimes, some studies showed that white students were more likely to use drugs and alcohol than their African American peers. Based on research conducted by federal agencies, Health and Human Services Secretary Louis Sullivan reported:

> white male high school seniors were almost twice as likely to use cocaine as were blacks (12 percent vs. 6.1 percent according to data from the government's National

High School Senior Surveys from 1985 to 1989). Forty percent of white male seniors had used marijuana, compared with 30 percent of black male seniors. . . . The studies also found that 88 percent of white male students said they had consumed alcohol in the last year, compared with 73 percent of black males.[33]

Other studies have questioned these findings, and it is clear that both drugs and alcohol represent a severe problem in depressed minority neighborhoods in cities where African American and Hispanic youth have a high rate of unemployment and harshly limited prospects for the future. The invasion of crack cocaine, beginning in the late 1980s, meant that whole areas of urban ghettoes and barrios were captured by drug dealers and gangs that terrorized law-abiding families. For many minority-group youth, a job in the underground drug economy, a businesslike, well-organized, and competitive operation, is a respected means of survival. A black minister, Cecil Williams, says that many teenagers are drawn to work in the cocaine trade simply because they want jobs. The drug business is seen as a "safety net," a place where it is always possible to make a few dollars.

"Money and drugs are the obvious immediate rewards," Williams adds. "But there is another strong motivating force, and that is the desire to show family and friends that they can succeed at something . . . and they see no chance to find a well-paying job with career possibilties."[34]

During the 1990s, there were a number of reports by the National Household Survey on Drug Abuse and other university research teams that the overall use of drugs in the United States was declining. However, in April 1993, a federally funded University of Michigan survey found that there was a significant increase in the use of marijuana, cocaine, LSD, and other illicit substances by eighth graders—confirmed in 1997 by a similar United Nations report.[35]

Efforts at Control

The major emphasis in government-funded programs is on interdiction and punishment, with approximately 70 percent of federal dollars being spent on efforts to prevent drug trafficking, to intercept shipments, and to punish offenders. With tougher enforcement laws, since 1980 the average sentence length for federal drug offenses has climbed 20 percent to about 5.5 years, and prisons and local jails are overcrowded with offenders. It is obvious that a major aspect of the drug problem involves the African American and Hispanic poor in American cities. However, authorities warn that the widespread myth of drugs as primarily a ghetto problem is misleading. It enables one to ascribe all the profound social problems of the inner city to drugs—blaming racial minorities for their involvement, while ignoring the deeper problems of unemployment and lack of education. Moreover, it permits middle-class white Americans to avoid responsibility for the widespread use of drugs among their own families and friends.

An example of how many white youth are involved in recreational drugs can be found in the Winter Olympics incident in February 1998 when a champion Canadian snowboarder had his gold medal taken back because of evidence of marijuana use. *Time Magazine* points out that among snowboarders and, by implication, other enthusiasts of stunt skiing, in-line skating competition, and other extreme "airborne" sports, who are predominantly white:

> . . . pot has been a common part of the life-style. Along with freedom, travel and the pursuit of that perfect powder day, marijuana is regarded by certain riders as traditional ritual. [One snowboarder says] "It's so common, nobody thinks about it."[36]

Despite such evidence, government figures showed that nearly three-quarters of inmates serving time in local jails on drug charges in the early 1990s were black or Hispanic. Nonprofit organizations like the Drug Policy Foundation have concluded that the drug war is racially biased on all fronts. A number of government officials and authorities on drug abuse have argued that the only way to attack the problem is to legalize narcotics under a tight control system, as a number of European nations have done with mixed success. However, there has been little support for this position, and it seems unlikely that Congress or the American public would approve it.

Linkage of Drug Abuse and Leisure

Relatively few research studies have explored the relationship of leisure and recreation with drug abuse. Iso-Ahola and Crowley conducted one study that examined the role of leisure in the lives of adolescent substance abusers. Surprisingly (since one might assume that drug abusers would have fewer recreational interests), they found that

> substance abusers had a tendency to participate more frequently in leisure in general and physical recreation activities in particular. . . . Because of their personality predisposition toward sensation-seeking and low tolerance toward [repetitious] experiences, substance abusers presumably prefer active leisure lifestyles. But if leisure activities fail to satisfy their need for optimal arousal, leisure boredom results and drug use may be the only alternative.[37]

A second study, by Ann Rancourt, explored the relationships among recreation, leisure, and substance abuse in a treatment program for women. It focused on two issues: the past attitudes and behaviors of the subjects with respect to leisure and the potential role of recreation in residential treatment programs. The subjects revealed that, while their use of drugs was recreational in that they thought of it as "partying," it was rarely enjoyable. Instead, some said: ". . . it was like a job; I had to get high . . . to feel normal." . . . abuse ultimately became "like medication, not like recreation."[38]

Rancourt found that many women felt that they had missed out on their childhoods and that taking part now in such experiences as roller or ice skating, visiting parks or beaches, bowling or picnics, gave them the intense feeling of being young again. While "normal" kinds of play had meant little to them while abusing drugs, now they began to realize that it could make a positive contribution to their lives.

A final important point with respect to substance abuse is that the most dangerous drug by far is legal—tobacco. Government reports through the 1990s have concluded that while heart disease and cancer may be listed as the nation's leading killers, the biggest underlying cause of death is tobacco use. Research by the American Medical Association, for example, has found that smoking contributed to the deaths of 400,000 persons a year—more than the deaths caused by drug use, guns, irresponsible sexual behavior, and automobile accidents combined.[39]

Commercialized Sex

A third important category of commodified, morally marginal leisure activity consists of sex. While sex for sale has been part of many societies through the ages, it has rarely been as systematically and widely exploited as it is today.

Edwin Schur points out that over the past several decades many Americans developed a *Playboy*-influenced mentality, in which sex came to represent a symbol of competitive striving and acquisition and an omnipresent element in the mass media, advertising, and varied forms of entertainment. He writes that the hallmark of the *Playboy*-influenced lifestyle is consumption.

> Women, much like the other fun-offering products, are to be consumed. The female is depicted as a concertedly sought and ultimately purchasable acquisition. [In *Playboy*] the issue was money. Men made it; women wanted it. . . . The message was simple: You can buy sex on a fee-for-service basis, so don't get caught up in a long-term contract.[40]

Playboy and other magazines like it encouraged men's tendency to view women primarily in sexual terms and to be preoccupied with detailed and heavily eroticized female body parts. Through their pictures, stories, and articles, these publications promoted a general lifestyle in which men "could have it all."

In America, Schur writes, entrepreneurs are constantly on the lookout for new business opportunities. The American obsession with sex presented many such opportunities. That sex—formerly viewed as an intimate and even sacrosanct activity—now can be seen as just another business field illustrates the degree to which all forms of leisure have been commodified in contemporary American life.

Sex for Sale

Probably the leading example of sex being used as a commodity for commercial gain is prostitution. In America's early history, prostitution flourished in frontier areas where there were many men and few women, but also in cities and towns where established "madams" and houses of prostitution were tolerated as necessary evils. In the 1820s, urban reformers in the United States declared prostitution a threat to municipal virtue and social order and conducted campaigns against brothels.

For a time, prostitutes were viewed primarily as victims of male predators. However, during World War I, with growing concern about venereal disease, the image of the prostitute was transformed from sex-victim to sex-villain. New laws against prostitution penalized women exclusively and frequently violated their civil rights. In describing this period, historian Barbara Hobson points out that men held all the power but took none of the responsibility for illicit sexuality or for the larger socioeconomic pressures that drove women into prostitution.[41]

In the modern era, prostitution is often permitted tacitly to exist in the form of call-girl rings or escort services, along with massage parlors that advertise openly in many cities and are often a front for prostitution. Nevada is the only state that permits legal houses of prostitution in a number of its counties. The feminist movement is divided regarding this social problem. For many feminists, it represents sexual slavery and a vivid representation of women's economic and social subservience. But for others, the growing ethic of sexual independence for women, plus the fact that some women who engage in prostitution have vigorously defended their right to choose their occupation, challenges the underlying assumption of female sexual passivity that underlies much condemnation of prostitution.

In many cities today, prostitution is tolerated, provided that it is limited to certain streets or downtown neighborhoods or to avenues leading to the city's outskirts. When the problem becomes too blatant, police may crack down by harassing prostitutes. In some cases, as in Portland, Oregon, police seize and impound the cars of men caught patronizing street prostitutes. During the mid-1980s, organized-crime groups with Far East ties began to import thousands of women from South Korea and Taiwan, moving them through a network of American brothels, according to federal and state law enforcement officials.

While it is difficult to measure the actual volume of spending on prostitution, a clue may be found in a 1998 International Labor Organization report on prostitution in Southeast Asia. In that report, it estimated that the annual income from prostitution in Thailand, a relatively small nation, was between $22 billion and $27 billion.[42] In major U.S. cities, as street crackdowns, along with the combined forces of AIDs and drug addiction, thin the ranks of street prostitutes, many professional "sex workers" today make use of the Internet, cellular phones, pagers, and other devices to make business arrangements.

Pornography

A second leading example of commercialized sex today is pornography—the manufacture and sale of books, magazines, and videotapes depicting sexual activity in all its varieties. In the past, fascination with this kind of material was regarded as a sick and shameful kind of obsession. Today, interest in sexual materials is so widespread that it is no longer regarded by most individuals as evidence of sinfulness or mental disturbance.

Writing in *The Christian Century*, Mary Ellen Ross points out that pornography is readily available to all, including children, and in the privacy in our own homes. She writes:

Pornographic images have been proliferating at a remarkable rate. What was a $5-million-a-year enterprise merely 25 years ago has boomed to a $7-billion to $10-billion-a-year industry today. . . . This surge is due in part to the discovery of new markets. While adult bookstores, peepshows and movie theaters still thrive, the fastest growing sectors of the industry are pornographic videocassettes, cable television, and phone sex.[43]

In recent years, radical feminists have tried to define pornography in law as an exclusively male phenomenon, in which women were invariably the victim of exploitation and brutality. However, this is clearly not the case, and there is evidence that a considerable number of women today enjoy pornography; 30 percent of those renting X-rated videos in a 1986 survey of retailers of "adult" films, for example, were women.

In the late 1980s, a federal Commission on Pornography issued a report that concluded that there was a causal link between pornography and aggressive or violent behavior toward women—contradicting the findings of an earlier commission that it was *not* a cause of sexual crime. At this time, growth in moral militancy in American society was evidenced in a series of restrictive Supreme Court decisions that enabled officials in a number of cities to close adult bookstores because of solicitation for prostitution or other offenses. Some cities enacted stricter ordinances controlling the display and sale of pornographic materials, or established "anti-porn" squads, putting pressure on real estate owners to shift their "sex-oriented" buildings to less offensive businesses.

In cities like New York, intensive efforts have been made to reduce the number of sex-oriented businesses such as topless bars, video stores, and "peep shows" by stricter zoning regulations and firmer enforcement—in some cases resulting in the dispersement of such businesses to scattered locations around the city.

In general, the X-rated industry has been in a slump since the late 1980s, with at least half of the nation's adult movie theaters closing down and the sales of magazines like *Playboy* declining sharply. Many forms of sex-oriented play, as described in Chapter 8, had been affected by growing fears of sexually transmitted disease, particularly the AIDS epidemic. Patronage of legal, health-inspected Nevada brothels was off by as much as 40 percent.

At the same time, other forms of exploiting sexual interest have continued to evolve. For example, in motion pictures there has been a distinct trend toward increasing nudity and the more open depiction or simulation of the sex act.

Some forms of erotic play rely on electronic means of communication. The use of 1-900 telephone lines for caller-paid conversations increased dramatically in the late 1980s, with revenues reaching several hundred million dollars each year. Barbara Rudolph writes:

So far, sex has been the best seller, generating more than a third of the industry's revenues. The dial-a-porn lines offer everything from recorded fantasies to lusty personal ads. Bawdy party lines have also proliferated, though their popularity is fading. Many of the numbers are far from erotic, providing legitimate dating services or outlets for gentle conversation.[44]

Since the mid-1990s, an increasing volume of pornographic material trading in sexual imagery on the computer by downloading pictures from the Internet has been investigated by a team of researchers from Carnegie Mellon University. In an 18-month study, they surveyed over 917,000 sexually explicit pictures, film clips, and other materials, with 83.5 percent of the digitized pictures classified as pornographic. According to their report, exchanging or purchasing such materials is one of the largest recreational applications of users of computer networks.[45]

Summing up the trend, in 1997, *U.S. News and World Report* concluded that the sex industry had been transformed from a minor subculture on the fringes of society into a major component of American popular culture. The number of hard-core-video rentals rose from 75 million in 1985 to 665 million in 1996. In the same year, Americans spent more than $8 billion on hard-core videos, peep shows, live sex acts, adult cable programming, sexual devices, computer porn, and sex magazines—an amount much larger than Hollywood's domestic box office receipts and all the revenues generated by rock and country music recordings.

> Despite having some of the toughest restrictions on sexually explicit materials of any Western industrialized nation, the United States is now by far the world's leading producer of porn, churning out hard-core videos at the astonishing rate of about 150 new titles a week.[46]

Recognizing the immense volume of pornographic materials that are created annually and the emergence of the sex "industry" as a field of employment involving huge numbers, some commentators refer to it and to prostitution as "victimless." In response to a *U.S. News and World Report* article that describes the porn field's financial impact and presents some of its star performers as happy-go-lucky exhibitionists, a Seattle family doctor argues that a depressing trail of human abuse underlies porn. In his practice, he writes:

> I have encountered multiple patients who were "exotic dancers" and who "acted" in porn films. Nearly all were survivors of childhood sexual abuse and lead lives of continued abuse, addiction, and depression. They "follow the money" and approval in their sexualized lives, just as their abusers taught them. The trauma of sexualizing a child leaves her bereft of skills with which to build a real career. . . . Had the story taken a closer examination of these depressing lives, you would have illuminated the reasons why "normal" people who view pornography need to boycott the industry.[47]

Within each of the kinds of morally marginal leisure activities described in this chapter—gambling, substance abuse and commercialized or exploitative sex—responsible leisure-service planners must determine what their proper role should be. In many cases, gambling is presented within a respectable recreation context in the form of a fund-raising Las Vegas night or planned trip to Atlantic City. Liquor is an accepted part of many social occasions or events. "Adult" films or sex-based magazines may be seen in varied settings—such as college film series or military Post Exchanges. Highly respectable hotel chains make millions of dollars by offering their patrons porn films on in-house television channels.

In each such setting, recreation, park, and leisure-service managers must make a judgment based both on their view of what desirable leisure experiences *should* be and on the kinds of values that they seek to express to the community they serve. The ultimate goal cannot simply be the number of participants attracted to a program or the revenues gained by program offerings. Instead, it must be to enhance and enrich the lives of participants, through creative and constructive recreation.

Technology's Role in Commodifying Leisure

Clearly, many of the forms of play and recreation that emerged in the twentieth century and became important elements in the growing recreation industry were made possible by advanced technology. For example, the invention of radio, motion picture, the phonograph, and television all dramatically reshaped the everyday leisure patterns of everyday American families and gave rise to huge new industries.

Within the realm of outdoor recreation, technologically innovative forms of play such as scuba diving, parasailing, skydiving, hang gliding, snowmobiling, and other kinds of off-road travel have opened up new environments for the play experience. New and costly forms of high-tech equipment for hunting and fishing include night-vision glasses, trail-monitoring devices, simulated hunter training units, and electronic fish finders, attractants, and depth gauges. In sports, electronic swing analyzers provide computer-generated tips for improving baseball or golf performance; innovatively designed equipment guarantees more power and accuracy in tennis play.

Toys of every sort reflect technological innovation. Yesterday's simple and inexpensive water pistol has been transformed into Super Soakers, Robo Blasters, Stream Machines, and other automatic weapons with powerful velocity and water capacity. Some are battery-powered with flashing lights and electronic sounds that taunt one's opponent in comic mimicry of military realism.

Of all forms of commercially produced technological play, many of the most popular and profitable are electronically based. Computers can be used to compose and play music, individually or in concert with other musicians, create art, and choreograph dances. But these uses pale in comparison with the proliferation of video games and the Internet as forms of leisure involvement.

At every level, from designing racing yachts to opening new windows to the world for disabled persons, and from grooming snow slopes at ski resorts to creating more-than-lifelike virtual "pets," technology has reshaped the leisure world. What will the future hold? It is impossible to predict, but all authorities and futurologists agree that the world of tomorrow will continue to produce exciting new forms of high-tech play and living possibilities.

A key force behind this prospect will be the drive to create profitable recreational enterprises. As this chapter has shown, not only traditional forms of play but the morally marginal pursuits of gambling, substance abuse, and commercialized sex, in one form or another, make use of modern technology. In so doing, they contribute immeasurably to the nation's less visible economy.

As Chapter 1 shows, spending on several major categories of recreational activity accounts for over $400 billion each year in the United States. To this, one must add a number of areas of spending such as major sectors of travel and tourism or sports participation that are not included in the *Statistical Abstract's* totals (see page 10). If one then adds the amounts spent on gambling—certainly over $500 billion—on illegal drugs, over $100 billion; alcohol, over $50 billion; and commercialized sex, probably over $40 billion; the total expenditure on commodified leisure amounts to well over a trillion dollars.[48]

While this presents only *one* way to judge the value or impact of recreation and leisure, it is an impressive sum. However, there are other equally important ways. One of them involves the quality of our lives—and here the idea of environment comes in. The chapter that follows discusses the relationship between leisure and the environment, not only in terms of forests, lakes, and mountains, but also the living environment that surrounds most people every day in the cities, towns, and villages where they live.

Summary

Uniquely, leisure has been transformed from an area of personal and social life marked by self-determination, freedom of choice, and creative expression to an immense industry in which many attractions are controlled by huge corporations with sophisticated marketing and promotional resources. This chapter explores the meaning of consumerism in modern society and the way in which major institutions have adopted commercial strategies. Through diversified offerings, product licensing, traditional holidays, and even the death of celebrities, the public is offered a host of leisure services and products. The Disney organization is cited as a leading example of creative development, in its theme parks, entertainment programs, and even sports sponsorship.

A critical area of commodified leisure involves morally marginal pursuits having to do with gambling, substance abuse, and commercialized sex—all immensely profitable enterprises that are offered either legally or illegally, but that attract a large segment of the population. Underlying all such developments, modern technology has assisted both in the creation of new kinds of pastimes and in their delivery to potential audiences.

Key Concepts

1. Commodification may be seen as a logical expression of the free enterprise system, in which varied social services or products become profit-oriented offerings controlled more by market forces than by individual wishes or self-expression.

2. Linked to this development, consumerism, in which people use the purchase of goods and services to frame their own identity and make an impression on others, becomes a way of life.

3. Many of the established fields of daily living, including religious practice, health care, higher education, or even the management of the prison system, have adopted commercial, profit-oriented tactics to ensure economic survival and public support.

4. In leisure itself, such types of agencies as public or nonprofit organizations, health and fitness clubs, or major restaurant chains have developed a wide range of different games, sports, services, and events to broaden their appeal.

5. A unique feature of the last decades of the twentieth century has been the formation of huge conglomerates that combine companies in the entertainment, communications, sports, and travel fields into powerful new enterprises that influence the public's leisure. Disney is cited as a leading example of such organizations.

6. The term "morally marginal" applies to those kinds of leisure experiences that have been generally disapproved by society in the past, but that today have a degree of social approval and acceptance. Often their legal status depends on the region in which they are offered, the age of those participating, and even whether government itself is the sponsor as opposed to a private party. In some cases, an activity is acceptable to a certain point—as in drinking—but regarded as an illness when carried beyond that.

7. Gambling is a leading example of an activity that consumes hundreds of billions of dollars of public spending each year, is approved or sponsored by government, has both harmful and beneficial effects, and is prosecuted as a crime when conducted privately.

8. Substance abuse is widely regarded as a harmful, self-destructive activity, although alcohol consumption as such is accepted as a popular pastime or form of social activity by the vast majority of the population. In contrast, because narcotic drugs are generally illegal, they form the basis for a huge criminal enterprise, both nationally and worldwide.

9. Commercialized sex, again, is generally disapproved by moral forces in society but is permitted to exist in many disguised forms in most communities. Pornography, once thought of as a morally shameful preoccupation, today enters millions of homes through adult films played on family VCRs.

10. Technology as a means of creating new kinds of leisure experiences or making them widely available underlies the growth of leisure as an industry to an estimated trillion-dollar annual expenditure in the United States.

Endnotes

1. Butsch, R. 1990. *For Fun and Profit: The Transformation of Leisure Into Consumption.* Philadelphia: Temple University Press, p. 3.

2. Kraus, R. 1996. Play's New Identity: Big Business. *Journal of Physical Education, Recreation, and Dance* (October): 36.

3. DeGrazia, S., cited in Shivers, J.S., and L.J. deLisle. 1995. *The Story of Leisure.* Champaign, IL: Human Kinetics, p. 3.

4. Corrigan, P. 1997. *The Sociology of Consumption.* London: Sage Publications, pp. 3–23.

5. Boxer, S. 1998. I Shop, Ergo I Am: The Mall as Society's Mirror. *New York Times* (March 28): B-7.

6. Henry, I. ed. 1990. *Management and Planning in the Leisure Industries.* London: Macmillan, p. 41.

7. Kelly, J. 1991. Commodification and Consciousness: An Initial Study. *Leisure Studies* (10): 11.

8. Trueheart, C. 1996. The Next Church. *Atlantic Monthly* (August): 37.

9. Manning, S. 1999. Classrooms for Sale. *New York Times* (Mar. 24): A-27.

10. Brooke, J. 1997. Prisons: A Growth Industry for Some. *New York Times* (November 2): 20.

11. State Prisons Go After New Source of Financing Their Inmates. 1996. *New York Times* (July 7): 14.

12. Crossley, J., and T. Ellis. 1988. An Entrepreneurial Application: Systematic Innovation. *Journal of Physical Education, Recreation and Dance* (October): 35.

13. Lyall, S. 1998. Britain's Diana-Mania, Anniversary Edition. *New York Times* (August 23): AR-29.

14. Sport The Power of Business. Advertisement in *Athletic Business* (June 1997): 15.

15. Sterngold, J. 1996. Muting the Lotteries' Perfect Pitch. *New York Times* (July 14): E-18.

16. Safire, W. 1997. Losers Weepers. *New York Times* (January 22): A-17.

17. See Stock, R. 1997. When Gambling Threatens a Nest Egg. *New York Times* (June 26): C-8; and Blakeslee, S. 1997. Suicide Rate Higher in 3 Gambling Cities. *New York Times* (December 16): A-16.

18. Miller, D., and P. Pierce. 1997. Lotteries for Education: Windfall or Hoax? *State and Local Government Review* (Winter): 34–42.

19. Nossiter, A. 1996. Ballot Losses Signal End of Gambling's Lucky Run. *New York Times* (November 19): A-22.

20. Ayres, R.D. 1997. In New Orleans, the House Loses. *New York Times* (October 14): A-18.

21. Genes with a Don't Drink Label. 1990. *U.S. News and World Report* (April 30): 15.

22. Public Policy Trends 1998. *NTRS Report* (February–April): 3.

23. Bandy, L. 1991. "Alarming Trend" in U.S. Teens. *Philadelphia Inquirer* (June 7): 18-A.

24. Goldberg, C. 1998. Little Drop in College Binge Drinking. *New York Times* (September 11): A-14.

25. Surgeon General Says Ads for Alcohol Ignore Danger. 1992. *Associated Press* (March 24).

26. Dwyer, T. 1991. Beer Hall, the Message from Sports: Alcohol Is Drug of Choice. *Philadelphia Inquirer* (May 9): 1-A.

27. Sessoms, H.D., and S. Oakley. 1969. Recreation, Leisure and the Alcoholic. *Therapeutic Recreation Journal* (Winter): 21–31.

28. Goode, E. 1971. Turning on for Fun. *New York Times* (January 9): 27.

29. Study: Heavy Drug Use Hurts Young. 1988. *Los Angeles Times Service* (July 21).

30. Blakeslee, S. 1997. Brain Studies Tie Marijuana to Other Drugs. *New York Times* (June 27): A-16.

31. Poll Measures Use of Drugs Among Doctors. 1986. *Philadelphia Inquirer* (September 25): C-1.

32. Database: Sales in Drug Trafficking Worldwide, $500 Million. 1994. *U.S. News and World Report* (November 28): 33.

33. Moore, A. 1992. Sullivan: Drug Use Less for Black Teens. *Philadelphia Inquirer* (May 14): A-2.

34. Kleine, T. 1991. A Portrait of the Drug Dealer as a Young Man. *Utne Reader* (May–June): 63.

35. Wren, C. 1997. U.N. Report Says Tens of Millions Use Illicit Drugs. *New York Times* (June 25).

36. Galbraith, J. 1998. Dazed and Confused: A Whiff of Pot Smoke. *Time Magazine* (February 23): 50.

37. Iso-Ahola, S., and E. Crowley, 1991. Adolescent Substance Abuse and Leisure Boredom. *Journal of Leisure Research* (23/3): 260.

38. Rancourt, A. 1991. An Exploration of the Relationships Among Substance Abuse, Recreation, and Leisure for Women Who Abuse Substances. *Therapeutic Recreation Journal* (3rd Q.): 15.

39. Tobacco Top Death Cause, Study Shows. 1993. *Philadelphia Inquirer* (November 3): 42.

40. Schur, E. 1989. *The Americanization of Sex*. Philadelphia: Temple University Press, pp. 86–87.

41. Hobson, B. 1988. *The Politics of Prostitution and The American Reform Tradition*. New York: Basic Books.

42. Olson, E. 1998. U.N. Urges Fiscal Accounting Include Sex Trade. *New York Times* (August 20): A-11.

43. Ross, M.E. 1990. Censorship or Education? Feminist Views of Pornography. *Christian Century* (March 7): 244.

44. Rudolph, B. 1988. Business: Who Ever Said Talk Was Cheap? *Time Magazine* (Sept. 19): 44.

45. Elmer-Dewitt, P. 1995. On a Screen Near You: Cyberporn. *Time Magazine* (July 3): 38–45.

46. Schlosser, E. 1997. The Business of Pornography. *U.S. News and World Report* (February 10): 43–44.

47. Bittenger, K., 1997. The Porn Industry (Letter to the Editor). *U.S. News and World Report* (March 3): 6.

48. Stynes, D. Leisure—"The New Center of the Economy," in Geoffrey Godbey, Ed., 1993. *Issue Papers*. University Park, PA: Pennsylvania State University and Academy of Leisure Sciences, pp. 11–17.

13 Environmental Trends and Issues

Environmental concerns and causes will continue to besiege the United States and Canada. Global warming, acid rain, losses related to biodiversity, and abandoned nuclear waste products will be health and environmental concerns of the decades. Participation in outdoor leisure pursuits will increase. Individuals seeking a return to nature and their roots will place an increased load on the natural world. Designated recreation areas, in particular, may see this factor impact resource quality. Parks will continue to move toward closing their entrance gates once a preestablished visitor capacity has been met. user and entrance fees to outdoor areas will increase and the concern about the rights of all users will mount. Many environmental trends and concerns will continue to be linked to leisure.[1]

More than a century later [the] philosophical and practical struggle continues—with higher stakes and fiercer fighting. There is little doubt that the preservationists are losing ground. The ills that beset the nation's first and still more magnificent park affect the park system as a whole: underfunding, overcrowding, pollution, encroaching commercial development, invasion of exotic species, and the decline of natural, historical, and cultural treasures. "We've crested: We can no longer offer the quality of experience we once did," says Yellowstone's resource chief, John Varley.[2]

From a preoccupation with the people who engage in recreational pursuits and the factors that influence their involvement, we now turn to an examination of the physical setting in which we live and play—the environment. This chapter deals with past and current efforts to set aside parks, forests, and waterways for outdoor recreation, as well as other efforts to counter air and water pollution, protect endangered species, and promote the sustainable uses of natural resources. It discusses a number of conflict areas, such as the ongoing struggle between those who favor fuller exploitation of outdoor resources for economic purposes and those who resist such policies. In so doing, it outlines a number of newer approaches to environmental protection, including ecotourism, partnerships between business and ecological groups, and changing practices of national land-management agencies.

Beyond this, however, the idea of environment must be extended to the urban, metropolitan, or small-town settings in which the majority of Americans live. Here, large and small parks, playgrounds, environmental centers, bicycle paths and trailways, riverfronts, and even streets and housing developments represent places critical to improving the quality of life. Thus, environment in both natural and urban locales is a key element in promoting societal well-being and enhancing the rich use of leisure.

The Environmental Movement: An Overview

The history of recreation and leisure in the United States was closely intertwined with the development of major federal and state parks, forests, and other sites for conservation purposes during the latter half of the nineteenth century. Accompanying and promoting this trend was the growing interest of many Americans in preserving the wilderness, both as a unique national heritage and as a venue for outdoor exploration and recreation. In the decades after the Civil War, many of the nation's wealthiest citizens carved out wilderness retreats for themselves in the Adirondacks or other scenic regions, spent vacations on Western cattle ranches, or mounted big-game hunting expeditions in the Rocky Mountains.

American attitudes toward wilderness changed markedly. Initially, it was often viewed as dangerous and meant to be conquered—by leveling forests, wiping out buffalo herds, or building dams to tame wild rivers. In the process of bringing "civilization" to the land, settlers had often wreaked havoc on the natural environment. The celebrated cowboy artist, Charles Russell, sums up an environmentalist's view of westward expansion:

> In my book, a pioneer is a man who turned all the grass upside down, strung bob-wire over the dust that was left, poisoned the water, cut down the trees, killed the Indian who owned the land, and called it progress.[3]

However, this attitude began to change as states and then the federal government set aside great scenic monuments, historic sites, and natural wonders, initially with the intention of preserving them as wildlands and gradually the goal of providing settings for camping, sightseeing, and active forms of outdoor recreation.

In the opening decades of the twentieth century, this linkage continued with the establishment of such important federal agencies as the National Park Service, Forest Service, Bureau of Land Management, Bureau of Reclamation, and other departments or offices concerned with fish and wildlife, dam and reservoir construction, and similar functions. Particularly in the Forest Service, administratively located within the federal Department of Agriculture, a multiuse concept prevailed that gave a high priority to cattle grazing, lumbering, and other economic uses of the environment.

Environmental Recovery Programs

Following World War II, there was growing public concern about the loss of wilderness areas and oceanfront beaches and the environmental degradation caused by industrial wastes, overuse of recreational sites, lack of sewage treatment plants, and similar causes. This concern, along with awareness of the impact of pesticides on wildlife, led to the work of the Outdoor Recreation Resource Review Commission and its report in 1962, with major recommendations for national environmental action. Powerful drives toward preserving or acquiring new open space and parkland, curbing pollution, and promoting natural beauty led to a host of federal and state legislative programs. The establishment of the Bureau of Outdoor Recreation, the Land and Water Conservation Fund, the Wilderness Act of 1964, and the later Urban Park and Recreation Recovery Program all represented major steps in the nation's becoming increasingly ecologically concerned.

At the same time, the role of recreation within federal land management programs was strengthened, and numerous new parks and recreation areas were established, many of them closer to the eastern or midwestern states where a major portion of the population lives.

However, during the 1980s, this process was slowed, as the rate of federal and state land acquisition declined, and policies shifted strongly toward favoring the commodity interests that profited from business uses of the West—mining, logging, and agriculture. A continuing battle ensued, with powerful business interests and many local citizens who depended for employment on these traditional industries on one side, and a coalition of organizations like the Sierra Club, National Wildlife Federation, and Wilderness Society on the other. Major new initiatives to develop new areas were delayed or defeated in order to protect threatened wildlife species. On-the-ground environmental activists chained themselves to giant redwood trees to protect them against logging or carried out other acts of sabotage to hamper commercial uses of public lands.

In response, organized groups of western landowners, city officials, company directors, and lobbyists joined together to charge that the more extreme environmentalists were hostile to new technology, capitalism, and industry, and unrealistic in terms of the need to maintain the economies of the western states. With growing political power in the mid-1990s, a determined faction of Congressional conservatives sought to cripple the U.S. Environmental Protection Agency and set up a virtual environmental "exemption bazaar" with bills that would:

> Open the Arctic National Wildlife Refuge in Alaska, the nation's largest protected natural region, to oil and gas drilling
>
> Prevent the Environmental Protection Agency from keeping toxic fill out of lakes and harbors by limiting its funding for sewage treatment programs
>
> Suspend the listing of new endangered species and slash funding for the Endangered Species Art programs
>
> Cut funding by two-thirds for the Agriculture Department to purchase wetlands from farmers to protect ecological systems

Other legislative efforts at this time sought to increase logging in the Tongass National Forest, shrink the boundaries of Shenandoah National Park in Virginia, open wilderness areas in Voyageurs National Park in Minnesota to motorized recreation uses, and slash funding for maintenance of the Mojave National Preserve in California. Joining those who supported such efforts to exploit the wilderness more freely were groups of outdoor recreationists whose interests—such as promoting the use of off-road vehicles or preventing gun-control legislation—coincided with those of the proponents of these measures.

Threats to Outdoor Environments

Although most of the proposals just described did not succeed, it was recognized during the mid- and late-1990s that the nation's wilderness system was in perilous condition. A 1997 article in *U.S. News and World Report* spoke to the problems afflicting the National Park Service, the agency responsible for most of the natural treasures and key outdoor recreation attractions. While uses of the national parks—as one key element in the nation's wilderness empire—had expanded steadily to over 270 million visitors each year, throughout the system:

> Reduced budgets have spurred the steady deterioration of roads, buildings, sewers, and other infrastructure. Campgrounds are being closed, operating hours shortened, interpretive programs trimmed, seasonal rangers laid off. Priceless natural and historical assets are deteriorating steadily. Base-line scientific knowledge vital to the parks' long-term protection is lacking, and the shortage of funds has drastically reduced research.[4]

In addition to problems within the parks themselves, uncontrolled commercial and residential development around them poses additional threats. Yellowstone, for example, contains the world's most unique geothermal features, varied and abundant wildlife, and spectacular scenery. However, within the 18-million-acre Greater Yellowstone Ecosystem, including Grand Teton National Park, seven national forests, three national wildlife refuges, and over three million acres of private property, there are massive threats of overcrowding and pollution. Ranchettes, subdivisions, motels, commercial strips, golf courses, and tourist attractions spread into lowland stream valleys, robbing wildlife of needed winter habitat. The planned expansion of eight ski resorts around the park and proposals to lease 2.7 million national forest acres for oil and gas development added additional threats.

Similar problems affect Everglades and Biscayne National Parks in Florida, Maine's Acadia National Park, the Grand Canyon, and Great Smoky Mountains National Park, the nation's most popular big park, now afflicted by bumper-to-bumper roads, insect infestations, and on many days a thick brown haze caused by nearby factories and power plants. Federal reports make it clear that the Environmental Protection Agency and state agencies have been systematically deficient in inspections, detecting violations of air and water quality regulations, and enforcing controls in factories, meat-packing plants, drainage system, and water-treatment facilities.

Preservation of the nation's wetlands, crucial to wildlife and fisheries and to filtering contaminants from drainage from agricultural areas, represents another vital concern. During the decade between 1985 and 1995, over a million wetland acres were lost; the lower forty-eight states have now lost more than half the wetlands that existed in colonial days.

In a harsh summary of the environmental crisis faced by the United States in the final decade of the twentieth century, Daniel Sitarz summed up the need to create and enforce policies that would lead to a "sustainable America." We are eroding the fertile soil that nourishes our crops, depleting the nation's groundwater, degrading the rangelands, destroying wetlands and wildlife habitat, and extinguishing species—some forever, he writes. He continues:

> Our chemicals are depleting the Earth's protective ozone layer. Our lifestyles are dramatically changing the Earth's climate. We are harvesting our fisheries to the point of collapse. We are producing toxic and radioactive substances that must be contained forever to be safe. . . . These acts cannot be considered environmentally sustainable. Yet they all occur in the United States today. To achieve a sustainable America, we must change them.[5]

Conflict in Land-Management Priorities

Resistance to ecologically based conservation drives is usually couched in economic terms. Local industries, residents, and pressures groups fight against new restrictions or conversion of privately owned land to parkland, with the claim that the lifeblood of employment in their regions is dependent on continuing or expanded activity—such as the clear-cutting of hundreds of thousands of acres of forest lands.

In response, environmentalists typically make the argument that while commercial exploitation of wildlands is finite—that is, when the trees are cut down, the jobs end—maintaining forests or other natural resources for controlled outdoor recreation use can continue indefinitely.

In a growing number of cases, different social or economic priorities come into conflict. For example, in New York State, just outside the borders of Adirondack Park, the largest state park outside Alaska, state officials planned to locate a new maximum-security, 750-cell prison, which would have created jobs and invigorated the local economy. While local residents supported the plan, vacation homeowners and environmental groups charged that it would severely pollute nearby Tupper Lake and damage wildlife in the region. The plan was abandoned. In California, a six-year effort to build the world's largest landfill in Riverside County, next to Joshua Tree National Park—a facility to be the size of 1500 football fields, providing 1300 jobs and substantial income to the region—was fought by conservationists on the grounds that the garbage dump would draw pests and predators and would damage the environment.

In many cases, the clash between commercial and environmental interests has led to vandalism, criminal activity, and violence. For example, on Lake Ontario west of Watertown, New York, cormorants nesting on islands in the lake were wiped out illegally by the hundreds in a mass shotgun slaughter—because they had come into conflict with local interests. Sport fishing in the lake, a thriving industry, had been damaged by the birds devouring smallmouth bass, and so the cormorants, a federally protected species, were surreptitiously killed.

In other cases, radical environmentalists have sought to force grazing cattle off public lands by cutting miles of barbed-wire fencing in Wyoming and other western states. Other activities have sabotaged lumbering equipment, plugged water pipes, damaged windmills, and fire-bombed mink-breeders' cooperatives.

In a dramatic example of such sabotage, in October 1998, arsonists set fire to and destroyed several ski lifts and other structures in Vail, Colorado, with an estimated $12 million in damages. This desperate criminal act came as the culmination of a lengthy effort by environmentalists to prevent commercial development for skiing within an 800-acre wilderness area outside Vail that was considered the best remaining habitat for lynx in Colorado.[6]

Role of Outdoor Recreation

As this example demonstrates, outdoor recreation obviously plays an important part in the ongoing struggle by environmentalists to protect wilderness areas. In some cases, recreation groups have opposed the transfer of properties that they felt would limit their leisure pursuits.

For example, the federally approved transfer of the western face of Sandia Mountain, just outside Albuquerque, New Mexico, from Forest Service ownership to the 490-member Sandia Pueblo tribe was vigorously resisted by local residents and organized outdoor recreation groups. The scenic mountain, rising 10,378 feet into the desert air, is used annually by one million hikers and picnickers, 275,000 cable-car riders, 50,000 bird watchers, 10,000 rock climbers, and 10,000 hang gliders. Recreationists feared that their use of the mountain would be restricted by the Sandia Pueblo Indians who, using casino profits, had hired Washington lobbyists, anthropologists, and prestigious legal firms to promote their claim.

Aside from such disputes, as Chapter 10 points out, there are continuing controversies among different groups of outdoor recreation enthusiasts who have conflicting ecological values and leisure interests. For example, drivers of off-road vehicles like motorcycles and four-wheel-drive trucks or jeeps are seen as destructive to the land and to wildlife. By their intrusive presence, they offend more conservative or ecologically conscious hikers, backpackers, and other wilderness visitors.

Similarly, boating and rafters floating down rivers often offend swimmers, fishing enthusiasts, or other nature lovers, by drinking, drug-taking, raucous behavior, yelling obscenities, or trespassing and using private property as lavatories. The use of personal watercraft, or jet skis, a national craze, has resulted in many vacationers on shores of lakes and rivers being upset by constant noise and dangerous maneuvering. In a number of cases, such as the Florida Keys or the waters around San Juan Island, Washington, their use has been banned or sharply restricted.

In still other cases, conflict has arisen between those using sailboats or canoes and others on powerful motor-driven craft, or between snowmobilers and cross-country skiers. Williams, Dossa, and Fulton have reported on numerous instances of disputes between downhill skiers and snowboarders and on the efforts of ski center managers to serve both groups of recreationists.[7]

Another land management issue centers around the growing popularity of golf, with open spaces being steadily converted into new 18-hole links. Many environmentalists decry this trend, pointing out that today's rolling fairways and greens require massive amounts of land, water, and chemicals, using far more fertilizers and pesticides than farmers do. Robbins writes:

> And when it rains, it pours. Runoff from golf courses has been found to have contaminated nearby groundwaters, lagoons, lakes, and wetlands. The golf boom is causing pollution and social dislocation [and] teed-off environmentalists and local-rights groups are starting to fight back.[8]

In response, many outdoor recreation, park managers, and golf professionals make a strong argument about the value of golf courses in preserving open space ad other ecological values. Strikingly, in Vail, Colorado, the development of eight golf courses in twenty miles of river valley meant that spring pasture land for sheep grazing disappeared and sheepherding, a traditional industry in the region, was sharply reduced during the 1990s. The conflict between golf, historically viewed as an upper-class sport, and sheepherding, a hardscrabble poorly paid occupation, was paralleled by life in Vail itself. A fashionable vacation region because of its scenic location and appealing winter sports, the community and surrounding Eagle County have an assessed real-estate value of $6.5 billion, for 29,000 residents. It requires many workers, often Mexican.

> Hotel and restaurant workers [in Vail] earn about $15,000 a year. By contrast, the Hyatt Regency Beaver Creek, a Vail valley resort, offers this winter an "extravagant honeymoon package"—a week-long stay that includes sauna, sleigh ride, dog sled ride and hot air balloon ride for the price of $13,999.[9]

New Strategies in Environmental Management

Recognizing the kinds of conflicts that have been described in this chapter, it is important to stress that major progress is being made in restoring and protecting the natural environment and making it available for intelligently managed outdoor recreation.

Changing Policies of Land-Management Agencies

In the late 1990s, for example, the National Park Service moved quickly to take advantage of two bills passed by Congress in 1996 to raise entrance fees substantially to support park operations and to seek assistance from major corporations acting as official corporate sponsors of individual parks, historic monuments, or other special projects.

In the following year, the Park Service announced a radical new plan to restore Yosemite's natural environment by tearing up roads and parking lots, removing buildings and bridges and all but banning cars from inside the valley by 2001. Day visitors to the park would leave their cars outside, boarding shuttle buses to enter the valley, while overnight visitors would leave their cars at hotels or campgrounds, rather than drive freely through the park. A regional transportation network would be set up; jammed roads would be converted to bike paths, and cluttered campgrounds to meadows.[10]

In a number of other parks and recreation areas, similar plans were set in motion. A year later, in 1998, Secretary of the Interior Bruce Babbitt announced a new program under which the Park Service would help local communities conserve and manage land and water resources, with annual funding of $250 million. Over 200 projects to be undertaken by local, county, and state governments in cooperation with nonprofit organizations would result in 1100 miles of new trails, 1200 miles of additional river corridors, and 35,000 acres of expanded parkland and open spaces:

> Projects include developing a recreational trails plan for Alaska's Kenai Peninsula Borough, securing public recreational facilities along the Connecticut River in Massachusetts, and creating a series of interconnected access and camping sites on islands and mainland bordering Lake Huron.[11]

In 1998, the Forest Service took action to suspend road building in the back country of most national forests—an action that would effectively preclude logging on about 33 million acres of roadless land that is not protected as designated wilderness. In addition, tens of thousands of miles of deteriorated logging roads that are no longer used would be closed. In the same year, the new chief of the Forest Service announced that it would be embarking on a series of reforms that environmentalists had demanded for decades, shifting away from pro-logging policies and toward more watershed restoration, wildlife conservation, and better recreational opportunities. He stated:

> Timber drove our budgets, our incentive and reward systems, and much of our ecosystem agenda. The times are changing, and a single interest can't have it all. We're simply taking a more balanced view of the public's demands.[12]

Underlying this change in policy is the nation's growing demand for outdoor recreation, with national forests becoming increasingly popular for camping, mountain biking, and other activities. People made 860 million visits to national forests in 1997, more than three times as many as those made to national parks. Beyond this, about 75 percent of Forest Service jobs now relate to recreation and only 3 percent to logging.

Restoration of Natural Habitats

A second shift in environmental management has involved systematic efforts to restore natural settings and reverse major changes that had been made by earlier government planning. For example, in the early 1960s, the Army Corps of Engineers diverted 103 miles of oxbows and marshes into a 56-mile canal that fed into lake Okeechobee in Florida as a major recycling project intended to halt the flood-and-drought cycle that had regularly damaged the Everglades. However, the project had its down side:

Lake Okeechobee became choked with algae. Its world-class bass fishery all but vanished. The Everglades' water supply shrank to a trickle. Unable to flush and filter pesticides and fertilizers, the great marsh began to dry up and die. Ninety percent of its brilliantly plumed wading birds disappeared. Pollution bleached coral reefs and wiped out fish in Florida Bay . . .[13]

Beginning in 1996, however, the Army Corps of Engineers undertook a $500 million project to put back the original kinks of the Kissimmee River, restore the wetlands, and permit controlled flooding. Similarly, in Glen Canyon, Arizona's hydroelectric dam, the Pacific Northwest, Maine, and California's Central Valley, dams are being dismantled or remodeled to eliminate their environmentally destructive effects and permit wildlife and natural settings to flourish again.

Heavily logged regions in New England and the mid-Atlantic states are being permitted to return to black cherry and oak groves and are alive again with animals once feared lost forever to the region: bear, beaver, elk, river otter, bobcats, and wild turkey. In states across the country, trash and solid waste landfills are now being converted into greenways and other sites for outdoor recreation.

Strikingly, one of the richest potential sources for developing healthy, natural ecosystems consists of using military bases that have traditionally had extensive land areas set aside as buffer zones for maneuvers or artillery practice. With the closing or shrinkage of several major bases, such as Fort Devens, Massachusetts, Fort Ord, California, or Eglin Air Force Base in Florida, a number of such properties are now being maintained as models of ecological conservation and biological diversity. In some cases, they are being turned over directly to the Fish and Wildlife Service or other nonmilitary federal agencies.[14]

Partnerships in Land Preservation

A major trend in the management of many different kinds of public service projects today involves the linkage of two or more organizations that share funding, personnel, or other resources to achieve shared goals. There are numerous examples of long-term alliances of environmental and outdoor recreation organizations to carry out major acquisition projects or planning studies. Partnerships frequently involve volunteer groups, conservancy organizations, "friends of parks," and similar bodies that take responsibility for managing directly or assisting in the operation of a single park, trail system, or other natural resource.

Role of National Corporations

Many major businesses have contributed to environmental programs and projects by assisting the National Park Foundation, the Congressional-chartered nonprofit fund-raising partner of the National Park Service. For example, Charles Schwab and Co., Mobil Foundation, the Fannie Mae Foundation, the Eureka Vacuum Cleaner Co., and Target Stores have all contributed funding support for Earth Day, National Park Week, and similar programs.

In other settings, Canon U.S.A. has given a $1.2 million "Expedition into the Parks" grant to support twenty natural resource conservation projects, and Lever Brothers Co. has donated over $400,000 worth of recycled plastic lumber for construction projects in nearly thirty national parks. Georgia-Pacific, the wood-products giant, has developed a partnership with the Nature Conservancy, the national environmental group, to oversee vast forest tracts in North Carolina—agreeing to cut no trees on one-third of a 21,000-acre property and to get Conservancy approval to cut on the other two-thirds, removing downed trees by the least destructive means. Other easement or conservation agreements reached in 1999 provided for the long-term protection of over 750,000 acres of wilderness in Maine and 10,000 acres of giant redwood trees in California's Humboldt County, involving partnerships between government and major lumbering concerns.

Similarly, alliances between long-time adversaries, cattlemen and environmental groups, are becoming more common, with the formation of "land trusts" that preserve open space for combined agricultural and scenic value—and bar the use of land for future resort, housing, or other development through conservation easements. On a larger scale, alliances of dozens of organizations from frequently feuding factions—hunters and anglers on the one side and conservationists on the other—have been achieved in the new umbrella organization, the National Resource Summit of America. In this group, "tree huggers," personified by the Sierra Club, and the "hook-and-bullet crowd," such as Buckmasters, Inc., which promotes hunting, are now working together to promote environmentally sound legislation and government policies.

In many municipal or state park systems throughout the United States, "friends" groups, conservation organizations, and foundations are now assisting in fund-raising, developing legislative support, and actually adopting specific parks or programs. Often several different kinds of organizations are joining in cooperative efforts, as in the New Hampshire Parks AmeriCorps Program, which links the federal Corporation for National Service, the Student Conservation Association, and the New Hampshire Division of Parks and Recreation. In Illinois, the Nature Conservancy, the state Department of Conservation, and Ducks Unlimited mobilized forces to establish the Cypress Creek National Wildlife Refuge.

Hundreds of other joint projects designed to promote the development of trailways, teach conservation principles, encourage the recreational use of rivers in nondestructive way, restore wetlands, or improve wildlife protection programs are carried out each year, often involving the cooperation of university departments. Many hundreds of volunteers have contributed to trail building or repair through the American Hiking Society's Volunteer Vacations programs, and hundreds of thousands work on local beach or park clean-up and other maintenance programs in cities and towns throughout the country.

Ecotourism and Sustainable Rural Tourism

While some of the policies just described have sought to limit the flow of outdoor recreationists or tourists into state parks and other natural environment, or to curb the intrusion of roads, buildings, and other commercial amenities into such settings, the reality is that many government agencies are forced to depend on the fees and revenues derived from such sources.

Typically, many state park systems rely heavily on parks with lodges and cottages, golf courses, marinas, and other profitable facilities to support their budgets. In 1996, two committees of Pennsylvania state legislators concluded that, since the present park system yielded only $9 million in user fees against an operating budget of $50 million—with a "red-ink" backlog of $150 million needed to make crucial repairs to park facilities—it would be necessary to exploit the parks' commercial potential more fully. To do this, they recommended that growing numbers of the state's 116 parks be opened to private development, including large lakefront hotels, conference facilities, restaurants, and similar commercial operations. When it came down to attracting tourists and paying bills, the legislators said, "plain old forests, bubbling brooks and pretty vistas" no longer did the job.

What values should prevail when such policies are considered? While the principle of protecting the environment and making it available to all is a powerful one, fee structures and commodification have entered into every area of public and nonprofit leisure-service agency management (see Chapter 12). At the same time that revenue-seeking facilities such as boating marinas, ski centers, and similar elements are introduced into state parks—which do not generally represent remarkable scenic attractions like Yosemite, Yellowstone, or Grand Canyon—every effort must be made to minimize their impact on the natural environment.

One solution is to clearly define the character of different elements of a park system, and to jealously protect from intrusion or overuse the natural areas or those in which wildlife or other ecological elements might be threatened. As much as possible, commercialized or developed facilities should be confined to limited, outer areas of a park and roads and motorized travel kept from interior or wilder areas.

Beyond this, the movement that has captured the imagination of many environmentalists and park managers is *ecotourism*. Known also as "resource-based tourism," "sustainable rural tourism," and even "agritourism," Ewert and Shultis define this in the following terms:

> . . . tourism activities and experiences dependent on the attributes associated with natural and relatively undeveloped settings. These activities generally involve small groups of tourists and often include learning opportunities related to the local culture and/or natural environment.[15]

While one aspect of ecotourism involves travel to other lands and exposure to other peoples, their customs and lifestyles, the approach also may be applied to visiting rural or countryside regions that are sparsely populated and where natural resources have traditionally provided the basis for the local economy. Unlike visits to park systems with huge expanses of natural territory, ecotourism in this sense is carried out in regions with limited forest areas, small rural communities, and settlements linked to fishing, mining, and forest products. Swinnerton and Hinch write:

> . . . rural areas are characterized by a cultural landscape reflecting the dynamic interrelationship between a community and its means of livelihood. Therefore a sense of history is imprinted on the landscape. It is precisely this mosaic of natural, cultural and scenic resources that makes rural areas attractive to tourists.[16]

Ewert and Shultis point out that ecotourism and resource-based tourism may include such recreational activities as hiking, kayaking, homestays in traditional villages, nature photography and observation, snorkeling, camping, and rafting. In some cases the attractions may be within a state or other park area. In others, such historical features as famous battlefields, old mines, mills, canal towpaths, or early settlements may be close by, with park campgrounds providing a temporary lodging place for visitors. What is important is that the ecotourism experience be respectful of both the physical, natural environment and the people who live there.

Whether domestic or international, ecotourism embodies the principle of stewardship for the land and people. Zeiger and McDonald write that it is not exploitive and must not change the local environment or culture in order to attract visitors. They continue:

> . . . the ecotourist must "take only pictures and leave only footprints" on the environment that he or she explored. . . . The tourism industry has destroyed numerous irreplaceable environmental areas, such as coral reefs and forests, because of the tourist's demand for modern luxuries when traveling. The ecotourist recognizes [and minimizes] the adverse effect of such tourism. . . . Ecotourism provides a unique opportunity to educate the tourist in a natural environment. Hands-on activities, information displays, and educational seminars offer the visitor a better understanding of the local environment [including] natural habitats and archaeological areas.[17]

As a variant of this approach, a growing number of families today prefer to visit farms or ranches, to become exposed to the realities of life in such settings, rather than the gloss and glitter of stays in expensive resorts with packaged entertainment and luxury accommodations. In Europe, this form of vacation travel is known as "agritourism," and it has been estimated that about $2 billion has been spent by European countries to promote and subsidize it through the 1990s. A variant of it in Canada is called "heritage tourism." This approach focuses on natural, cultural, and historic attractions such as national and provincial parks, nature reserves, museums, galleries, cultural festivals, and historic sites that highlight Canadian identity.

Leisure and the Urban Environment

While the term *environment* usually suggests the natural surroundings of the outdoors—mountains, forests, prairies, streams, and lakes—a second kind of environment must also be considered. This is the urban or metropolitan environment, the cities, towns and suburban areas where most people live most of the time. From a leisure perspective it is essential to understand how parks, playgrounds, sports and cultural facilities, and, beyond them, even housing developments, streets, plazas, and waterfront areas affect the quality of daily life.

In the early 1990s, census reports confirmed that more than half the nation's population resided in metropolitan areas of a million or more people, resulting from decades of movement from small towns and towns to urban centers and their suburbs. Census findings also showed that there had been a dramatic shift in population from the Northeast and Midwest to the South and West.

Within this overall picture, there have been other shifts due to external and internal migration patters. In 1998, the Census Bureau confirmed that several metropolitan areas, such as New York, Los Angeles, Chicago, and other western and southwestern centers had gained heavily from immigration from other countries.

At the same time, other migration trends are influencing the ethnic and socioeconomic makeup of the nation. Retirement patterns have seen many older persons move from northern states to Sunbelt areas. The decline of family farming and other rural employment opportunities resulted in smaller towns and villages losing the bulk of their population in such areas. In some cities, such as Minneapolis, which was 93 percent white in 1970, the minority population—consisting heavily of blacks and Asian Americans—rose to 21 percent during the 1980s. On the other hand, a University of Michigan study showed in 1998 that many African Americans were reversing a half-century exodus from the South, by returning to a region that offered an improved economy and a more favorable racial climate.

Obviously, regional differences have a strong influence on the recreational patterns of the residents of metropolitan areas. For example, there are marked differences in the amount of vacation travel by Americans to national parks. Studies have shown that 37 percent of residents from the Mountain region (states such as Arizona, Colorado, or Nevada) visit these attractions, while only 12 percent of residents in the mid-Atlantic region (Pennsylvania, New Jersey, and New York) do so.

Expansion of "Sprawl" Cities

There has been immense growth in the size and population numbers of metropolitan areas in a number of western states. In Scottsdale, Arizona, for example, barely 2000 people lived on the single square mile that the city represented in 1950. By the mid-1990s, 165,000 people lived in a megalopolis three times the physical size of San Francisco. In cities like Las Vegas, Nevada, Salt Lake City, Utah, or Denver, Colorado, flourishing economies and appealing climates have drawn millions of new residents. Surrounded by vast vistas of mountains, deserts, and scenic open spaces, these areas also suffer today from traffic congestion, labor shortages, overcrowded schools, and many of the same social problems that affect older cities.

In flourishing Scottsdale, for example, many schools are:

> . . . short of textbooks and a Federal court has ordered the system to get more state financing. And something called the "inner city," built about 30 years ago, is an urban orphan—denounced for its crime, racial conflict, and abandonment.[18]

Within this overall picture, a number of major cities have adopted aggressive policies, both to meet pressing social challenges and to improve and protect their natural environments. In Phoenix, for example, the municipal department of Parks, Recreation and Library has initiated a battery of innovative programs designed to serve "at-risk" youth. At the same time, Phoenix, the sixth largest city in the United States, has set aside large tracts of land acquired during the 1960s and 1970s as regional parks administered by the Maricopa County Parks and Recreation Department. Parks both within and on the borders of the city offer an immense range of outdoor settings and recreational opportunities, including innovative new environmental and outdoor education centers.

The Wildland-Urban Interface

A major concern linked to the expansion of such cities has to do with the wildland-urban interface. While the relationship between settled communities and suburban development and their surrounding countryside has been a long-standing phenomenon, today it is receiving greater attention because of concern about the impact of recreational use on close-by natural environments.

Environmental critic Mike Davis cites as a negative example the patterns of exploding urban development in southern California where, in Los Angeles, the city fathers failed to set aside adequate public parkland for the growing metropolis as private developers gobbled up beachfront, canyon, and ranchland. Davis notes that by the late 1920s, barely half an inch of publicly owned beach frontage was left for each citizen of Los Angeles County. He concludes that for generations, market-driven urbanization has transgressed environmental common sense, with the result that:

> Historic wildfire corridors have been turned into view-lot suburbs, wetland liquefaction zones into marinas, and flood plains into industrial districts and housing tracts. Monolithic public works have been substituted for regional planning and a responsible land ethic. As a result, Southern California has reaped flood, fire and earthquake tragedies that were as avoidable, as unnatural, as the beating of Rodney King and the ensuing explosion in the streets.[19]

From an outdoor recreation and environmentalist perspective, Alan Ewert points out that the wildland-urban interface in many regions represents an important concern for resource management and research. First, he writes, wildland areas in close proximity to large urban centers offer a natural resource with unique attributes and easy accessibility for millions of people. Second, he continues:

> . . . these interface areas serve important social and ecological functions for society while simultaneously being extremely vulnerable to human impact and pressures. As a result of these impacts, interface areas deserve a higher level of research and management efforts in order to preserve the natural resource while meeting the demands of a diverse set of users.[20]

The Challenge in Older, Central Cities

Moving more directly to the role of parks and recreation within older, central cities, particularly in the Northeast, mid-Atlantic and Midwest regions of the United States, earlier chapters have shown how networks of leisure-service facilities and agencies were developed over the past century in such communities.

Many formerly thriving industrial cities have suffered major economic losses due to the decline of traditional manufacturing businesses, aggravated by rising costs of government linked to infrastructure breakdown, the demands of welfare and related social services, crime, and similar problems. The role of parks and recreation in meeting such challenges during the post–World War II era was described in Chapter 2.

Beyond such economic and social changes, many of the problems encountered by older central cities stemmed from the planning strategies that had been followed during the past few decades. In her influential book, *The Death and Life of Great American Cities*, Jane Jacobs challenged the prevailing practice of building immense high-rise private apartments with narrow streets and huge, impersonal public housing projects that in effect destroyed neighborhood life and became infested with drugs, crime, and other social pathologies. Jacobs made recommendations that many cities sought to follow, including new, lower, and more open public housing designs and the inclusion of more playgrounds and small parks promoting neighborhood life.

Since that time, however, many cities have continued to be constricted by the flow of cars, using highways and access routes that artificially divide sections of the city and encourage travel to malls and employment centers outside the central cities themselves. Gratz and Mintz write:

> Speeding traffic, the absence of curbside parking, the cutting down of flowering shade trees, and the elimination of sidewalk furniture and plantings—engineering prescriptions—have degraded downtown streets [and resulted in] a continuous stream of moving vehicles. . . . Everywhere in this country, the automobile has been eroding the public realm.[21]

In response to this challenge, a growing number of cities have closed streets to traffic, encouraging retail stores, galleries, sidewalk cafes, plantings, and the opportunity for greater civic engagement for residents and visitors. The related problem of suburbanization and the emergence of so-called Edge Cities—satellite centers of high-tech businesses, expensive housing developments and often gated communities, and privatized services—have continued to draw vitality from the central cities themselves. However, recent reports by the federal Department of Housing and Urban Development indicate that the city/suburban dichotomy continues to grow.

> [In the late 1990s] suburbs contained 75 percent more families than cities, compared with 25 percent more in 1970. For every American who moved to a city in that period, four relocated to a suburb. As those with means flee the city's high taxes and poor schools and services, urban poverty has worsened; in 1990, 14 percent of city census tracts were classified as high poverty, more than double the figure of two decades before.[22]

While the ring of older suburbs immediately around the central cities has developed many of the same social and economic problems affecting inner-city neighborhoods, hidden subsidies in terms of transportation, sewer construction, and other forms of government service or subsidies often favor the residents of newer suburban developments. Recent research shows that most ordinary Americans, although still preferring detached, single-family homes, are disenchanted with the traffic and commercial congestion that often surround their suburban developments and would prefer more traditional neighborhoods clustered around smaller shopping and village-type centers.

There is also growing evidence that the cities themselves retain an identity and appeal that more isolated, outer housing areas cannot provide. Based on analysis of leading cities in other countries, Anton Zijderveld comments that there is a distinct pattern of preferring either city or suburban life, depending on age and family makeup:

> . . . families with young children prefer to live in the suburbs for obvious reasons (affordable housing, better schools, family-oriented facilities, safety, etc.), young professional couples without children and single managers and professionals often prefer to live in the center of the big city (cultural events, etc.) Moreover, there are urban governments these days which design policies to attract young families and senior citizens to the inner city again to restore the demographic balance.[23]

The importance of the physical environment in reinforcing the attractiveness of city neighborhoods cannot be overestimated. Varied studies have shown the importance of green spaces—involving trees, grass, places for friends and family to meet—to a sense of neighborhood belonging and relaxed living. Such settings offer places to play, relief from tenement crowding, and the opportunity for inner-city residents to join together in planning and developing landscaped areas, organizing community celebrations and picnics, and carrying out cleanup projects.

Neighborhoods continue to retain an important place in civic life, with many cities having experienced success in encouraging neighborhood revitalization. Community groups have been increasingly successful in fighting unwise demolition for "urban renewal," displacing long-term middle- or working-class residents for wealthier new tenants, and in similar causes. Street fairs, crime watch, and neighborhood service centers, along with fuller support given to local parks and playgrounds, have been part of this trend.

Fuller Government Concern with Environment

On a broader scale, major efforts have been made to enrich city environments and enhance the appeal of urban living. In the early 1970s, the federal government established national parks in major metropolitan areas: Golden Gate National Recreation Area in San Francisco and Gateway National Recreation Area in New York and New Jersey. In the years that followed, other federally sponsored urban parks included Cuyahoga Valley National Recreation Area in Ohio, the Santa Monica National Recreation Area in Southern California, and the Jefferson National Expansion Memorial in St. Louis, Missouri. More recently, the U.S. Forest Service has initiated tree-planting and other environmental projects in a number of eastern cities. However, the large-scale programs that were sponsored by federal agencies during the 1960s and 1970s to assist disadvantaged neighborhoods and racial minority groups—many of which included environmental and recreation programs—no longer are in vogue.

Instead, many cities have embarked on aggressive, entrepreneurial ventures to promote their own identity, encourage business relocation, and gain revenues through varied cultural, sports, and environmental ventures.

Entrepreneurial City Management.   Hall and Hubbard argue that a new kind of western city has evolved in recent years. The post-industrial, post-modern metropolis, in their terms, is usually dramatically different from its predecessors, in terms of revitalized city centers with impressive high-rise office buildings, improved transportation networks, and elaborate new sports facilities and waterfront complexes. But the key difference, they argue, is in a new approach to urban politics and planning, in which city leaders adopt such business-based approaches as risk-taking, inventiveness, and high-pressure self-promotion.

They describe the concept of entrepreneurship in city management as emphasis on running cities in a more businesslike way, stressing bottom-line outcomes, and making use of public-private partnerships to attract funds, build facilities, and find other proactive ways of promoting company relocations and investment in civic enterprises. Within this effort, "boosterism" is a critical function. Hall and Hubbard write:

> . . . most city governments are allocating increasingly high budgets for the advertising and promotion of the city as a favorable environment for business and leisure. . . . Almost every city now has its requisite series of promotional pamphlets, posters and other cultural products communicating selective images of the city as an attractive, hospitable and vibrant international city in which to live and work. What is also increasingly evident is that this marketing of place seldom restricts itself to extolling the existing virtues of the city, but seeks to redefine and reimage the city, [and to] erase the negative iconography of dereliction, decline and labor militancy associated with the industrial city.[24]

Changing the image of the city is therefore seen as a key component of entrepreneurial government, akin to the promotional methods evolved by the Disney theme parks, known as "imagineering." To achieve this end, many major cities have constructed prestigious projects that serve as symbols of their rejuvenation. Baltimore's Inner Harbor, Vancouver's Pacific Place, Atlanta's Peachtree Center, and New York's Battery Place are all examples of such ventures.

Baltimore's Inner Harbor.   To illustrate, Baltimore's downtown revitalization strategy included such projects as Charles Center, Harbor Place, the National Aquarium, new hotels, a convention center, and a widely acclaimed new baseball stadium, Oriole Park at Camden Heights. Supporting these projects, aggressive programs of activities and free entertainment in the Inner Harbor area—including flea markets, fireboat displays, concerts, boat races, parades, city fairs, international festivals, and other performing arts events—drew many visitors to the semicircle of parkland around the Inner Harbor through the 1980s and 1990s.

While such developments are clearly successful in attracting tourists, some critics argue that this thrust can ultimately be self-defeating. They point out that most jobs involved in serving tourists are low-level—in hotels and restaurants, for example, consisting chiefly of maids, janitors, front-desk help, cooks, food servers, bartenders, and the like. Based on this, they argue that to seek to revitalize a city based on the hospitality industry alone is dubious.

Buzz Bissinger cites the example of Newark, New Jersey's new Performing Arts Center, a $180-million structure hailed for its architectural splendor and acoustics. Critics, public officials, and planners alike say that it is more than just an attractive place to hold operas, concerts, and plays; instead, it serves as a symbol of urban resurgence in a community that had long been viewed as an example of inner-city decline. However, Bissinger suggests that it is both misguided and psychologically dangerous for Newark and other cities like it to believe that recovery depends on

> . . . transforming themselves into entertainment satellites for suburbanites and tourists and conventioneers. Such projects are based on a premise that seems ultimately defeatist: that the only way to save the American city is to build it and shape it for those who don't live there and never will.[25]

Instead of relying on their cultural and environmental attractions to draw pass-through visitors, modern metropolitan areas must also focus on the less glamorous task of meeting the needs of residents of every class: the wealthy, the middle-class, and low-income groups.

Features of Live-In Cities

In so doing, the urban environment again becomes critical, in physical terms. The provision of safe, well-kept parks and playgrounds is essential, particularly in view of studies in the 1990s, which indicated that many urban playgrounds were not properly equipped or supervised.

In larger parks, greenways or trailways, hiking paths, or bicycle trails appeal to a growing number of residents, young and old. Many cities now have nature reserves or environmental centers used for conservation education for school classes, or "adventure gardens" or "discovery parks" where children can engage in self-directed exploration of the natural world. Increasingly, marshes and wetlands are being preserved for such purposes, and in some cities efforts are being made to reintroduce native animal and bird species that have disappeared over time.

Sports facilities are essential to host children's and youth leagues, adult competition, and self-directed fitness activities. Swimming, as the most popular outdoor activity, needs to be available inexpensively and safely, along with instruction. Winter sports and boating activities are important ingredients for communities whose climate permits construction of needed facilities.

Greenery and gardening pastimes can be developed even in the heart of crowded city neighborhoods, through the use of vacant city lots or small areas set aside for cooperative gardening projects. In many cases, greenery flourishes today on the rooftops of city apartment buildings, or in small, tucked away sites near major transit lines.

While such environmental provisions are not glamorous and rarely serve to attract tourists or gain revenues, they contribute significantly to the quality of life in the central city and deserve support and encouragement, along with more spectacular and impressive amenities.

Often, support for such environmental features involves a trade-off among conflicting priorities. As an example, until the mid-1980s, four vacant lots in a Hispanic neighborhood on the lower East Side in New York City's Manhattan were dumping grounds for old furniture, appliances, car parts, and even bodies. Then, neighborhood residents began to clean up the lots, getting rid of the refuse, planting flowers, vegetables, and herbs and building makeshift shelters called *casitas*. Over time, Jane Lii writes, the gardens flourished and turned into:

> . . . unofficial community centers, where weddings, birthday celebrations and block parties were held. On hot and muggy summer evenings, some residents of the Lower East Side fled their apartments to relax with friends in the casitas.[26]

However, it was too good to last. In 1997, driven by the demand for affordable housing, the city government gave a private developer the right to clear the gardens and to build 98 condominiums for middle-income families. As bulldozers scooped out vines, shrubs, and little fruit trees from what had been the Chico Mendez Garden, the 10th Street Garden, Maria's Garden, and Angel's Garden, neighborhood gardeners and their supporters stood by and chanted, "Shame! Shame on you!"

Which need was greater?

Summary

Apart from changes in the makeup of the population and trends in many areas of leisure participation, a third important concern of leisure planners today has to do with environment—both the natural setting of forests, mountains, lakes, and rivers and the closer-to-home environments for urban, year-round play.

This chapter traces the history of environment-related policies in the United States from the nineteenth century to the post–World War II period efforts to expand and protect the nation's natural resources. It outlines the ongoing conflict between business interests pressing for fuller commercial uses of wilderness and prairie and conservationists who would maintain strict control on such practices and on many forms of outdoor recreation as well. Citing the role of partnerships among environmental groups and businesses and the trend toward ecotourism, the chapter concludes with a discussion of the urban environment as part of the recovery of older, central cities.

Key Concepts

1. Environment in both natural and urban settings is an important factor in promoting national well-being and is an integral element in the broad leisure spectrum.
2. From a period when the wilderness was feared and meant to be conquered, the United States gradually shifted to a determination to protect great, national scenic treasures and to make the setting aside of open spaces an important priority.
3. Over the past four decades, there has been a continuing struggle between business interests linked to ranching, grazing, logging, and oil drilling and local residents dependent on these fields for jobs, and others' concern with the nation's ecological well-being over appropriate regulations governing the use of natural resources. Sim-

ilar conflicts have affected industries and agriculture with respect to air and water pollution and have resulted in considerable progress during this period.

4. Apart from such problems, the national parks and forests themselves have suffered from overdevelopment, crowding and destructive outdoor recreation uses, and a lack of adequate fiscal support for maintenance and supervision.

5. In other settings, the disappearance of wetlands and beach frontage, depletion of the Earth's ozone layers, overharvested fisheries, and overbuilding of resorts and other structures close to natural areas have contributed to an environmental crisis and the need for stronger national policies.

6. Increasingly, many of the issues affecting wildlife, such as the reintroduction of wild species and the conflict between recreationists and wild animals, as well as specific hunting and fishing practices, are calling for a reassessment of public values and practices.

7. In response to such needs, land management agencies are imposing new controls on recreational uses of the nation's major parks, and in some cases eliminating roads, structures, or other civilized amenities in them. Efforts are also being made to correct past engineering mistakes that have been destructive to the environment and to wildlife and to restore natural habitats.

8. Increasingly, civic and conservation groups, along with major businesses and hundreds of thousands of volunteers are joining together in partnership alliances to protect and maintain natural resources.

9. Ecotourism and sustainable rural tourism serve as an important new strategy that links respect for the physical and human environment to efforts to provide economic benefits for rural regions and develop nondestructive uses of the outdoors.

10. A new approach to promoting the image of older cities through aggressive design of facilities and activities that will appeal to visitors is part of a larger entrepreneurial approach to overcome decay and economic decline.

11. While such efforts and cultural or recreational complexes can do much to promote tourism, ultimately, if cities are to succeed, they must also provide healthy, quality-of-life settings for residents of all classes—including parks, playgrounds and opportunities for varied forms of recreation and social interchange.

Endnotes

1. Clark, R. 1997. In Clark, R. and L. Canter, eds. *Environmental Policy and NEPA: Past, Present, and Future.* Boca Raton, FL: St. Lucie Press, p. 16.

2. Satchell, M. 1997. Parks in Peril. *U.S. News and World Report* (July 21): 24.

3. Russell, C., cited in Foote, T., review of Egan, T. *Lasso the Wind: Away to the New West* (New York: Alfred Knopf). Book Review in *New York Times* (Sept. 6, 1998), p. 5.

4. Satchell, *op. cit.*

5. Sitarz, D., ed. (with Preface by Vice President Al Gore). 1990. *Sustainable America.* Carbondale, IL: Earthpress, pp. 7–8.

6. Obmascik, M. 1999. Out of the Ashes. *Mountain Sports and Living* (January/February): 20.

7. Williams, P., K. Dossa, and A. Fulton. 1994. Tension on the Slopes: Managing Conflict Between Skiers and Snowboarders. *Journal of Applied Recreation Research* (19/3): 191–213.

8. Robbins, E.1996. Golf War Syndrome. *Utne Reader* (March–April): 22.

9. Brooke, J. 1995. Golf Replaces Grazing in Vacation-Rich Vail. *New York Times* (September 16): A-3.

10. Lelyveld, N. 1997. Yosemite: Help for Mother Nature. *Philadelphia Inquirer* (November 16): A-3.

11. National Park Service Lends a Helping Hand. *Parks and Recreation* (July 1998): 31.

12. Satchell, M. 1998. Mountain Bikers Over Corporate Loggers. *U.S. News and World Report* (May 18): 36.

13. Satchell, M. 1996. To Restore Nature, A Turn of the Spigot. *U.S. News and World Report* (April 8): 5.

14. Stevens, W. 1996. Wildlife Finds Odd Sanctuary on Military Bases. *New York Times* (Jan. 2): B-9.

15. Ewert, A., and J. Shultis. 1997. Resource-Based Tourism: An Emerging Trend in Tourism Experiences. *Parks and Recreation* (September): 95.

16. Swinnerton, G., and T. Hinch. 1994. Sustainable Rural Tourism: Principles and Practices. *Trends* (31/1): 4.

17. Zeiger, J., and D. McDonald. 1997. Ecotourism: Wave of the Future. *Parks and Recreation* (September); 85.

18. Egan, T. 1996. Urban Sprawl Strains Western States. *New York Times* (December 29): 1.

19. Davis, M. 1998. Cited in review of book, *Ecology of Fear: Los Angeles and the Imagination of Disaster* (New York: Henry Holt), in *New York Times* (August 21).

20. Ewert, A., in Ewert, A., D. Chavez, and A. Magill, eds. 1993. *Culture, Conflict and Communication in the Wildland-Urban Interface.* San Francisco: Westview Press, p. 8.

21. Gratz, R.B., and N. Mintz. 1998. *Cities Back From the Edge: New Life for Downtown.* New York: John Wiley, p. 89.

22. Koerner, B. 1998. Special Report. *U.S. News and World Report* (June 8): 28.

23. Zijderveld, A. 1998. *A Theory of Urbanity: The Economic and Civic Culture of Cities.* London: Transaction, p. 128.

24. Hall, T., and P. Hubbard, eds. 1998. *The Entrepreneurial City.* New York: John Wiley, pp. 6–7.

25. Bissinger, B. 1997. Drive-Through Cities. *New York Times* (November 6): A-15.

26. Lii, J. 1997. Bulldozers Flatten the Islands of Green. *New York Times* (December 31): B-3.

14 Charting the Future: Challenges for the Leisure-Service System

The technological innovations taking place in the banking industry [and in the wholesale and retail sectors] are indicative of the kinds of sweeping changes that are redefining every aspect of the white-collar and service work. . . . Many observers wonder how an increasingly under-employed and unemployed global workforce, displaced by new technologies, is going to be able to afford all of the products and services being turned out. . . .

The new professionals—the so-called symbolic analysts or knowledge workers—come from the fields of science, engineering, management, consulting, teaching, marketing, media, and entertainment. While their number will continue to grow, it will remain small compared to the number of workers displaced by the new generation of "thinking machines." Drucker says quite bluntly that "the disappearance of labor as a key factor of production" is going to emerge as the critical "unfinished business of capitalism."[1]

The delegates [to the National Curriculum Conference on Parks and Recreation] were in general agreement that a proliferation of specializations and options within the undergraduate program tended to weaken the core curriculum and the undergraduate's commitment to the profession at large. . . . Dr. Marilyn Jensen challenged the delegates to be aware of the changes in higher education that affect and will continue to affect our programs of professional preparation. She spoke of the relevancy and problems associated with new technologies and new approaches—such as distance learning—and their implication. She also reminded those in the profession at large that universities are in the mood to consolidate programs and that our identity could be lost unless we have strong professional support and our faculties demonstrate the uniqueness of our knowledge and our relevance to the mission of the institution.[2]

We turn now to a more focused look at America's future and the role that leisure and the organized recreation, park, and leisure-service field will play in it. This chapter presents some of the alternative visions of the future and the probable impact of technology, the emerging information society, and population change on leisure. It summarizes the findings of the 1998 survey of leisure-service educators with respect to challenges facing this profession in the century ahead.

The chapter then discusses each of the fourteen challenges that constituted the survey, pointing out that two of the statements that received the lowest ratings of importance by respondents may potentially have great significance for the leisure-service field.

Forecasting the Future: Alternative Views

Earlier chapters in this text have summarized a number of the predictions that social scientists have made about probable trends for the future. They include such elements as the emergence of an increasingly interactive society, based on the growth of electronic information processing and communication; the creation of numerous new kinds of technology; the globalization of the business world and its impact on travel and tourism and the spread of cultural and entertainment products; growing gaps between the rich and poor; and increasing concern about environmental well-being.

Obviously, experts do not always agree on the directions that the nation's economy is likely to take in the years ahead, or on its effect on peoples' lifestyles. One economist writes:

> We've never had it so good. . . . on the eve of a new millennium we are living in an age of unparalleled economic prosperity and material comfort, in the most affluent civilization that this long-suffering planet has known.[3]

On the other hand, another authority writes:

> . . . the tenor of public discussion is persistently gloomy. Surveys routinely show a populace increasingly worried about its future prospects and the future prospects of its children. . . . Even well-educated professionals—the "knowledge elite" who are mostly thriving in today's global economy—are worried and fearful.[4]

Despite such different views of the future, there is general agreement that it will be heavily influenced by new technologies in all areas of national life: education, business, health care, environment, and leisure.

Technology's Influence on Leisure

The impact of continuing high-technology developments on leisure falls under three headings: (1) the emergence of new kinds of leisure pursuits; (2) the use of technological processes in the management of recreation, park, and leisure-service agencies; (3) the potential effect of changing patterns of employment and job opportunity on the nation's free time.

New Kinds of Leisure Pursuits

New forms of communication, entertainment, or manufacturing processes have already transformed many of our traditional leisure pursuits in such areas as outdoor recreation, sports, home-based entertainment, and even social relationships. With respect to leisure-service programming, computer-based activities are likely to become a much fuller part of classes, hobby activities, or guidance of participants.

The variety of new kinds of pastimes that may appear can only be guessed at. Elmer-Dewitt suggests that such pursuits may fit into familiar forms over the years immediately ahead. However, after a few decades, they will begin to blend together and lose their distinct identities. TVs, VCRs, CD players, computers, telephones, video games, newspapers, and mail-order catalogues will merge to create new products and services that can only be dreamed about today. New versions of transportation, communication, game-playing, and even love-making, Elmer-Dewitt writes, will all be transformed by emerging technologies.

Popular entertainment is likely to diversify in a bewildering way in the years ahead. Fiber-optic cable will bring hundreds, even thousands, of TV channels into the home, and interactive computer technology will give viewers almost total control over what they wish to see.[5]

Within this vision of a new high-tech world, some of the possibilities for future change are not altogether appealing. For example, the proliferation of waves of pornography on the Internet and its potential for sexual predators reaching possible victims has aroused considerable concern. Beyond this, we are beginning to ask questions about the impact of extreme levels of involvement with computer-based leisure pursuits. A study conducted by researchers at Carnegie Mellon University, financed in part by the National Science Foundation, found that heavy use of the Internet appeared to be linked to higher levels of depression and loneliness by those using the computer network:

> Participants who were lonelier and more depressed, as determined by standard questionnaires at the outset of the two-year study, were no more drawn to the Internet than those who were originally happier and more socially engaged. Instead, Internet use itself appeared to cause a decline in psychological well-being, the researchers said. . . . on average, for those who used the Internet most, things got worse.[6]

Increasingly, people become so enthralled with computer work that is part of their professional lives that they allow it to dominate their leisure lives as well, with disturbing consequences for personal relationships. William Macklin writes:

> . . . all along the data-glutted continuum where smart machines and intelligent people interface, there is deepening concern that as computers are functioning more like people, humans are working more like machines—logging longer hours at tireless devices, relying more and more on electronic communication instead of face-to-face contact.[7]

High-Tech and Leisure-Service Management

Clearly the adoption of advanced technological processes has had a major impact on recreation, park, and leisure service operations. Computers are used at every level of program development and implementation, from target-marketing analysis to scheduling, registering, and monitoring classes, sports tournaments and leagues, or special events. They are essential today in personnel and fiscal management, and in many specific program sectors, such as outdoor recreation and travel, in guiding participants to appropriate destinations.

Computer classes and workshops are increasingly part of program offerings for youth and adults, and special computer classes are now being marketed for children and youth. More and more institutions are experimenting with "distance" learning, through which electronic communication can be used to serve large numbers of individuals in scattered locations.

For example, information technology is proving invaluable in the field training of professional personnel serving special populations. Anderson, Brown, and Soli describe the use of interactive video technology in a project carried out jointly by the University of North Dakota and the North Dakota Parks and Recreation Department, partially funded by the U.S. Department of Education/Rehabilitation Services Administration. Using two-way, voice-activated video systems to transmit live, high-quality audio and color video between several sites, this collaborative effort is used to train personnel across a large geographical area to facilitate the physical and social integration of persons with disabilities into recreation and leisure services and settings.[8]

Boon or Bane?   Numerous other examples of the use of information technology in recreation programming and management operations appear in the professional literature. At the same time, there is an ongoing controversy as to whether the ultimate impact of exploding information technology on the overall society is positive or negative.

At the World Future Society's Eighth Annual General Assembly in 1996, this question brought such negative responses as the charges that "infotech" is "shriveling and shredding" the society, creating growing gaps between the rich and poor, destroying millions of jobs, speeding the pace of work, and making time increasingly scarce.

On the other hand, those seeing information technology as a boon rather than a bane argue that it represents the critical resource of the future, creates wealth, and is helping to build a single global economy.[9]

Impact of Information Technology on Work and Leisure

The third way in which the growing use of electronic communication and data-processing methods affects leisure services has to do with its critical impact on the job market and patterns of employment today and tomorrow. Within the powerful new, interactive "information society," Winslow and Barmer write that knowledge and knowledge work dominate the operation of all sorts of organizations, whether in education, human services, manufacturing, or fiscal affairs:

Knowledge work includes research and development, process design, product design, logistics, market research, marketing, advertising, sales, distribution, legal, public relations, accounting, personnel, finance, health care, and so on.[10]

They conclude that managing knowledge-based assets and workers has become the key element in company profitability or organizational success. Through the 1990s, this trend has had a radical impact on patterns of employment. In the middle of the decade, it was predicted that in just one service industry, commercial banking and thrift institutions, technological changes and restructuring would eliminate 30 to 40 percent of jobs—almost 700,000 jobs—within the next seven years. Sweeping changes are redefining every aspect of white-collar and service work. The nation's secretaries are among the first casualties of the electronic office revolution, as personal computers, electronic mail, and fax machines replace typewriters, paper files, and routine correspondence. Jeremy Rifkin writes:

It's not just low-level jobs that are disappearing. A growing number of companies are deconstructing their organizational hierarchies and eliminating more and more middle management. . . . the men and women in "garden-variety middle management jobs" are "getting crucified" by corporate re-engineering and the introduction of sophisticated new information and communication technologies. Eastman Kodak, for example, has reduced its management levels from thirteen to four.[11]

The implication of this growing trend, as the concluding section of this chapter will show, is that great numbers of men and women will find their job situations increasingly precarious. While one sector of employees will have good jobs and in many cases will be overworked, many others will be forced to hold two or three jobs to make a reasonable livelihood. In each case, their ability to enjoy rich leisure lives will be affected in terms of money, free time, and emotional needs.

Effect of Population Changes

Moving beyond issues of technology and the oncoming information society, other predictions during the 1990s involved population growth, shifting age groups, and changes in regional and residential patterns of living. In addition to the trends cited in Chapter 6, demographers and futurologists have identified the following probable shifts in population makeup.

Fortune Magazine summarized a number of changes expected to occur over the next few decades: (1) Life expectancy for both men and women is likely to increase steadily, with a dramatic rise in Medicare costs; (2) by 2010, New England and Florida will have the highest proportion of elderly citizens, with baby-boomers reaching 65 and the number of retirees rising to 33 million citizens, compared to 25 million in 1991; and (3) the cost of Social Security payments would reach $558 billion in 1991 dollars in 2020, almost double the level in 1995.

Male/Female and Family Relationships

Other predicted demographic changes will affect the male/female balance in American society in the years ahead. In the late 1980s, it was reported that the scarcity of American males of marriageable age and the abundance of females that had characterized the 1970s and 1980s was shifting, and that through the twenty-first century there would be a surplus of adult males and an undersupply of females. This change is likely to affect the social behavior of men and women. According to University of Houston social scientists, when eligible males are comparatively rare, there is a tendency for them to exploit the situation.

> In such a society, men have multiple relationships with women and become less willing to commit themselves to one woman in marriage. But when young males are more numerous than females, the situation turns around and men are more eager to pursue marriage.[12]

During the late 1980s, the average age at first marriage for women began to drop, and the number of family households increased. With the expected rise in the birthrate and a leveling off of divorces, the growing number of families with young children will have important implications for recreation and leisure. Many other families in the twenty-first century will be divided by divorce, multiplied by remarriage, expanded by new birth technologies—or perhaps all of the above. Single parents and working mothers will be more common, as will out-of-wedlock babies, although the concept of the "illegitimate" child will diminish as the patriarchal nuclear family becomes less prevalent.

The number of never-married individuals increased steadily from 1970 to 1991, according to a 1992 Bureau of the Census report. About one-fourth of American adults eighteen and older—41.5 million—have never married, and the total number of single persons, including divorced, widowed, and never married, rose from 38 million to 71 million, proportionately from 28 percent to 39 percent.

Life may become more difficult for middle-aged couples who will be part of extended family networks of crisscrossing loyalties and obligations. As life spans lengthen and marriages multiply, they could find themselves caring all at once for aging parents, frail grandparents, children still in school, and perhaps even a step-grandchild or two. It is predicted that the number of Americans 65 and older will reach 65 million by the year 2030, compared with 30 million in the early 1990s. As the number of those who are 85 and older increases fivefold to 15 million within the next three decades, there will be a boom in the number of retirement communities for the affluent and nursing homes for many others.

Where People Will Live

Linked to these predictions are new expectations of where many Americans will live. The post–World War II years saw major shifts in residential patterns, with millions of middle-class families moving from central cities to suburbs and many others from the older, colder Rustbelt states to Sunbelt areas in the South, West, and Southwest.

While attention has chiefly been focused on the social problems of large cities, the reality is that close-in suburbs also are experiencing many of the same problems. Many smaller communities are suffering as well. Long-term poverty is more severe in rural areas, with a substantial underclass of both blacks and whites in southern states, from Appalachia to the Mississippi Delta. Throughout the Midwest and the plains states, many small towns have lost substantial numbers of their populations, and rural organizations like the Grange, which typically offered rich leisure opportunities to farm families, are declining in number.

At the same time, a new kind of American living environment has been steadily emerging—the so-called edge city. In *Edge City: Life on the New Frontier*, Joel Garreau describes the new kind of community that has resulted from the mushrooming office-corporate-shopping mall-residential development encircling many of America's largest cities. In these new urban centers, we see "the culmination of a generation of individual American value decisions about the best ways to live, work and play." Edge cities usually do not fall within a single governmental unit's control, but operate under quasi-nongovernmental associations that act as "shadow governments." Heavily dependent on automobile access, and with enforcement policies that keep out the homeless, the poor, the beggars, and others who are unattractive or "inconvenient," these new American "Main Streets," contrast sharply with older cities. At the same time, they lack the grand parks, boulevards, concert halls, museums, and other amenities of central cities—and are described by many residents as "plastic," a "hodgepodge," or "sterile."[13]

Challenges Facing the Leisure-Service Field

Having reviewed several of the major social, economic, or technological changes that are predicted to occur in the years ahead, we now turn to the specific focus of this chapter—challenges facing the field of recreation, park, and leisure services, as viewed by a large sample of leisure-service educators. Table 14.1 summarizes the findings of the *1998 Trends and Issues Survey* regarding the challenges that respondents believed would be most critical to this field of service in the years ahead. Fuller details of the survey and of the first section of findings (see page 96) are given in Appendix A.

The concluding section of this chapter presents an analysis and discussion of each of the fourteen challenges, based on the background presented throughout this text. In each case, the questions raised and recommendations offered relate chiefly to the work of public and nonprofit leisure-service agencies. However, they also have implications for other types of organizations, since the needs of community groups often are served by several different kinds of agencies.

Challenge 1. Need to Serve Increasingly Diverse Society

As earlier chapters have shown, the makeup of American society has changed radically over the second half of the twentieth century and will continue to change dramatically in the years ahead. One of the key ways in which transformation is occurring has to do with the racial and ethnic makeup of the population and the forecast that within a few decades, people of color will outnumber the present white majority.

If the leisure-service profession is to live up to its mandate, it must be proactive in serving *all* populations effectively and in using recreation and allied social services as a tool

TABLE 14.1   Ranking of Challenges Facing Leisure-Service Field in Twenty-First Century. Each item should be preceded by phrase, "Need to —"

	Weighted Score
1. Serve increasingly diverse society (race, age, gender, etc.).	453
2. Emphasize key social purposes of recreation: working with at-risk youth, serving persons with disabilities, promoting community development, etc.	437
3. Achieve fuller public understanding of value of recreation and parks and of leisure-service profession.	434
4. Upgrade recreation and park programs and facilities, particularly in inner cities and for minority populations.	417
5. Adopt a benefits-based management approach, researching, proving, and publicizing positive outcomes of recreation.	411
6. Promote recreation's identity as health-related field.	392
7. Develop partnerships with environmental organizations to protect and restore wildlands, waterways, etc.	386
8. Employ marketing approach to achieve fiscal self-sufficiency and gain public respect and support.	378
9. Expand and improve family-centered programs and facilities.	373
10. Promote higher values and ethical practices in youth sports competition.	363
11. Strive for fuller mainstreaming of persons with disabilities in community recreation programs.	360
12. Plan for long-term role of recreation and leisure in potentially job-scarce economy.	341
13. Develop higher levels of professionalism, through accreditation, certification, continuing education, or program standards.	340
14. Unify separate branches of leisure-service field (public, nonprofit, commercial, therapeutic, etc.) in common programs and projects.	298

Note: As in Table 5.1 (page 96), challenges are ranked in importance by respondents, with 1 being the highest, and 14 the lowest.

to build intergroup understanding and positive community relationships. In general, the need to serve major racial or ethnic minorities in American society today will involve the following priorities: (1) to provide enriched programs of leisure services and to overcome past inequities with respect to facilities and leadership; (2) to promote intercultural understanding through programs that represent the traditions and customs of minority groups; (3) to strive to overcome patterns of racial or ethnic segregation—including self-segregation—in community life; (4) to recruit members of minority groups into leadership roles and to encourage career development leading to professional advancement; and (5) to serve generally as advocates and spokespersons not simply for "tolerance," but for whole-hearted acceptance and respect.

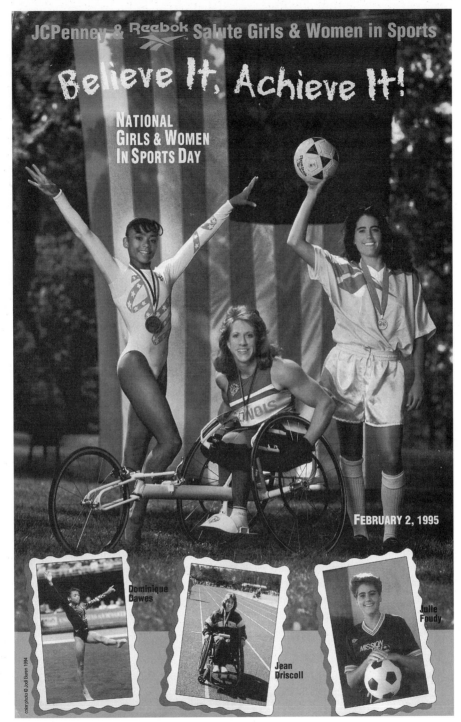

FIGURE 14.1 Vivid illustration of diversity in American life. This poster shows the growing role of women in sport, inclusion of racial minorities and persons with disability, and involvement of major corporations in supporting leisure-related programs.

To achieve such goals, it will be essential to involve members of minority groups heavily in planning, decision making, committee and council work, and other forms of input. Beyond this, recreation, park, and leisure-service agencies may serve as mobilizing agents to bring other community elements—business, religious, educational, and social service—together to solve problems related to racial or ethnic divisiveness and achieve higher levels of cooperation and social harmony.

Gender Equity.   Chapter 8 has shown how much progress has been made in providing fuller opportunities for girls and women in sports, outdoor recreation and other active pursuits, and in leadership positions. Clearly, the trend has been toward breaking down past gender-based discrimination. In many youth organizations, both sexes are now served equally in joint male/female memberships and program activities.

However, it is still abundantly clear that in professional recreation and park service, as in other areas of public service, business, or political life, women still are hampered by the "glass ceiling" that prevents all but a few from rising to higher levels of responsibility and compensation. The support of school and college sport is still biased in favor of male participants, and administrators of joint male and female athletic programs are disproportionately male. In other types of settings, such as private membership or golf clubs, women are still frequently discriminated against, and the task will be to overcome all such inequities.

With respect to the issue of serving those with alternative sexual lifestyles, most leisure-service agencies have barely begun to consider what their responsibilities might be. In many cases, gay and lesbian individuals form their own recreational clubs or associations, and in many others they simply take part in ongoing community programs without attention being paid to their special identity. However, some school districts and other agencies have formed special groups to serve homosexual youth or adults, and this may represent a growing trend. A second issue facing many leisure-service administrators has to do with the employment of youth leaders who are gay or lesbian—a matter that has come before the courts in a number of settings.

Age and Family Factors.   A third component of the "diversity" challenge involves the need to serve each of the major age groups effectively, recognizing the changes that are occurring in population makeup, such as the dramatic increase in the number of elderly persons. Similarly, all the changes that have taken place with respect to family structures present a powerful challenge to recreation, park, and leisure service professionals.

Challenge 2. Emphasize Key Social Purposes of Recreation

As earlier chapters have shown, public and nonprofit leisure-service organizations have traditionally been regarded not simply as providers of light amusement, but rather as sponsors of significant community services.

The report of the National Symposium Committee on the recreation and park field's agenda for the twenty-first century, published by the National Recreation and Park Association, stressed that leisure-service agencies generally—and public recreation and park agencies in particular—needed to provide more than "fun and games." Their recommendations stressed the urgency of serving all social classes with significant program elements:

> We [in the public recreation and park movement] tend to justify and provide parks and recreation in terms of attendance and dollars generated instead of on the improvement of society. We must provide leadership in meeting social issues as well as economic and community development needs.
>
> Parks and recreation must join forces with other social and human service agencies to develop networks vital to the delivery of all programs addressing and serving the needs and concerns of all people.
>
> The fact is that parks and recreation has become very middle class, operated by middle-class people who plan and provide services to the middle class. Our responsibility is to provide opportunities for a better quality of life through parks and recreation. Parks and recreation professionals must have as their major concern, the individual, family and community at all socioeconomic levels.[14]

Earlier chapters have outlined a number of the important social contributions that may be made by organized recreation, park, and leisure-service agencies. As a single example, many organizations have taken on the task of working with at-risk youth—young people who because of dysfunctional families or neighborhoods, the lack of desirable models, or other economic, personal, or environmental influences are at high risk for gang involvement or delinquent behavior that may ultimately lead to more serious criminal activity.

In recent years, social scientists have tended to downplay the role of recreation in meeting the needs of problem youth. However, many organizations, such as the Boys and Girls Clubs of America, the Salvation Army, or the Police Athletic League, that work intensively in depressed urban communities, *do* regard recreation as a vital element in antidelinquency programs—along with other needed family services, tutoring and vocational guidance, substance-abuse clinics or support services, and the use of outreach workers with juvenile gangs. Much of their funding support, whether from government grants or foundation or private giving, expresses the conviction that their programs, which are *heavily* based on recreation activities, do achieve many of the objectives linked to overcoming juvenile delinquency.

In part, their contribution consists not only of working with "problem" youth, but with the bulk of children and youth who need positive leisure outlets that build self-esteem, habit of self-control and self-discipline, creative and athletic outlets, respect for others, trust in adults, and acceptance of important societal values—as well as appealing alternatives to other forms of pleasure-seeking activities.

In the mid-1990s, Schultz, Crompton, and Witt conducted a survey of public recreation and park agencies to determine whether they offered special programs and services for at-risk youth and to learn the nature of these programs. Of 628 responding agencies, 55 percent targeted some part of their programs to serve at-risk children and youth—in many cases in collaboration with the business community, foundations, nonprofit agencies, school districts, and law enforcement agencies.[15]

A detailed study of actual practices in nineteen public recreation and park agencies across the United States showed that these departments offered such services as: "latch-key"

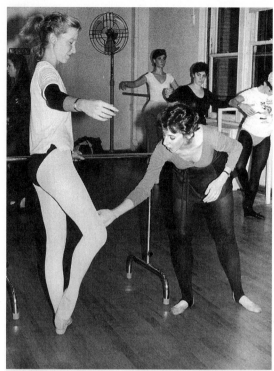

As an example of benefits-based programming, the New York City YWCA offers a huge range of recreation, vocational, and cultural activities, including such classes as ballet instruction, health and fitness programs, and computer skills classes.

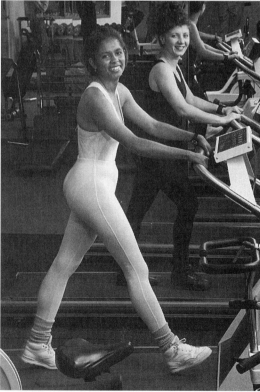

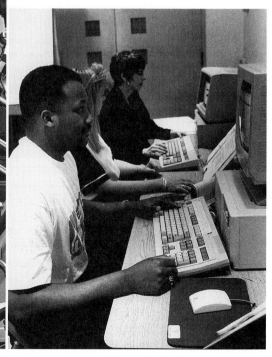

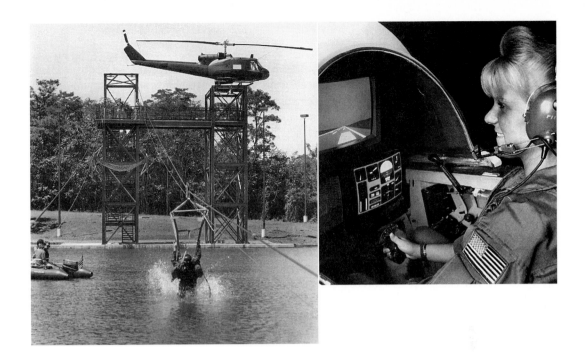

It is essential to provide children and youth with meaningful and challenging leisure experiences that will help them gain needed adult skills and contribute to community life. Here, teenagers gain realistic skills in pilot training and "helicopter survival" sessions in the U.S. Space Camp in Huntsville, Alabama. In Long Beach, California, and in many other cities, young children volunteer to take part in beach cleanup and other environmental projects.

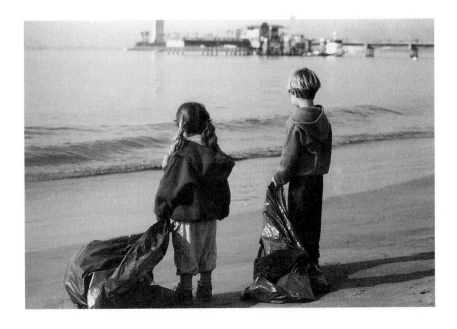

programs for children; day care services; substance abuse prevention; mental health and family counseling; teen pregnancy services; gang, violence, and family abuse programs; career development; and numerous other recreation and cultural activities. Within many other areas of social service, public and nonprofit leisure-service agencies offer equally important programs to meet individual, family, and neighborhood needs. Clearly, this responsibility represents a major challenge for leisure-service organizations, today and in the years to come.

Challenge 3. Achieve Fuller Public Understanding of Recreation, Parks, and Leisure Services

As a relatively new field of public service, having expanded significantly only since World War II, recreation, parks, and leisure services have nonetheless achieved a relatively high level of public understanding and support. This is evidenced both in the degree to which people engage in varied forms of recreation on a personal or private level and the extent to which they take part in organized, community-based programs. In 1998, Harper, Godbey, and Foreman summarized the findings of several research studies that confirmed this picture of positive public support. They reported the following:

> Approximately two-thirds of North Americans say that leisure is of equal or more importance to them than work.
>
> Despite report of declining free time, North Americans average about 40 hours of free time per week.
>
> Recreation and park services, as a percentage of local government spending, have remained constant during the last few decades.
>
> In terms of age groups served, while the impression in that programs are chiefly for children, older persons are more likely to use local parks more frequently than any other age group.[16]

Despite these findings, there are several areas in which public understanding and support of leisure services should be strengthened. First, there is the long-standing suspicion of play that originated centuries ago, linked to the Protestant work ethic. To counter this negative attitude, it is important that the positive values of play and recreation be consistently documented and made known to the public—both through scholarly research, application of the benefits-based approach, and effective public relations.

Realistically, it has also been true that when fiscal crises compelled many government agencies to slash their budgets, those services most closely linked to public safety or health tended to maintain the highest level of support, while others, like recreation, libraries, or social services, tended to be cut. The solution to this problem, again, is to make sure that recreation programs *do* serve significant social goals.

Beyond this, simply because the overall leisure-service field is so diverse, with many different types of organizations and program offerings, the public at large may not recognize it as a specific area of service. One strategy that may be useful in this regard would be for recreation, park, and leisure-service practitioners to play a fuller role in community development. This has been defined as follows:

> [Community development involves] a group of people in a locality initiating a social action process (i.e., planned intervention) to change their economic, social, cultural, and/or environmental situation. International strategies of community change vary widely from programs that target a specific problem (e.g., irrigation projects, nutrition for children) to [broader strategies involving] political and social structures (e.g., the human rights movement, women's movement).[17]

Community development encourages people to take action to improve their life conditions in a process that encompasses personal involvement and growth, indigenous leadership, and heavy reliance on local resources for solving local problems. Recreation, parks, and leisure services provide an ideal area of community development. Clearly, the field cannot afford to let itself be narrowly defined as an isolated amenity. Instead, leisure-service practitioners must develop ties of common purpose with other professionals concerned with public health and health care, environmental protection and recovery, education on all levels, law enforcement, and economic development. Only in this way can it continue to receive and build public support and gain fuller recognition as a vital community service.

Challenge 4. Upgrade Recreation and Park Programs and Facilities, Particularly in Inner Cities and with Minorities

Obviously, this challenge is closely tied to two of the preceding challenges: the need to serve an increasingly diverse society, and to emphasize key social purposes of recreation. As earlier chapters have shown, the harsh fact is that, while many public and nonprofit leisure-service organizations have developed impressive new facilities and rich program offerings, recreational opportunities in inner-city neighborhoods are often barren and run-down.

The growing "have" and "have not" gap in American society is vividly reflected in the leisure-service field. Tom Goodale points out that spas, resorts, and clubs serving the wealthy are obviously not available for those not "well-heeled." Beyond this, government heavily subsidizes various cultural facilities and organizations that benefit the wealthy primarily—such as museums, galleries, concert halls, and theaters, which are often tax-exempt. He goes on to describe the decline of tax dollar support in

> . . . poor communities and comparative abundance of tax dollars in rich ones. Compare per capita open space, athletic fields, indoor facilities, classes and programs, or library hours, holdings and programs in any poor community with any rich one. More than race or religion, this apartheid state is based on money.[18]

How can this disparity be remedied? Obviously, in addition to its racial and economic bases, it is also linked to issues of political influence. Residents of wealthier communities or neighborhoods tend to be politically active, to have their voices heard, to serve on committees and councils—and to fight to have their needs met—more than the poor, who historically have not played active political roles in local government.

What is essential is that civic officials, planners, heads of nonprofit agencies and others come to grips with the problem and place the leisure needs of the poor and inner-city

table of contents

SUMMER SCHEDULE 1998, volume 12, issue 1

LONG BEACH
PARKS·RECREATION·MARINE

Check This Out

ANNUAL COASTAL CLEANUP

September 19, 1998

Registration: 8-8:30 a.m.
Cleanup: 8:30 a.m.-Noon

See pg. 37 for details or call Eileen Fortin @ 570-3165

All programs subject to change without notice

partners of parks

Long Beach Parks, Recreation & Marine wishes to thank Partners of Parks for their continued support of recreational services for the outdoor enthusiast in Long Beach. Their efforts are much appreciated.

PARTNERS OF PARKS

Betty L. Davenport, Chairman
Bea Antenore, Vice-Chairman
Bob Lamond, Treasurer

Partners of Parks, 2760 Studebaker Rd., Long Beach, 90815-1697

Schedule Layout & Design:
Gabriel Daigle

CITY OF LONG BEACH
Department of Parks, Recreation and Marine

2760 Studebaker Road,
Long Beach, CA
90815-1697
Phone (562) 570-3100
Fax (562) 570-3109

◆

Parks, Recreation & Marine wishes to thank the following people for their support:

RECREATION COMMISSION
Gladys A. Gutierrez, *President*
William R. Clark, *Vice-President*
David Sanchez
William Marmion
Jonathan S. Monat
Wanda Draper
Bea Antenore

◆

The Long Beach Parks, Recreation & Marine Department (LBPRMD) prohibits discrimination on the basis of race, color, national origin, age and handicap in all of its programs.

◆

The information in this publication is available in an alternative format by request to Jane Grobaty at 570-3232. The City of Long Beach intends to provide reasonable accommodations in accordance with the Americans with Disabilities Act of 1990. If a special accomodation is desired, please call Jane Grobaty 48 hours prior to the event at 570-3232.

FIGURE 14.2 Contents page of Long Beach, California, Parks, Recreation & Marine summer brochure. Many programs and facilities serve important social and environmental needs and involve partnerships with varied community organizations.

minority populations higher on the scale of priorities. Both as an ethical responsibility and as a practical approach to providing stability in the community, countering antisocial forces, and enriching the quality of life generally, there should be a *minimal* standard of recreational opportunity in *all* neighborhoods. Joint planning and cooperation by all agencies, including public departments, Ys and Boys and Girls Clubs, Police Athletic Leagues, school systems, police departments and other groups, will be essential in meeting this challenge.

Challenge 5. Adopt a Benefits-Based Management Approach

The key principle of the benefits-based management approach is that the traditional method of justifying recreation programs and services by listing the numbers of those who attend or the revenues derived from particular facilities or events is not sufficient. Instead, if the recreation, park, and leisure-service field is to gain a fuller degree of public understanding and support, and if individual agencies are to gain the same level of priority and funding as other community services, it is essential that the actual outcomes and benefits of leisure-service programs be measured and publicized.

As described by Lawrence Allen and other leisure-service educators at professional conferences and in national publications, the benefits-based approach has four major steps: (1) Recreation, park, and leisure-service agencies should develop clearly defined goals and objectives, in terms of the outcomes and benefits they intend to achieve; (2) all program elements should be carefully designed to achieve these benefits; (3) programs, special projects, or other services should be systematically monitored and evaluated to determine the benefits that have been gained; and (4) varied forms of public information media should be used to make sure that all elements of the public—taxpayers, organization members, civic groups, and officials—realize the positive benefits of agency activities.[19]

Eckhart and Allen point out that growth of support and interest in benefits-based management (BBM) of recreation, park, and leisure service agencies over the past several years has been remarkable. They state that

> . . . the profession has totally embraced this philosophy and management strategy. There are now numerous national projects attempting to advance the profession's understanding of BBM and document the benefits of recreation programs that utilize the Benefits-Based Programming (BBP) model, which supports the BBM philosophy. The National Recreation and Park Association has been a leader in promoting and supporting these efforts.[20]

In addition to focusing on human-service or economic outcomes, the benefits-based approach can also be invaluable in addressing other important needs of the leisure-service profession that were ranked in a 1998 survey of educators. The challenges include such elements as the promotion of recreation's identity as a health-related field, developing partnerships with environmental organizations, encouraging higher and more humanistic values in sports competition for youth, or facilitating mainstreaming for disabled persons. All such goals can and should be clearly defined and consciously worked toward, monitored, and evaluated.

Challenge 6. Promote Recreation's Identity as Health-Related Field

There are two components to the case that can be made for recreation, parks, and leisure-services as an important health-related field. First, there is extensive evidence showing that regular, moderate exercise, which is carried on most consistently within a framework of social support or recreational interest, is a key factor in promoting physical health throughout life. The effect of such exercise—whether gained through fitness programs, sports, gardening, swimming, or other leisure pursuits—is to help prevent heart disease but, beyond that, also help deter cancer, diabetes, obesity, or other illnesses or unhealthy conditions.

However, physical health and the prevention of disease is only part of the broader concept of wellness, which embraces one's social, emotional, intellectual, and work life, and which contributes significantly to total life satisfaction. The role of improving one's lifestyle through desirable, diversified leisure activity is important not only in a positive sense. It also reinforces one's ability to withstand other, harmful leisure involvements, such as the use of tobacco, alcohol, or narcotics; gambling addiction; or obsessive involvement in high-risk forms of play.

As earlier chapters point out, over the past three decades, numerous studies have documented the personal, social, environmental, and economic benefits derived from organized recreation programs. Specifically, research studies have established the direct physiological, psychological and lifestyle-modification benefits for different age groups, such as the elderly, from carefully planned and directed programs of physical activity. Similarly, there are impressive reports from major corporations that show how physical recreation and fitness programs for employees have succeeded in reducing job absenteeism, accidents and injuries, and employee turnover, with substantial savings in health insurance costs.

The challenge for leisure-service agencies with respect to strengthening this field's identity as a health-related discipline is threefold: (1) to design programs wherever possible to achieve desirable health and wellness benefits, both for the population at large and for specific subgroups with special health or fitness needs; (2) to develop precisely framed goals and objectives to measure the outcomes of such programs and to monitor them systematically; and (3) to communicate positive findings and benefits in a creative and systematic way to the public at large.

Challenge 7. Develop Partnerships with Environmental Organizations to Protect and Restore Wildlands and Waterways

As Chapter 13 has shown in detail, over the past three decades, federal and state efforts to enhance air and water quality have been remarkably successful. Many lakes and rivers, for example, that had been almost totally lifeless as a result of years of uncontrolled pollution are now thriving with recovered water quality and healthy fish populations. Similarly, federal assistance to local authorities has resulted in major acquisition programs to set aside open-space and parkland areas, wetlands, and other natural resources.

In all such efforts, the recreation and park profession, along with thousands of individual practitioners and state or local societies, has worked closely with environmental organizations to support needed legislation or carry out specific projects of land acquisition, environmental education, or park development. In city after city, volunteer groups of citizens are rehabilitating parks and playgrounds; cleaning up vacant lots; planting trees and restoring beachfronts, hiking trails, and other natural areas.

However, the harsh reality is that many forms of outdoor recreation are harmful to the natural environment and need to be more carefully controlled. The development of an environmental ethic that will help to guide the practices of recreation and park planners and administrators in this area is a crucial priority. To achieve such goals, leisure-service professionals cannot operate in a totally independent way. Through both structured and informal alliances and partnerships, they must work closely with other governmental and private groups to sustain a higher level of environmental health.

Challenge 8. Employ Marketing Approach to Achieve Fiscal Self-Sufficiency and Gain Public Respect and Support

Initially, the provision of recreational services like parks, playgrounds, and community center activities was regarded as an essentially free public function comparable to highways, police and fire protection, or the public schools—paid for through taxes, but without charges at the point of service delivery. Gradually, as more varied and elaborate facilities began to be built—such as swimming pools, tennis courts, golf courses, indoor skating rinks, and marinas—it became customary to charge modest fees for their use. Throughout the decades after World War II, the use of fees and charges—for registration, admission, instruction, use of equipment, and other services—was the subject of an ongoing debate. Those opposed to them argued that they represented a form of double taxation and that they tended to exclude children, the elderly, the disabled, and the poor from participation. Those in favor of fees and charges argued that they were essential to maintain and expand programs in an era of fiscal austerity.

In time, the argument became moot, as most public recreation and parks systems on local, state, and federal levels imposed fees and charges on a wide range of program activities. Community residents tended to accept such policies without objection. For example, in a study conducted by Economic Research Associates in the mid-1970s, most citizens interviewed felt that more recreation services should be on a pay-as-you-go basis. Recreation and park administrators reported that although initial resistance to new or increased fees was reflected in a short-term decline in usage, this effect tended to disappear in two or three years.

In city after city, where the slogan of "reinventing government" was increasingly heard, pressure to use revenue sources to support recreation and park budgets mounted throughout this period. In New York City, for example, where the public park and recreation budget was found to be the lowest of eighteen major American cities as a percentage of the overall municipal operating budget in the mid-1990s, financial cuts had a devastating effect:

> Years of disproportionate budget cuts have taken their toll. Playing fields and equipment are in disrepair. Local parks programming has been virtually eliminated. Our

urban forest is not being pruned, sick trees are not being cared for and dead trees are not being replaced. Parkland is being privatized at an alarming rate. . . .

The social contract that provided outdoor spaces in our crowded city has been broken, forcing children to play indoors in crowded tenements that parks were built to relieve.[21]

In response, to offset dwindling financial resources, New York's Parks and Recreation Department embarked on a new path: an aggressive pursuit of profits. It hired its first marketing director, whose responsibility was to find money-making opportunities and corporate sponsors. In 1996, Douglas Martin wrote:

Last fall the Parks and Recreation Department turned Central Park's drives into a test road for BMWs. It is renting out DeWitt Clinton Park to a dinner theater production. Last week, it signed a deal allowing a sporting goods company to advertise on basketball backboards. It is looking into endorsing a soft drink—the Official Beverage of City Greenswards?—and is even imagining its own credit card, complete with a holographic image of the park of your choice.[22]

An example of contemporary marketing approaches of public recreation and park departments may be found in Prince William County, Virginia, where the Chinn Aquatic and Fitness Center offers a huge, spectacular indoor pool with whirlpools, saunas, and an outdoor sunbathing deck, along with a large gymnasium and fitness room equipped with the latest weight-training technology. Services provided at the Chinn Center include aerobic classes, dance programs, computerized fitness assessments, child care, birthday parties and facility rentals, youth activities, and other family program features. Built at a cost of $10.4 million, the complex makes use of varied fee structures, including youth, senior, and couple discounts; daily admissions charges; and six-month and one-year pass plans. In the mid-1990s, annual membership charges in the publicly owned facility ranged from $160 for senior residents of Prince William County to $655 for nonresident couples.

Such efforts were not unique to public recreation and park agencies. Many organizations, like voluntary youth associations, religious federations, and others, began to use high-powered promotional techniques to gain public support and increase their revenue sources. For example, in the past, armed forces recreation programs had been financed by a combination of appropriated funds (tax moneys allocated by Congress) and nonappropriated funds (derived from on-base revenues from messes, vending machines, and post exchange stores). Gradually, during the 1980s, the level of appropriated funds for recreation in the military was cut back. In 1991, Bill Mullins wrote:

Few of us could have predicted a decade ago that military recreation programs would obtain additional operating funds by literally turning trash into cash, soliciting corporate sponsorships, or promoting, administering and operating leisure travel services. These enterprises, among other initiatives, are helping military recreation professionals manage their fiscal transition into the twenty-first century.[23]

Recreation and park educator John Crompton rejects the notion that the term *marketing* is a euphemism for *hucksterism*, and that it is concerned only with "selling" programs or gathering revenues. In his view, the key benefits of marketing-oriented revenue-generating approaches to recreation and park management are that they:

- Provide increased resources that can be directed to favored projects for which there would otherwise be no funds.
- Are lauded by elected officials because tax support is reduced (or services are increased/enhanced without a tax increase).
- Offer a wider range of services to citizens without increasing taxes, which increases the department's citizen/political constituency support.
- Enhance political strength, which may be associated with generating revenues from non-tax sources.
- Enhance reputation for being an innovator/leader in the city.
- Increase incentive for staff to offer high quality and relevant services. Pricing services builds in accountability. The services have to meet a real need and their quality has to be high or people will not pay for them.
- Offer staff a new challenge and thus induce an atmosphere of vitality, energy, and excitement in the agency.[24]

With the newer approach to city management that relies on aggressive promotional efforts, "boosterism" that builds a positive image of the metropolis, linkage with business and industry, and "bottom-line" management, the entrepreneurial and marketing emphasis just described is extremely appealing to many public leisure-service agencies. However, the challenge it presents to leisure-service managers lies in the fundamental conflict between marketing approaches that are aimed chiefly at middle- and upper-class community residents and the need of public and nonprofit agencies to fulfill their social mission by serving disadvantaged populations.

Over the past decade, a number of critics have expressed concern about the implications of the leisure-service field's having moved so sharply into an entrepreneurial mode. For example, Dustin, McAvoy, and Schultz argue strongly that the chief purpose of the recreation and park profession must be to promote human growth and development. When the need for profitability takes over, they write: "We are concerned about the possibility that the values and purposes underlying the traditional public delivery of park and recreation services will be undermined by the values and purposes underlying business practices."[25]

Challenge 9. Expand and Improve Family-Centered Programs and Activities

As earlier chapters have shown, the need to strengthen family life in the United States represents a widely shared concern. To accomplish this, it is necessary for leisure-service agencies to recognize many of the changes that have taken place in family structures and lifestyles over the past several decades.

Typically, many public and nonprofit leisure-service agencies, as well as religious organizations, the armed forces, and commercial businesses provide clubs and special events, hobby classes, weekend outings, camping, and sports activities that enrich and strengthen family relationships. Instead of focusing solely on traditional family units through "Father and Son Nights," or "Mother and Daughter" programs, family-directed programming today takes into account the impact of divorce and separation, children born out of wedlock, children with adoptive or foster parents, extended families, or other non-traditional family units.

Community sports have served as a valuable medium for encouraging positive parent-child relationships. Soccer in particular has become an extremely popular youth sport, and Little League, ice hockey, and other sports involve parents in coaching, transporting, and rooting for their sons and daughters. The kinds of attachment and trust built by such shared participation are particularly relevant today, in view of recent research showing that a major factor in helping youth withstand the temptations of drug experimentation or other delinquent behavior consists of having close ties with their parents.

Organizations like the YMCA or YWCA in a number of cities have been particularly active in developing family-service programs, including activities that meet high-priority social needs. As a single example, the YMCA in Sarasota, Florida, sponsors a range of services for families, such as a youth center for teen runaways, housing services for pregnant adolescents, a home instruction program featuring parent-child play serving preschool children, administration of foster-care services in the Y's region, family-conflict consultants, and numerous other special events for families.[26]

Similarly, within the armed forces, the Department of Defense offers extensive community and family-support programs including advocacy services that address the prevention, treatment, and rehabilitation services needed to counter child abuse and neglect, along with child care and child development programs on several levels. Recreation is an important element within this overall battery of services.

Challenge 10. Promote Higher Values and Ethical Practices in Youth Sports Competition

As Chapter 9 makes clear, one of the most popular and valuable areas of leisure involvement in modern society consists of sports participation and spectatorship. On every level, from youth or school leagues, to adult and special sports programs for the elderly, or to college and professional sports, competitive play represents a major recreational interest.

However, sport is also riddled by problems of conflicting values and ethical management on many levels. Although we profess to believe that athletic competition helps to build positive character traits, such as self-discipline, commitment to a cause, team loyalty and sportmanship, and respect for one's opponent, often other values prevail as winning becomes overemphasized.

In college sports, rules are constantly broken in terms of recruiting practices, the coddling of nonstudent athletes, or the subsidization of star players. In big-time professional sports, the impact of free-agentry that moves players from team to team, the shifting of team franchises, the immense salaries paid players, the arrogant behavior of many athletes, and the struggles between players and their unions and team owners all have undermined fan loyalty in recent years.

While most such problems are beyond the control of recreation, park, and leisure-service professionals, they *do* have an important role to play in helping to organize and direct youth sports on the community level. In a variety of settings, such as community leagues for different age levels, competition sponsored by the Police Athletic League, Catholic Youth Organization, or hundreds of other organized programs, it is essential to follow the guidelines formulated by leading coaches' and parents' sports associations. Real sportsmanship, obeying the rules, and keeping winning and losing in proper perspective can help to ensure that the sports experience is a positive one for young people—and that they will carry it on through life, rather than quit at an early point, as many teenagers do.

Challenge 11. Strive for Fuller Mainstreaming of Persons with Disabilities in Community Recreation Programs

An important thrust in community recreation programming today involves providing leisure services for persons with disabilities. There are well over 40 million individuals today in the United States with disabilities that limit them significantly in one or more areas of daily life. Together with their families—whose lives are affected by their disabilities—they comprise a major segment of the nation's population.

Apart from therapeutic recreation services in residential or other institutional treatment settings, many community organizations today have accepted the challenge of working with persons with disability. Such special recreation programs are immensely varied. In some cases, they may consist of an organization that offers a single type of activity, such as wheelchair basketball. In other situations, they may focus on persons with a single type of disability, such as the developmentally disabled or those with visual impairment. Still other special-recreation organizations provide a wide range of activities—including educational, counseling, vocational, and rehabilitative services—for persons with different types of disabilities.

Within this field of service, the strongest thrust today is toward mainstreaming persons with disability. Numerous public and nonprofit community organizations have accepted this as a mandate and make the inclusion and full or partial integration of persons with disability within the larger population a key priority. It is important to recognize that such programs do more than provide the ability to make friends, raise self-esteem, improve mental or physical fitness, or contribute to the quality of life of disabled persons. Often the success of disabled athletes or their performance in other areas of leisure involvement helps the nondisabled population recognize their real potential more fully. Extending this point, fuller inclusion in community recreation programs can serve as a channel for broader empowerment or life opportunities for persons with disabilities in other areas of life—in education, career development, community life, or political roles. As in the case of dealing with racial or ethnic diversity, recreation agencies may serve as a fulcrum around which other community groups may organize their efforts.

Challenge 12. Plan for Long-Term Role of Recreation and Leisure in Potentially Job-Scarce Economy

Those responding to the Leisure Educators' Survey did *not* assign this challenge a high level of importance, compared to most of the other needs listed in the survey form. Nonetheless, from a long-term perspective it may present one of the most difficult problems facing society in the coming century, and a particularly critical one for leisure-service professionals.

Changes in the Workforce.   During the 1970s and 1980s, the U.S. Bureau of Labor Statistics predicted a continuing but gradual rise in the size of the labor force, with women becoming an increasingly larger segment of job holders. The nature of work itself was expected to be influenced by a proliferation of "knowledge workers," who prepare newsletters, tapes, information transmission materials, and similar products for education, training, and other business uses. In general, a long-term trend from blue-collar to white-collar jobs was expected, along with a decline in farm work and manufacturing employment and an increase in service industries.

Other trends that were predicted at this time included the growth of part-time jobs and job-sharing, particularly for men and women who sought to combine paid work with family responsibilities. Moonlighting—the holding of more than one position—was expected to remain fairly constant, with multiple jobholders about 4.5 percent of the work force. Because of technological changes, it was anticipated that there would be a high rate of job obsolescence, compelling many individuals to seek new jobs or enter second, third, or even fourth career fields during their working lives.

Potential Impact of Automation.   During the 1970s and 1980s, it was widely predicted that employment patterns in the future would be sharply affected by the degree to which automation would supplant human effort. Each year, there were accounts of new industrial automatons—or, to use the more popular term, *robots*. Unlike the versions portrayed in science fiction, industrial robots are not strange, exotic beings. Instead, they are machines that can be programmed to carry out simple, repetitive tasks that are usually performed by human workers.

In an article on "The Workless Society" in *The Futurist*, it was predicted that in the twenty-first century, intelligent machines will replace almost all workers, and people will get paid for doing nothing, in a life of ease and abundance. Of course, the use of automation will apply to some fields, such as manufacturing, agriculture, mining, and transportation, more fully than it will to service fields that involve working directly with people.

Despite *The Futurist's* predictions, the wholesale replacement of human workers by machines is still not an immediate threat in the United States. Apart from their widespread use in automobile manufacturing, robots have not been widely introduced to the American workplace. The National Service Robot Association had about 250 individual and corporate members in 1992, most trying to develop machines that would clean hazardous-waste sites, deliver food in hospitals, or assist the disabled. However, as new functions for the application of artificial intelligence are discovered and machines to carry them out are created, it seems probable that economic reasons for applying them will outweigh social concerns about displaced workers.

If this occurs, and if large numbers of working men and women are displaced from the nation's economy, it is clear that American society will face a critical choice. Historian Christopher Lasch points out that the prospect of universal abundance made progress a morally compelling ideology in the past. But, writes Lasch, affluence for all now appears unlikely, even in the distant future; the emergence of a global economy, far from eliminating poverty, has widened the gap between rich and poor nations, and poverty is spilling over into the developed nations from the Third World. The increase in the numbers of homeless, unemployed, illiterate, drug-ridden, and other effectively disfranchised people is a clear indication of this trend in America.[27]

Lasch asks whether we can afford to continue the trend of the 1980s, which saw the rich get richer and the poor get poorer. Similarly, Hess, Markson, and Stein suggests that if work tasks are not distributed more evenly, a society could arise made up of a busy elite of professionals and a "useless" majority unable to master the critical skills of the job world.[28] To a degree, such fears are reflected in real life today, in terms of the large numbers of inner-city residents, often men and women of racial minority background, with limited education and job skills, who are simply unable to obtain meaningful work in a highly technological age when most jobs have moved away from the city. In a recent book, *When Work Disappears: The World of the New Urban Poor,* William Junius Wilson documents this problem as it exists today in Chicago's inner city.[29]

Job-Cutting in the 1990s.   A new trend in the work/leisure relationship appeared in the 1990s, when hundreds of major corporations restructured themselves, "terminating" millions of employees—often white-collar or middle-management professionals. This dramatic shift came about for several reasons: (1) the influence of growing information-processing technology that helped make business operations more efficient; (2) the merger of huge companies that led to heavy cutbacks in employees or transfer of their work locations; and (3) more than anything, a new determination to downsize companies, making them more efficient and yielding greater profits to company executives and stockholders.

Again and again through the decade before century's end, headlines repeated the same "downsizing" story:"

Job Cuts at AT & T Will Total 40,000, 13 Percent of Its Staff

Lockheed to Eliminate 12,000 Jobs; Reflects Cutbacks by Military

Travelers and Citicorp Plan to Cut 8,000 Jobs

Chase and Chemical Agree to Merge in $10 Billion Deal: 12,000 Job Cuts Seen[30]

Similar job slashes were carried out by IBM, Sears, Xerox, McDonnell Douglas, RJR Nabisco, Dupont, General Motors, 3M, and numerous other major corporations. Overall, it was reported by the U.S. Labor Department in 1998 that 8 million employees had been downsized during the period from 1995 to 1997—with most cuts involving permanent layoffs.[31] A new wave of layoffs was announced in the two years that followed, making it clear that the downsizing trend would continue.

Since many laid-off employees were unable to find new jobs at comparable levels of responsibility and pay, and since more companies were unwilling to hire new permanent workers, several job patterns became increasingly evident in the United States during the late 1990s.

Outsourcing.   As part of the trend toward a global economy, many manufacturing concerns shifted key parts of the their operations overseas to undeveloped countries with cruelly low pay scales—as a single example, athletic shoe assembly plants in Asia and Indonesia.

A second example of outsourcing involved companies having major functions carried out by other concerns on a subcontract or special-project basis that could be easily terminated on short notice, so the company would have no responsibility for a large, full-time, "permanent" staff with health benefits or other "perks."

Heavier Workloads.   With many employees unable to find new jobs that were close to their original positions or pay scales, millions of men and women were forced to take two or more jobs to eke out needed income. In the companies that downsized, often the employees who remained were expected to carry heavier workloads. During the mid- and late-1990s, there were a number of cases of labor unions protesting or actually calling strikes to resist the excessive overtime job schedules imposed on their members. While sharing the work would obviously have created more jobs, it would have reduced these companies' profit margin, and so they were reluctant to do this.[32]

Temporary and Part-Time Workers.   Great numbers of employees were placed on temporary status or given part-time jobs, without benefits or security, which often amounted to full-time work at substantially less pay.[33] This pattern is vividly illustrated in many universities today that employ considerable number of graduate students—or even men and women holding the doctorate—for part-time teaching assignments, rather than hire full-time faculty members on tenure tracks.

The impact of these trends has been to create a sense of insecurity and lack of faith in the nation's economic system. With companies increasingly disavowing a sense of social responsibility or commitment to their employees, and with work often becoming more pressured, stress and job-related anxiety have become widespread. At an early point, *Time Magazine*'s Lance Morrow summed up the situation:

> A transformation that [is] merciless and profound is occurring in the American workplace. These are the great corporate clearances of the '90s, the ruthless, restructuring efficiencies. The American work force is being downsized and atomized. . . . Millions of Americans are being evicted from the working worlds that have sustained them and the jobs that gave them not only wages and health care and pensions but also a context, a sense of self-worth, a kind of identity.[34]

Implications for Leisure.   These trends have the following implications for leisure: (1) For many families with both parents working, or for individuals with two jobs or excessive work hours, there will be less free time to engage in leisure pursuits; and (2) for many others, with little or no work in a job-scarce economy, there will be excessive free time—but neither the fiscal ability nor the will to enjoy such free time *as* leisure.

To deal with the first concern, some leisure-service agencies are experimenting with flexible program designed to serve individuals with heavy, unusual, or rotating job schedules. Others have developed more short-term programs so that individuals with limited free time can still engage in recreational pursuits. For the second group, the continuing trend toward relying on fees and charges to support program expenses means that many leisure-service organizations have relatively few program offerings that do not require participants to pay their way. The option of developing special programs to serve the unemployed or underemployed has been explored in only a few settings, but may represent an important tactic for the future—as it was during the Great Depression of the 1930s.

Beyond this, the most rewarding uses of leisure depend heavily on the attitudes of participants. It will be difficult for many individuals who are unemployed or underemployed to enjoy their free time in creative and constructive ways without a nagging sense of guilt.

Impact of Telecommuting. A unique effect of the growth of computer-based communication systems has been that, with the Internet, e-mail, fax machines, and similar aids, the location of work settings has been made far more flexible.

In some cases, this has meant that small towns and rural areas in states like Maine, Nebraska, Wyoming have become the sites for company operations making use of telecommunications for such tasks as processing credit-card calls or other post-industrial work functions. On a broader scale, millions of American workers have begun to seek the flexibility of working all or part of the time away from their office or plant, using home computers to maintain communication and carry out their assignments. Kirk Johnson points out that there are numerous possible arrangements. Some individuals "steal" an occasional half-day or two at home, while others live a thousand miles or more from the office and are rarely seen in person. Increasingly major corporations are developing systems to impose structure and supervision on telecommuting workers. For example, the Wall Street giant, Merrill Lynch, has set up a

> ... "Telecommuting Simulation Lab," to teach people to work at home the Merrill Lynch way. That means everything from a formal application process and regular work hours to a company approved chair. ... The company has extended its reach into aspects of telecommuters' lives that had been the realm of personal choice, including rules for how to work at home, and when to work, and how to work safely.[35]

A negative aspect of telecommuting is that at-home employees may feel isolated and fear that they will drop out of the loop and be overlooked when key assignments are passed out. Beyond this, the lack of interchange with others in the office or plant setting may mean that telecommuting workers have a greater need for social programs in their communities geared to individual, couple, or family groupings.

Although the notion of office romances has become increasingly perilous with a surge of lawsuits or other claims involving sexual harassment, based on short- or long-term relationships between co-workers, the reality is that many American men and women meet each other at work, date, and even marry. *U.S. News and World Report* estimates that between 6 million and 8 million Americans enter into a romance with a fellow employee each year.[36] As telecommuting becomes more prevalent on a part- or full-time basis, how will it affect the nation's marriage rate?

On the other hand, the advantage of telecommuting for many distance employees is that it permits them to live in rural or isolated areas where skiing, hunting, or other outdoor sports are readily available to them.

Challenge 13. Develop Higher Levels of Professionalism Through Accreditation, Certification, Continuing Education, or Program Standards

Curiously, although the survey examined the views of leisure studies department chairpersons or other leading faculty members, who presumably would be strongly in favor of measures to promote higher levels of professionalism in this field, this challenge statement received the next-to-lowest level of support.

It is possible that many college and university educators, whose curricula have not sought or gained formal accreditation status, believe that accreditation standards are too high, or that the process itself is too cumbersome or expensive. They may also believe that tying professional certification to one's having graduated from an accredited higher education program is too restrictive. In their view, denying certification to individuals who have been educated in other specialized fields than recreation and leisure may prevent talented people from entering this field.

Possibly also, many educators may believe that there is an overload of professional societies in different areas of specialization—each with its own publications, agendas, conferences, and workshops. Despite such views, the overwhelming position of men and women who have been leaders in this field over a period of years is that professional advancement in terms of basic and continuing education, affiliation with national and state societies, and other initiatives that improve services and promote public understanding is absolutely essential. The steady growth of continuing education programs is evidence of this strong conviction held by recreation, park, and leisure-service professionals throughout the United States.

These issues are particularly important in view of several major trends affecting higher education in the United States. Tim Luke, for example, writes in *Telos*, a journal of higher education, that many colleges and universities are being crippled by funding reductions, confusion over curricula goals and content, redefinitions of relevance, and pushing and pulling over practicality. He continues, pointing out that intellectual excellence is rarely the target of higher education reforms:

> Instead, operating efficiency, understood along the lines of industrial input-output models, becomes the new gold standard of educational performance as financial resources devoted to tertiary education continue to shrink.[37]

Michael Taves agrees, pointing out that there have been attempts by many colleges and universities to deal with the fiscal crisis by "reengineering," "restructuring," and "downsizing," while desperately trying to remain competitive in the marketplace for students. Sometimes, he writes, this is done by devising innovative new programs, but more often through more forceful marketing and especially by investing in physical and technology infrastructure to strengthen the perception of institutional modernity and competitiveness. Within this framework, the tradition of a liberal arts education is linked to an industrial age that is fast disappearing. Instead, colleges and universities are becoming increasingly attentive to market needs, becoming service-oriented and community-responsive, often developing strategic partnerships with the private sector.[38]

How does this relate to higher education in recreation, parks, and leisure studies and services? Many institutions have already experienced major shakeups, with leisure-service units being disbanded or assigned to other administrative units, such as travel, tourism and hospitality, public health, sport management, schools of business, or social work administration. Given this background, it is essential that college and university leisure-service curricula affirm the linkage of their courses to the primary goal of preparing leisure-service professionals as a unifying thrust within these separate, specialized programs.

Beyond this, as Jensen suggests (see page 347), every evidence of professionalism, such as certification, accreditation, continuing education, and encouragement of a high level of research and published scholarship, will be invaluable in helping university administrators understand the importance of this field and its validity as an area of academic specialization.

The history of every other specialized profession in American society, including such fields as medicine, nursing, law, accountancy, social work, and education, shows inevitably that as educational and certification requirements are strengthened and as higher education programs become more advanced, the field itself becomes more widely respected and its performance more effective. Certainly, in terms of the major changes that will take place in the oncoming decades of the twenty-first century, such public recognition and advanced levels of performance will be essential for those in the leisure-service field.

Challenge 14. Unify Separate Branches of Leisure-Service Field in Common Programs and Projects

As in their response to the preceding challenge dealing with the need to promote professionalism in the leisure-service field more fully, survey respondents gave a low level of support to this statement of need.

To put it in perspective, the field of professional leisure service is immensely diversified and complex today. Chapter 4 describes all the different kinds of organizations—public, nonprofit, commercial, therapeutic, and others—that provide major segments of recreational opportunity to the public. Realistically, of these, the only type of agency that regards the provision of recreation as its *primary* responsibility is the public, governmental recreation and park department. In each of the other types of sponsoring organizations, recreation represents a *secondary* function—that is, a means to a broader end.

As a consequence, the recreation and park establishment correctly views itself as the primary spokesperson for the field and its members as prototype recreation professionals. By far the highest proportion of the members of the National Recreation and Park Association are men and women working in the public recreation and park field. Those with other specialized interests, ranging from water-park management to athletic administration, tend to be members of other associations with their own publications, workshops and conferences, and promotional campaigns. In some cases, as in the National Employee Services and Recreation Association (NESRA), they have their own well-defined certification plans.

The question posed by Challenge 14 is, "Would it be possible or desirable to bring a fuller degree of unity and common effort to the fragmented leisure-service field by developing more partnerships and alliances among different types of sponsors?" Earlier chapters have shown that this trend has brought positive results in many community programs, as in the broad field of outdoor recreation and environmental protection. The benefits that might be achieved by such an effort would mean that public needs for constructive, creative recreation could be met much more fully.

Through joint planning and the sharing of priorities and resources, the overall recreation, park, and leisure-service field might better be able to avoid unnecessary duplication and to fill gaps in the provision of needed recreational programs. Beyond this, although they would not result in the formal unification of the various elements in the field—which would not be possible or desirable—such cooperative efforts might help the public gain a fuller understanding of the value of recreation and leisure in meeting personal and social needs of all citizens, today and tomorrow.

Summary

Forecasting the future, it is clear that advancing technology will continue to have an increasingly important impact both on the overall society and on the specific role of recreation and leisure in American life. This chapter examines several aspects of this development, including the kinds of innovative uses of leisure that may be influenced by new technology in the "information society," as well as the uses of electronic forms of communication and data-processing in the management of recreation agencies. It focuses heavily on the restructuring of the job world in the United States, with many corporations and other organizations downsizing, cutting hundreds of thousands of employees loose, and burdening others with excessive workloads.

The concluding sections of the chapter examine the responses of leisure-service educators to the *1998 Leisure Trends and Issues Survey*, with emphasis on priorities for the field in reconciling conflicting marketing and social-service management approaches. The need for continuing and strengthened professional development and partnerships among different elements in the field is stressed.

Key Concepts

1. Apart from the varied innovations in leisure pursuits provided by new technologies that were described in Chapter 12, the emergence of the information-based, high-tech society will have major implications for recreational planning and service delivery.

2. Although such sweepingly popular developments as the Internet have aroused great interest, there is growing concern among social scientists and futurists that they may have harmful, as well as positive, outcomes.

3. A major outcome of information technology has been the transformation of work patterns in industry and government and the rapid decline of many occupations and career fields. At the same time that job scarcity represents a problem for many white-collar and middle-management employees, many other "knowledge-workers" or skilled technicians are experiencing a heavy overload of work.

4. Among the challenges listed in the educators' survey that received the highest levels of support were the need to serve an increasingly diverse society, to emphasize the key social purposes of recreation, achieve fuller recognition of the field, and to strengthen its identity as a health-related social service.

5. Three dominant thrusts in organized recreation service in the years ahead will include the entrepreneurial/marketing emphasis, the human-services mission, and the benefits-based management approach.

6. Family-centered programming and the effort to promote positive values and outcomes in youth sports competition represent other important program emphases for the years ahead, along with increasing mainstreaming for persons with disabilities.

7. Although survey respondents gave a low level of priority to concern about the long-term role of recreation in a potentially job-scarce society, this clearly represents a problem that will have to be faced in the future, in terms of "have" and "have-not" population groups.

8. Finally, although respondents also gave little support to challenges involving professional development and unity among different branches of the leisure-service field, these too were seen as significant challenges for the future.

Endnotes

1. Rifkin, J. 1995. After Work: A Blueprint for Social Harmony in a World Without Jobs. *Utne Reader* (May–June): 55.

2. Sessoms, H.D. 1998. The National Curriculum Conference on Parks and Recreation. *Parks and Recreation* (June): 22, 24.

3. Polman, D. 1998. Prosperity. *Philadelphia Inquirer Magazine* (September 20): 5.

4. Mandel, M. 1996. *The High-Risk Society.* New York: Random House/Times Business, p. 4.

5. Elmer-Dewitt, P. 1992. The Century Ahead: Dream Machines. *Time Magazine* (Fall, special issue): 39–40.

6. Harmon, A. 1998. Sad, Lonely World Discovered in Cyberspace. *New York Times* (August 30): 1, 22.

7. Macklin, W. 1997. Face-to-Face or Interface. *Philadelphia Inquirer* (July 27): H-1.

8. Anderson, L., C. Brown, and P. Soli. 1996. The Rural Recreation Integration Project: Reaching Out with Interactive Video Technology. *Parks and Recreation* (May): 38–43.

9. Information Technology Revolution: Boon or Bane? 1997. *The Futurist* (January–February): 10–14.

10. Winslow, D.C., and W.L. Bramer. 1994. *Future Work: Putting Knowledge to Work in the Knowledge Economy.* New York: Free Press/Macmillan, p. vii.

11. Rifkin, *op. cit.*

12. Guttenberg, M., and P. Secord. 1988. In J. Fowles, Coming Soon: More Men Than Women. *New York Times* (June 5): F-3.

13. Garreau, J. 1991. *Edge City: Life on the New Frontier.* New York: Doubleday.

14. Mobley, T. and R. Toalson, eds. 1992. *Parks and Recreation in the 21st Century.* Arlington, VA: National Symposium Committee and NRPA.

15. Schultz, L., J. Crompton, and P. Witt. 1995. National Profile of the Status of Public Recreation Services for At-Risk Children and Youth. *Journal of Park and Recreation Administration* (Fall, 13/3): 1–25.

16. Harper, J., G. Godbey, and S. Foreman, 1998. Just the Facts: Answering the Critics of Local Government Park and Recreation Services. *Parks and Recreation* (August): 78–81.

17. Arai, S. 1996. Benefits of Citizen Participation in a Healthy Communities Initiative: Linking Community Development and Employment. *Journal of Applied Recreation Research* (21/1): 27.

18. Goodale, T. 1996. Taking Stock at Millennium's End. *Parks and Recreation Canada* (May/June): 9.

19. Allen, L. and T. McGovern. 1997. BBM: It's Working! *Parks and Recreation* (August): 48–55.

20. Eckhart, A., and L. Allen. 1998. Benefits-Based Programming: Improving the Health of Seniors. *Parks and Recreation* (July): 21.

21. *NYC's Parks in Peril.* New York City Neighborhood Open Space Coalition, 1994, p. 1.

22. Martin, D. 1996. This Time, Parks Mean Business: Aggressive Pursuit of Profit. *New York Times* (February 16): B-1.

23. Mullins, B. 1991. Managing Fiscal Transition. *Parks and Recreation* (October): 38.

24. Crompton, J. 1988. Are You Ready to Implement a Comprehensive Revenue-Generating Program? *Parks and Recreation* (March): 56.

25. Dustin, D., L. McAvoy, and J. Schultz. 1990. Recreation Rightly Understood. In Goodale, T.L., and P.A. Witt. 1990. *Recreation and Leisure in an Era of Change.* State College, PA: Venture Publishing, pp. 97–105.

26. Carson, M. 1997. Friends of the Family. *Discovery YMCA* (Spring): 20–25.

27. Lasch, C. 1992. Is Progress Obsolete? *Time Magazine* (Fall, special issue): 71.

28. Hess, B., E. Markson, and P. Stein. 1988. *Sociology.* New York: Macmillan, p. 619.

29. Wilson, W.J. 1996. *When Work Disappears: The World of the New Urban Poor.* New York: Alfred Knopf.

30. Headlines drawn chiefly from *New York Times* in mid-1990s.

31. Uchitelle, L. 1998. Survey Finds Layoffs Slowed in Last Three Years. *New York Times* (August 19), pp. 1, 19.

32. Meredith, R. 1997. 3 Strikes Threaten Spring Car-Sales Season: Workers Want Less Overtime; Companies Cite Competition. *New York Times* (April 24): A-22.

33. Abelson, R. 1998. Part-Time Work of Some Adds up to Full-Time Job. *New York Times* (November 2): A-1, A-18.

34. Morrow, L. 1993. The Temping of America. *Time Magazine* (March 29): 40.

35. Johnson, K. 1997. Limits on the Work-at-Home Life. *New York Times* (December 17): B-1. See also Polsky, W. 1995. Telecommuting: Creating a Nation of Isolates. *Employee Services Management* (May/June): 28–29.

36. Lardner, J. 1998. Cupid's Cubicles: Office Romance Is Alive and Well . . . *U.S. News and World Report* (December 14): 47.

37. Luke, T. 1998. Miscast Canons? The Future of Universities in an Era of Flexible Specialization. *Telos* (Spring): 15.

38. Taves, M. 1998. The New Fragmentation in Higher Education. *Telos* (Spring): 55–61.

APPENDIX A

Survey of Leisure-Service Educators

The purpose of this survey was to determine the views of leading college and university leisure-service educators with respect to the trends, issues, and challenges facing this field in the century ahead. Two sections of a survey instrument were developed, with 18 and 14 items respectively, based on a search of the literature in the field (professional journals, research publications, programs of professional conferences, reports of planning studies, and articles in related subject fields).

A sample of 195 educators was drawn from four sources: (1) the 1997 Curriculum Directory of the Society of Park and Recreation Educators (SPRE); (2) a larger, international directory published in Canada; (3) a 1998 listing of accredited recreation, park, and leisure-studies departments; and (4) the 1997–1998 SPRE Leadership Directory. With the exception of the last source, surveys were addressed to department or curriculum chairpersons, who were asked to identify their institutions, but were not requested to give their own names or titles. The SPRE Directory was the primary source for the sample; the others were used to supplement it, without duplication.

The survey was sent out in early September 1998. By October 15, 107 completed forms were returned, and tabulation was begun. Several surveys were returned after this date, but were not analyzed. The surveys were scored by having respondents rate each item as "high," "medium," or "low" in importance for the leisure-service field. A "high" rating was given a 5 score, a "medium" rating 3, and a "low" 1. The totals are shown on pages 96 and 354, with the items placed in ranked order.

In addition to rating the survey items, a number of respondents made additional comments, some at length. These fell under several headings:

Changing Societal Needs: Increased racial and ethnic diversity, growing gap between rich and poor; need to strengthen family-directed programs; need to serve special populations, such as the homeless or recent immigrants; problems concerned with the number of obese and unfit children; and need to reduce barriers for women and girls, particularly related to safety issues and freedom from violence.

Role and Image of Recreation and Leisure: Need to promote better leisure education in schools and community programs; fuller concern with "inverted" societal values (i.e., huge rewards for professional athletes and little concern about disadvantaged youth); desire for more "spirituality" in leisure programs, linked to resurgence of religion and religious-sponsored services; growing recognition of leisure as major economic force, including role of equipment manufacturers and retailers in outdoor recreation.

Environmental Issues: Concern about commercial exploitation of wildlands; impact of tourism on host communities; growth of high-risk outdoor recreation; trend toward global interdependence, with increased tourism in other countries, including short-term travel; population shifts, particularly toward coastline regions, with implications for pressure on water-based resources.

Professional Needs: Strong emphasis on need for expanded continuing education; fuller concern with ethical issues in the field; better methods of evaluating program effectiveness; roles of professionals in contracting services or consultant functions; need to build more public/private partnerships; need to strike sensible balance between "business-oriented" and "human-service" professional orientations; need to maintain leisure focus in specialized fields (such as sports management or travel and tourism) that have developed independent identities; and needed strategies for more effective lobbying and fund-raising efforts to support public recreation and park agencies.

Other trends and issues mentioned by individual respondents dealt with the impact of communications technology and its potential threat for promoting social "isolation" among many computer and Internet enthusiasts; a growing move toward simplifying one's lifestyle by many individuals and families; and concern about the impact of legalized gambling on many children, families, and communities.

The overall findings of the two sections of the study are discussed more fully in Chapters 5 and 14. A number of respondents who sent helpful comments were credited in the Preface (page xii). While not all respondents named their institutions, additional survey returns came from the following colleges and universities:

Arkansas State University at Fayetteville; Arizona State University West in Phoenix; California State University Colleges at Dominguez Hills, Hayward, Long Beach, Marysville, and San Diego; University of Connecticut at Storrs; University of Miami, West Florida, and Florida International Universities, and Florida State University at Tallahassee; Georgia Southern University at Statesboro and University of Georgia at Savannah; Eastern Illinois University; University of Indiana, Bloomington, Indiana State at Terre Haute, and Ball State University; University of Northern Iowa; Kansas State University at Topeka; Western Kentucky State College; University of Maine at Machias; University of Massachusetts at Amherst and Boston University; Western Michigan, Central Michigan, and Michigan State at Grand Rapids, and Michigan State University, East Lansing; University of Minnesota; Western State College in Missouri; University of New Hampshire; and Ithaca College and State University of New York at Cortland.

Also: North Carolina University at Chapel Hill, Mt. Olive and Elon Colleges, and Appalachian State, Rocky Mount, and Asheville State Universities; Minot College in Bottineau, North Dakota; Bowling Green, Kent State, Ohio State University, and University of Akron and Ohio University; in Oklahoma, Oral Roberts University and University of Tulsa; Slippery Rock, East Stroudsberg, Lincoln, and Temple Universities in Pennsylvania; Clemson University in South Carolina; University of South

Dakota and Sioux Falls State College; University of Tennessee at Memphis, and Middle Tennessee State College in Nashville; Baylor University and West Texas State College; Brigham Young University, University of Utah, and Utah State at Logan; Green Mountain College and University of Vermont; Old Dominion University in Virginia; Marshall College and Shepherd College, West Virginia; La Crosse State in Wisconsin; and the University of Waterloo, Ontario, and Concordia College in Montreal, Canada.

APPENDIX B

Suggested Course Materials

This appendix contains two types of materials to be used in conjunction with the text: (1) suggested topics for class discussion or essay examination questions and (2) possible individual or group assignments or projects to supplement readings and class discussion.

Topics for Discussion or Essay Examinations

1. Traditionally, leisure has been thought of primarily as time free from work or other pressing obligations. What are some other important ways of conceptualizing leisure, and what are some of its values in community life?

2. What were some of the key predictions regarding the expected role of leisure in American life in the decades immediately following World War II? To what extent have they been realized as the century has drawn to a close?

3. During the 1960s and 1970s, the counterculture movement represented a rebellion against many of the traditional values of American society. What were some of the key elements of this rebellion, and how did they affect recreation and leisure?

4. Later, in the last two decades of the century, Chapter 3 suggests that American society went through several important changes, including a shift in work/leisure values and time availability, an era of austerity, a conservative social trend, and growing emphasis on privatization in personal life and government operation. What were these changes and trends?

5. The public recreation and park movement has dominated the overall leisure-service field in the past, in terms of identity and professional education. Yet, several other major types of organizations today provide major elements of public recreational opportunity. Which are the most important of these, and what is their degree of interaction with public agencies?

6. As in other areas of public service, there has been a powerful thrust toward professionalization in the recreation, park, and leisure-service field. What are some of the key elements in this drive, and how successful do you feel it has been in terms of the public's view of the leisure-service field?

7. At century's end, a number of major demographic shifts have altered the makeup of the United States, in terms of age, population numbers, ethnic/racial identity, and similar factors. Describes these changes and their implications for leisure services in the decades ahead.

8. Of the four major age groups described in Chapter 7 (children, youth, adults, and the elderly), which do you feel have the most pressing need for expanded, purposeful recreational programs? Why? How can these best be met?

9. There has been a long-standing, idealized view of the American family as close-knit, affectionate, and stable, in contrast to the image of the family today, marked by divorce, the prevalence of single parents, lack of sound parental models, and abuse. How accurate is this view? What is the role of recreation and leisure in promoting positive family relationships?

10. Recognizing the long history of racial prejudice and discrimination in the United States, many individuals claim that today the "playing field" is equal for all, in terms of social and economic opportunities. How true is this? How can organized recreation services contribute to better interracial or interethnic relations?

11. Women and girls have also been discriminated against historically, in family, social, economic, and other spheres of daily life. Considerable progress has been made since World War II in overcoming past barriers, with sports representing a major area of increased opportunity. Why was this important, and what still remains to be done with respect to recreation and leisure?

12. Although homosexuality has gained a measure of acceptance in American society, there still exists widespread disapproval of gay and lesbian identity and lifestyles. What are some of the evidences of this, and what are its implications for recreational involvement? What are some of the issues facing leisure-service agencies with respect to homosexuality?

13. Obviously, sports represents a major area of leisure interest and involvement in the United States, although professional athletes and others sometimes minimize their importance as "playing a kid's game." Can you make a strong case for the social and economic importance of sports in modern society?

14. Sports are often justified as an ideal medium for building positive personality traits—loyalty to a goal or to a team, self-discipline, good sportsmanship, and obedience to rules. In what ways do we not live up to such expectations? How can directors of youth sports help to change negative values and behaviors?

15. Outdoor recreation, particularly in major federal or state parks, represents a major leisure involvement and economic value. Yet it also has the potential for harming the natural environment. Discuss this point and some of the more recent trends and policies to preserve that nation's wildlands.

16. Travel and tourism are also extremely popular forms of recreation. What are the primary motivations for pleasure travel and the various attractions that are offered tourists? How can public, private, and other types of agencies collaborate in promoting desirable forms of tourism?

17. The mass media of communication and entertainment represent another major sphere of leisure activity, with potential for both positive and negative outcomes. Discuss the role of television, video games, and other electronic forms of play from this perspective.

18. In the late twentieth century, leisure was transformed into a major industry, with giant conglomerates formed that controlled sports, television, movies, popular music,

and other pursuits and that programmed the American public into varied forms of participation. What are some of the important implications of this trend with respect to leisure's role in personal life?

19. An important element of the commodification of leisure has been the expansion and growing acceptance of varied forms of "morally marginal" play. Explain and illustrate this point and discuss the role of public, nonprofit, and other types of community leisure-service agencies in offering alternatives to this trend.

20. The term "environment" applies not only to wilderness or natural settings for play, but also to the urban and metropolitan regions in which most people live. How have recreation, parks, and leisure services contributed to urban renewal, particularly in older industrial cities that have suffered serious decline in recent years?

21. A key economic trend of the 1990s, projected to continue into the twenty-first century, involves massive downsizing, outsourcing, and the disappearance of millions of middle-management, white-collar, and even technical jobs as a result of technological development and the new "information society." How will this affect leisure-service planning and participation in the years ahead?

22. An important conflict in the leisure-service field involves the conflict between the marketing/entrepreneurial thrust that views recreation primarily from a businesslike, revenue-oriented field, and the human-service perspective that places key emphasis on achieving social goals. How can this conflict be resolved, and what will the impact of the benefits-based management approach be, in promoting public support for recreation, parks and leisure services?

Note: Topics 1 through 12 apply primarily to Chapters 1 through 8, while Topics 13 through 22 are chiefly relevant to Chapters 9 through 14. As such, they would be useful for midterm and final examinations, or to class sessions at different points of the semester.

Individual or Group Assignments or Projects

The following tasks may be undertaken by individuals or small groups of students as term reports or presentations before the class. Ideally, they should involve bibliographic research or more active data-gathering and should, if possible, encourage class participation. Students should have the option of being involved in one or more such activities during the semester.

1. *Historical.* Select a given period of history or a specific topic, such as the development of a particular type of pastime or other leisure-related theme, and carry out a detailed historical analysis of it. This may be submitted as a written report, or it may be presented to the class at a relevant class session.

2. *Leisure Factors.* Select a theme relevant to the course, such as the influence of race/ethnicity, gender factors, disability, socioeconomic class, and research its past

and present status, using text, periodical, and other sources. This might be done as a group project, with a shared presentation to the class.

3. *Agency Analysis.* Analyze a specific leisure-service agency in the community (public, nonprofit, commercial, therapeutic, etc.), visit and analyze it, giving details of its mission, organization or sponsorship, funding, program content, and populations served, for class presentation in a session when the leisure-service system is being examined.

4. *Debate Format.* Identify a controversial leisure-related issue and form two small teams or opposing class members, to debate the subject before the class. Possible subjects might be: (a) the pros and cons of legalized gambling; (b) the marketing/entrepreneurial approach to leisure-service management, opposed to the human-service approach; (c) positive versus negative aspects of sport as a major field of leisure involvement; (d) whether prostitution, drugs, or other "morally marginal" activities should be permitted, under controlled circumstances; or (e) whether the overall impact of television is beneficial or harmful, particularly for children and youth.

5. *Leisure Enthusiasts.* Have one or more members of the class, *or* a visiting speaker, who is a highly involved participant in some form of leisure activity, such as drama, painting, sports, high-risk outdoor recreation, hunting or fishing, drag racing, collecting, travel, etc., make a presentation describing his or her involvement in the activity, motivations, satisfactions, triumphs, or failures.

6. *Interest Inventory.* Within the class itself, make up a detailed leisure involvement survey form, covering various types of popular activities, their costs, and the time devoted to them, and have the form filled out anonymously by all students. This might include not only generally approved pursuits, but also such subjects as gambling, drinking, or drug use, etc. Have the findings tabulated and reported to the class for discussion.

7. *Current Topics.* Over a period of several weeks, systematically comb major newspapers, news magazines, and similar sources, for news stories or articles dealing with topics related to leisure, the environment, social trends, etc. Summarize these and discuss their implications.

Note: For several of these tasks, the footnotes following chapters in this text will provide useful background information or may lead to other sources. When assignments or projects are presented to the class, they should be done in as interesting a way as possible, using visual materials and involving other students, rather than simply reading reports.

BIBLIOGRAPHY

Andrew, Judith, and David James. 1991. *Rethinking College Athletics*. Philadelphia: Temple University Press.

Argyle, Michael. 1996. *The Social Psychology of Leisure*. London: Penguin.

Austin, David. 1996. *Therapeutic Recreation: Processes and Techniques*. Champaign, IL: Sagamore Publishing.

Baker, William. 1988. *Sports in the Western World*. Urbana, IL: University of Illinois Press.

Barnett, Lynn. 1995. *Research About Leisure: Past, Present, and Future*. Champaign, IL: Sagamore Publishing.

Bullaro, John, and Christopher Edginton. 1986. *Commercial Leisure Services: Managing for Profit, Service, and Personal Satisfaction*. New York: Macmillan.

Bullock, Charles C., and Michael J. Mahon. 1997. *Introduction to Recreation Services for People with Disabilities*. Champaign, IL: Sagamore Publishing.

Butsch, Richard, ed. 1990. *For Fun and Profit: The Transformation of Leisure into Consumption*. Philadelphia: Temple University Press.

Charlesworth, J.D., ed. 1964. *Leisure in America: Blessing or Curse?* Lancaster, PA: American Academy of Political and Social Science.

Compton, David, ed. 1996. *Issues in Therapeutic Recreation: A Profession in Transition*. Champaign, IL: Sagamore Publishing.

Cordes, Kathleen, and Michael Hilmi. 1996. *Applications in Recreation and Leisure: For Today and the Future*. St. Louis, MO: Mosby.

Corrigan, Peter. 1997. *The Sociology of Consumption*. London: Sage Publications.

Cross, Gary. 1990. *A Social History of Leisure Since 1600*. State College, PA: Venture Publishing.

Dumazedier, Joffe. 1974. *Sociology of Leisure*. Amsterdam: Elsevier.

Dustin, Daniel, Leo McAvoy, and John Schultz. 1995. *Stewards of Access, Custodians of Choice*. Champaign, IL: Sagamore Publishing.

Edginton, Christopher, Debra Jordan, Donald DeGraaf, and Susan Edginton. 1995. *Leisure and Life Satisfaction: Foundational Perspectives*. Dubuque, IA: Brown and Benchmark.

Findlay, J. 1986. *People of Chance: Gambling in American Society from Jamestown to Las Vegas*. New York: Oxford University Press.

Frank, Robert H. 1998. *Luxury Fever*. New York: Free Press.

Frank, Robert H., and Philip J. Cook. 1995. *The Winner-Take-All Society*. New York: Free Press.

Garreau, Joel. 1991. *Edge City: Life on the New Frontier*. New York: Doubleday.

Godbey, Geoffrey. 1997. *Leisure and Leisure Services in the 21st Century*. State College, PA: Venture Publishing.

Godbey, Geoffrey. 1994. *Leisure in Your Life: An Exploration*. State College, PA: Venture Publishing.

Goodale, Thomas, and Geoffrey Godbey. 1988. *The Evolution of Leisure: Historical and Philosophical Perspectives*. State College, PA: Venture Publishing.

Goodale, Thomas, and Peter Witt. 1990. *Recreation and Leisure: Issues in an Era of Change*. State College, PA: Venture Publishing.

Graham, Peter, ed. 1994. *Sport Business: Operational and Theoretical Aspects*. Dubuque, IA: Brown and Benchmark.

Guttmann, Alan. 1991. *Women's Sport: A History*. New York: Columbia University Press.

Hacker, A. 1992. *Two Nations: Black and White, Separate, Hostile, Unequal*. New York: Charles Scribner's Sons.

Hall, Tim, and Phil Hubbard, ed. 1998. *The Entrepreneurial City*. New York: John Wiley and Sons.

Henderson, Karla, M. Deborah Bialeschki, Susan Shaw, and Valeria Freysinger. *Both Gains and Gaps: Feminist Perspectives on Women's Leisure*. 1996. State College, PA: Venture Publishing.

Hine, Thomas. 1999. *The Middling of the American Brow: Social Change and the 20th Century*. New York: Alfred A. Knopf.

Hunnicutt, Benjamin. 1988. *Work Without End: Abandoning Shorter Hours for the Right to Work.* Philadelphia: Temple University Press.

Kelly, John. 1996. *Leisure.* Boston: Allyn and Bacon.

Kelly, John, and Geoffrey Godbey. 1992. *The Sociology of Leisure.* State College, PA: Venture Publishing.

Kelly, John, and Rod Warnick. 1996. *Recreation Markets: Trends Toward the Year 2000.* Champaign, IL: Sagamore Publishing.

Kraus, Richard. 1997. *Recreation Programming: A Benefits-Driven Approach.* Boston: Allyn and Bacon.

Kraus, Richard, and Lawrence Allen. 1997. *Research and Evaluation in Recreation, Parks and Leisure Studies.* Scottsdale, AZ: Gorsuch Scarisbrick.

Kraus, Richard. 1997. *Recreation and Leisure in Modern Society.* Menlo Park, CA: Addison Wesley Longman.

Lasch, Christopher. 1979. *The Culture of Narcissism: American Life in an Age of Diminishing Expectations.* New York: Warner.

Mandel, Michael. 1996. *The High-Risk Society.* New York: Times Business/Random House.

Mannell, Roger, and Douglas Kleiber. 1997. *A Social Psychology of Leisure.* State College, PA: Venture Publishing.

McFarland, Elsie. 1970. *The Development of Public Recreation in Canada.* Vanier City, Ontario, Canada: Canadian Parks/Recreation Association.

McGuire, Francis, Rosangela Boyd, and Raymond Tedrick. 1996. *Leisure and Aging: Ulyssean Living in Later Life.* Champaign, IL: Sagamore Publishing.

Mobley, Tony, and Robert Toalson, eds., 1992. *Parks and Recreation in the 21st Century.* Arlington, VA: National Recreation and Park Association.

Mundy, Jean, and Debby Smith. 1996. *Leisure Education: Theory and Practice.* Champaign, IL: Sagamore Publishing.

Murphy, James, E. William Niepoth, Lynn Jamieson, and John Williams. 1991. *Leisure Systems: Critical Concepts and Applications.* Champaign, IL: Sagamore Publishing.

Nelson, Mariah. 1991. *Are We Winning Yet? How Women Are Changing Sports and Sports Are Changing Women.* New York: Random House.

Oxendine, Joseph. 1988. *American Indian Sports Heritage.* Champaign, IL: Human Kinetics.

Rader, Benjamin. 1984. *In Its Own Image: How Television Has Transformed Sports.* New York: Free Press.

Rossman, J. Robert. 1994. *Recreation Programming: Designing Leisure Experiences.* Champaign, IL: Sagamore Publishing.

Royal, Robert, ed. 1995. *Reinventing the American People: Unity and Diversity Today.* Washington, DC: Ethics and Public Policy Center.

Russell, Ruth. 1996. *Pastimes: The Context of Contemporary Leisure.* Dubuque, IA: Brown and Benchmark.

Samuel, Nicole, ed. 1996. *Women, Leisure and the Family in Contemporary Society: A Multinational Perspective.* Wallingford, UK: CAB/International.

Schor, Juliet. 1991. *The Overworked American: The Unexpected Decline of Leisure.* New York: Basic Books.

Schleien, Stuart, M. Tipton Ray, and Frederick Green. 1996. *Community Recreation and People with Disabilities: Strategies for Inclusion.* Baltimore, MD: Paul Brookes Publishing.

Searle, Mark, and Russell Brayley. 1993. *Leisure Services in Canada: An Introduction.* State College, PA: Venture Publishing.

Sessoms, H. Douglas, and Karla Henderson. 1994. *Introduction to Leisure Services.* State College, PA: Venture Publishing.

Shivers, Jay S., and Lee J. DeLisle. 1996. *The Story of Leisure: Context, Concepts, and Current Controversy.* Champaign, IL: Human Kinetics.

Sitarz, Daniel, ed. 1998. *Sustainable America: America's Environment, Economy and Society in the 21st Century.* Carbondale, IL: Earthpress.

Wiggins, David. 1997. *Glory Bound: Black Athletes in a White America.* Syracuse, NY: Syracuse University Press.

Winslow, Charles, and William Bramer. 1994. *Future Work: Putting Knowledge to Work in the Knowledge Economy.* New York: Free Press.

Wolfe, Alan. 1998. *One Nation, After All.* New York: Viking.

PHOTO CREDITS

INDEX